The Rehabilitation and Management of Long COVID

This ground-breaking volume provides the first comprehensive resource for health professionals managing the rehabilitation of people experiencing Long COVID.

Founded on therapeutic principles and evidence from other chronic conditions, and informed by clinician and lived experience expertise, this book advances the narrative of Long COVID from "what do we know" to "what can we do." It skilfully integrates the latest evidence of the condition with practical therapeutic tips, supporting readers to develop the knowledge and skills needed to provide effective and respectful care for people with Long COVID. The lived and living experience of those with the condition is embedded in every chapter.

Written by clinicians, researchers, and lived experience experts, this book is an invaluable resource for health professionals in all services and settings.

Danielle Hitch is an Associate Professor of Occupational Therapy and Health Economist in a joint position shared between Deakin University, Geelong and Western Health, Victoria, Australia. Her professional life is founded on an enduring commitment to health equity and social justice, and her own lived experience as a carer and person with disability.

Joanne Wrench is a Clinical Neuropsychologist and Director of Psychology at Austin Health and an Honorary Fellow at the University of Melbourne, Victoria, Australia. She is a steadfast believer in equitable access to healthcare and the public health system, in which she has worked for over 20 years.

W0234715

"Long COVID is a global health issue that impacts the functional status and quality of life for millions living around the world. There are currently no cures for Long COVID. Therefore, resources such as this, which have been developed with patients, can be effective in increasing the knowledge and understanding of healthcare workers. Simultaneously, the tools provided here can support practitioners in recognising, assessing, developing and implementing appropriate interventions for Long COVID patients that can improve patient outcomes."

Professor Mark Faghy, Professor in Clinical Exercise Science,
Derby University, United Kingdom

"This is a comprehensive and concise account of the rehabilitation and management of Long COVID. It elegantly weaves lived experience in with the latest science and clinical experience to provide a compassionate resource for all health professionals. Long COVID is the sort of condition our siloed health systems struggle to care for – this book contains the keys to integrated person-centered care that have wider application to post-infectious syndromes and chronic conditions in general."

Andrew Baillie, The University of Sydney, Australia

The Rehabilitation and Management of Long COVID

A Handbook for Clinical Practice

EDITED BY
DANIELLE HITCH
AND JOANNE WRENCH

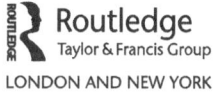

Routledge
Taylor & Francis Group

LONDON AND NEW YORK

Designed cover image: Getty Images

First published 2026
by Routledge
4 Park Square, Milton Park, Abingdon, Oxon OX14 4RN

and by Routledge
605 Third Avenue, New York, NY 10158

Routledge is an imprint of the Taylor & Francis Group, an informa business

British Library Cataloguing-in-Publication Data
A catalogue record for this book is available from the British Library

ISBN: 978-1-032-86559-1 (hbk)
ISBN: 978-1-032-86558-4 (pbk)
ISBN: 978-1-003-52810-4 (ebk)

DOI: 10.4324/9781003528104

Typeset in Vectora
by codeMantra

This book is dedicated to everyone with lived or living experience of Long COVID. We recognise and respect your ongoing resilience, persistence, and courage. We also acknowledge the care and support provided by health professionals and other caregivers to people with Long COVID.

May this book provide all readers with the knowledge, insights, and skills they need to enable people with Long COVID to live their best lives.

We stand with you, we support you, and we are committed to working together to ensure better outcomes for people with Long COVID.

Contents

Acknowledgements

The editors acknowledge the traditional custodians of the unceded lands, skies, and waterways on which this work was produced. We pay our deep respect to the Ancestors and Elders of Wurundjeri and Wadawurrung country in recognition of the deep history and culture of these lands.

Danielle Hitch sincerely acknowledges the love and support of her family – Nan, Dad, Mum, Chris, Freya, Orrin, and April. You are my reason for everything. She would also like to acknowledge the support of her colleagues at Deakin University and Western Health, who make her working life such a pleasure.

Joanne Wrench would like to thank her family – Mum, Dad, Richard, Ben, and Florence for their unwavering support and patience. She also extends her gratitude to her colleagues at Austin Health whose steadfast support made it possible to bring this idea to life.

Contributors

Miquette Abercrombie is a Long COVID sufferer surviving each day on her own with this debilitating illness.

Emily Alexander is a senior physiotherapist working in a major tertiary hospital in Victoria and a Long COVID survivor who is keen to share her experience and advocate for Long COVID sufferers.

Luna Amine is a single mother of two healthy kids who has lived experience of Long COVID, along with a bit of research and physical therapy experience.

Mary Rose Angeles is an early career researcher and health economist at Deakin University, Victoria, Australia. She specialises in economic evaluation methods, data analysis, and cost-effectiveness modelling.

Sarah Annesley is a senior research fellow and laboratory head at La Trobe University, Victoria, Australia. Her laboratory investigates neurological diseases including Long COVID and Myalgic Encephalomyelitis/Chronic Fatigue Syndrome and aims to identify biomarkers, understand the underlying disease mechanisms, and test the efficacy of therapeutic agents.

Emily Armstrong is a research coordinator at the University of Alberta, Canada. She enjoys reading whenever her cats move their heads out of the way.

Henry Barker is a young person who's been living with the Long COVID "giant" for over two years.

Tara Barton has a professional background in infectious diseases and sexual, reproductive, and women's Health. She is also a Long COVID advocate and lived experience educator.

Catherine M. Bennett is a Distinguished Professor and Chair in Epidemiology at the Faculty of Health and Institute of Health Transformation at Deakin University, Victoria, Australia.

Raeya Bognar (She/Her) is an Accredited Exercise Physiologist with first-hand experience of invisible illness, underpinning the clinician she is.

Sarah Booth is a qualified social worker at Western Health, Victoria, Australia, with over 20 years' experience in healthcare.

James Boyd is a digital health expert and inaugural Chair of Digital Health at La Trobe University, Victoria, Australia. He is dedicated to leveraging innovative technologies to address healthcare inefficiencies and improve patient outcomes through data-driven insights and virtual care solutions.

Bruce James Brew is a neurologist at St Vincent's Hospital, New South Wales, Australia. He is the director of the Peter Duncan Neurosciences Unit at St Vincents's Centre for Applied Medical Research and Professor of Medicine (Neurology) at the University of New South Wales and University of Notre Dame, Australia.

Melanie Broadley has been living with Long COVID since 2022 and has prior research experience in cognitive and health psychology.

Nathan Butler is an Associate Professor of Exercise Physiology and Director of the Active Health Clinic, Victoria, Australia.

Gemma Carey was a Professor of Public Health in the Centre for Social Impact, University of New South Wales, Australia.

Kerrie Clarke is a Clinical Psychologist who worked in the Long COVID Clinic at Austin Health, Victoria, Australia.

Brìghde Collins is a linguist with lived experience who most recently worked in Groot Island.

Darcie Cooper is an associate research fellow at the Centre for Innovation in Infection Disease and Immunology Research (CIIDIR) and the Institute for Mental and Physical Health and Clinical Translation (IMPACT), Deakin University, Victoria, Australia.

Rebecca Corva is an associate research fellow with the School of Medicine, Deakin University, Victoria, Australia and an Occupational Therapist at Western Health, Victoria, Australia.

Angela Crombie is an Associate Professor and Director of Research at Bendigo Health, Victoria, Australia. She has around 20 years of experience in health service research and is a passionate advocate for improving the health and wellbeing of regional communities.

Erica Crome has lived experience of Long COVID, with prior experience in clinical psychology, research, and public health policy.

Sandy Davies is a positive ageing advocate from the remote reaches of Northern Australia who hopes sharing her Long COVID lived experience will lead to better outcomes for others in the future.

Elle Defèin is a public health graduate and has continued working practically in the mental health and disability support space.

Farhana Dewan is a Speech Pathologist at Joan Kirner Women's & Children's Hospital, Western Health, Victoria, Australia.

Karen Dickinson manages her Long COVID with medication, meditation, pacing, prioritising time in nature and enjoying her family and friends. She's been medically retired from her career in environmental policy, but is grateful to have the capacity to share her experiences with practitioners and others living with Long COVID.

Fy Dunford is a Health New Zealand senior cardiorespiratory physiotherapist who co-developed the staff Long COVID clinic in Taranaki and works with patients with Long COVID in the community.

Steven Faux is a conjoint Professor of Rehabilitation and Pain Medicine at University of New South Wales and Notre Dame University, Australia. He co-leads the St Vincent's Sydney Long COVID Clinic.

Karen Felder is a former executive recruitment professional who had her active life upended by Long COVID and ME/CFS. She shares her experience to highlight the devastating impact of this illness and advocate for those still struggling.

Martin Ferguson-Pell is a physicist come biomechanical engineer and co-Principal Investigator of the Rehab Robotics Lab at the University of Alberta, Canada. He researches the use of technologies in accessible healthcare.

Karlie Flannigan is a COVID Intensive Care Unit survivor and has lived with Long COVID for four and a half years.

Gerard Flannigan has lived with Long COVID for four and a half years and has been involved with steering committees focused on Long COVID issues.

Melissa Frankcomb has a background in clinical nursing and is adapting to life with the challenges and changes that have come with Long COVID. She loves to seek beauty in all things.

Andrew Georgiou leads the diagnostic informatics research team at the Centre for Health Systems and Safety Research at the Australian Institute of Health Innovation at Macquarie University, New South Wales, Australia. Professor Georgiou's research areas include outcome measurement, quality and safety, and organisational communications research.

Sumitha Gounden is the Medical Director of Rehabilitation Services at Orange Health Service, Western New South Wales Local Health District, Australia.

Nada Hamad is a Senior Staff Specialist in Transplant and Cellular Therapies at St Vincent's Hospital, Sydney, Australia. She is also a Fulbright Scholar and conjoint Professor at the University of New South Wales, New South Wales, Australia.

Ali Harrington is a fun-loving female currently stuck in energy-saving mode, who has been living with Long COVID for over two years.

Martin Hensher is a Professor and the Henry Baldwin professorial research fellow in Health Systems Sustainability at the Menzies Institute for Medical Research at the University of Tasmania, Australia.

Danielle Hitch is an Associate Professor of Occupational Therapy and Health Economist in a joint position shared between Deakin University, Geelong and Western Health, Victoria, Australia. Her professional life is founded on an enduring commitment to health equity and social justice, and her own lived experience as a carer and person with disability.

Lynette Hodges is a Clinical Exercise Physiologist and Senior Lecturer in Sport and Exercise at Massey University, Palmerston North, Aotearoa, New Zealand.

Alex Holmes is head of Consultation Liaison Psychiatry at Royal Melbourne Hospital and an Associate Professor at the University of Melbourne, Victoria, Australia.

Sara Holton is a senior research fellow in the Health and Social Care Unit, School of Public Health and Preventive Medicine, Monash University, Victoria, Australia.

Julie Hughes is an Occupational Therapist with over 30 years of experience, including clinical and research work with people with ME/CFS. She is currently a Lecturer in Occupational Therapy at the Australian Catholic University, Queensland, Australia.

Louis Irving is a Professor and Respiratory Physician at the Royal Melbourne Hospital, and Director of the Lung Tumour Stream at the Peter MacCallum Cancer Centre, Victoria, Australia.

Nicole Jackson (she/her) is an Allied Health Assistant focused on helping people overcome obstacles between them and their dreams, drawing on personal experience from her own challenges due to Long COVID.

Sophie Julian is a small-business owner and confirmed Long COVID sufferer learning to live with the debilitating impact of the disease.

Victoria Lai is an Advanced Clinician Intensive Care Unit physiotherapist, currently working as an Allied Health Critical Care educator in the Northern Region of

Aotearoa, New Zealand. She is also a Lecturer in Physiotherapy at Auckland University of Technology, Aotearoa New Zealand.

Jessica Lee is a well-being writer, speaker, coach, and owner of The Spark Effect. She is currently living with Long COVID.

James Lewis is a Clinical Neuropsychologist and clinician researcher at The Royal Melbourne Hospital, Victoria, Australia.

Deborah Lupton is SHARP Professor in the Centre for Social Research in Health and Social Policy Research Centre, University of New South Wales, Australia.

Angela Ma is a Doctor of Physiotherapy graduate from The University of Melbourne and has worked as a Physiotherapist and Emergency Department Coordinator at two tertiary hospitals in Victoria, Australia. Angela is a second-generation immigrant passionate about equitable healthcare for diverse communities.

Mary Mangos is an abstract artist, creating expressive works inspired by nature and her personal journey with Long COVID (since September 2022). Previously, she worked as a consulting psychologist, speaker, and author of Finding Your Well-Being.

Tom Marwick is a professorial research fellow at the Baker and Menzies Institutes, Victoria, Australia. He is also Staff Cardiologist at the Royal Hobart Hospital, Tasmania, Australia.

Kevin Masman is a project manager, data manager of the COVIDthon, and statistician at Bendigo Health, Victoria, Australia.

Angela Maxwell-McRae lives with Long COVID and hopes sharing her experience of PEM will help other Long COVID patients.

Jodie McGregor is a Senior Clinical Neuropsychologist at Austin Health, Victoria, Australia, with experience working with people with Long COVID.

Elyse McInerney is a programme manager and policy adviser specialising in social justice and inclusion. She has been living with Long COVID since September 2022.

Jennifer Mepham is a Senior Cardio-Respiratory Physiotherapist at The OxyJen Physio clinic and a Professional Practice Fellow at the School of Physiotherapy, University of Otago, Aotearoa New Zealand.

Chantal C. Mitvalsky is a Senior Speech Pathologist in the Department of Speech Pathology at Austin Health, Victoria, Australia.

Michael Muleme is an Epidemiologist in the Barwon South West Public Health Unit in Geelong, Victoria, Australia.

Sharon Neale is an Occupational Therapist at Western Health, Victoria, Australia. She has 24 years of experience specialising in inpatient subacute care.

Elle O'Brien is a Long COVID lived experience advisor based in Melbourne, Victoria, Australia.

Kylie Ovenden is a Digital Health lecturer at La Trobe University, Victoria, Australia with extensive experience in health innovation. She was instrumental in establishing the regional health innovation hub and the COVIDThon at Bendigo Health, Victoria, Australia.

Elisa Perego is a researcher and disability activist with a special interest in Long COVID.

Thomas Ponissi was diagnosed with Long COVID in 2022. He was a university student at the time and has since graduated and commenced work. He writes in a personal capacity.

Kieva Richards is a Lecturer in Occupational Therapy with over 20 years of experience in healthcare and education across Canada and Australia.

Kristy Riley is a passionate mother and psychologist. Living with Long COVID has deepened her perspective on compassion and strength.

Hayley Scott is an Occupational Therapy lecturer specialising in rehabilitation and is passionate about enhancing patient recovery and professional education.

Michelle Scoullar is a paediatrician, international health specialist, and senior research fellow. She leads the paediatric component of a Long COVID specialist clinic, and her research focuses on issues of health equity and improving child health outcomes.

Leigh Seidel-Marks is a Dietitian with over 17 years of clinical experience and an advocate for people living with Long COVID. She was the clinical lead for multidisciplinary allied health-led ReCOVery service, Austin Health, Victoria, Australia.

Bernard Shiu is an Associate Professor at the School of Medicine, Deakin University. He is also a General Practitioner and Founder and Clinical Director of Geelong Long COVID Clinic.

Jennifer Smallridge is an Accredited Exercise Physiologist and director of Invisibly Brilliant, an online clinic serving the chronic illness population through validation, pacing, and problem-solving. She is also a professional speaker and co-founder of Connection Medicine, which educates healthcare professionals on chronic illness management.

Julie Taylor has lived experience of Long COVID with varied unfolding health conditions including a very dramatic need for brain surgery to clip an enlarging aneurysm! With the support of her GP, a team of nine multidisciplinary specialists and the Long COVID Clinic, she is still on the journey of recovery.

Judith Thomas is a research fellow within the Centre for Health Systems and Safety Research in the Australian Institute of Health Innovation at Macquarie University, New South Wales, Australia. Her research focuses on diagnostic informatics, including the impact of the COVID-19 pandemic on general practice.

Emma Tindill (she/her) is an Occupational Therapist who is passionate about supporting people with chronic "invisible" illnesses and established PivOT Health Occupational Therapy, a largely telehealth-based service located in Victoria, Australia.

Emma Tippett is an infectious diseases physician who established Clinic Nineteen, a telehealth-based service specifically to improve the health of people with Long COVID in Victoria, Australia.

Krishna Vakil is a casual research fellow with the School of Medicine, Deakin University, Victoria, Australia.

Paige van der Pligt is an Advanced Accredited Practising Dietitian, experienced clinician, and Senior Lecturer in Nutrition and Dietetics at Deakin University, Victoria, Australia. She also holds an honorary research appointment at Joan Kirner Women's and Children's Hospital, Western Health, Victoria, Australia.

Marlies Wanasili (she/her) is an Occupational Therapist with over 20 years of experience working with neurological clients in community rehabilitation.

Tanya Ward is a PhD candidate and casual research fellow at the School of Health and Social Development, Institute for Health Transformation, Deakin University, Victoria, Australia.

David A. Watters is a Distinguished Professor of Surgery at University Hospital Geelong, Barwon Health and Deakin University, Victoria, Australia.

Jenean Whitman is a Long COVID patient, contributing her lived experience in the hope this will help others with Long COVID.

Naomi Whyler is a General Medicine and Infectious Diseases Physician with expertise in managing Long COVID, Postural Orthostatic Tachycardia Syndrome, and dysautonomia.

Jane Willcox is a carer for people with Long COVID and dietetic clinician researcher with appointments as a senior research fellow at the Royal Children's Hospital, Victoria, Australia and Adjunct Associate Professor at Charles Darwin University, Northern Territory, Australia.

Joanne Wrench is a Clinical Neuropsychologist and Director of Psychology at Austin Health and an Honorary Fellow at the University of Melbourne, Victoria, Australia. She is a steadfast believer in equitable access to healthcare and the public health system, in which she has worked for over 20 years.

Charissa J. Zaga is a Senior Speech Pathologist and Acute Stream Leader in the Department of Speech Pathology at Austin Health, and a post-doctoral researcher in the Implementation Science Unit at the Institute of Breathing and Sleep, Austin Health.

Figures

Tables

Chapter 1

Introduction

Danielle Hitch, Joanne Wrench, Elyse McInerney, Jessica Lee, and Karen Felder

---

BOX 1.1   LEARNING OBJECTIVES

By the end of this chapter, readers should be able to:

- Explain how Long COVID emerged as a recognised condition and give a general description of its ongoing public health implications.
- Identify general principles for evidence-informed, high-quality Long COVID rehabilitation.
- Reflect on diverse meanings and perspectives about Long COVID terminology and consider their impact on working with patients.

1.1 FROM PANDEMIC TO PERSISTENT SYMPTOMS: THE EMERGENCE OF LONG COVID[1]

The first confirmed case of a new and mysterious respiratory illness was identified in Wuhan, China on 8 December 2019.[1,2] Three weeks later, an infectious disease surveillance system using artificial intelligence raised an early alert about rising case numbers. The virus was identified as Severe Acute Respiratory Syndrome Coronavirus 2 (SARS-CoV-2) in early January 2020, and the disease it causes was named 'COVID-19' by the World Health Organization (WHO) on 11 February 2020. By then, cases had been reported across 25 countries,[3] as the infectiousness and virulence of COVID-19 became increasingly apparent. On 11 March 2020, case numbers had escalated to the point where WHO declared COVID-19 to be a pandemic.[4]

Unlike many other illnesses, conditions, and disabilities we encounter as health professionals, COVID-19 is something everyone has experienced first-hand.

DOI: 10.4324/9781003528104-1

A significant proportion of the global population has experienced at least one COVID-19 infection,[5] and many people who are seropositive for COVID-19 are unaware they have been infected.[6] Those fortunate enough to avoid infection most likely know someone affected or have been subject to public health measures designed to stop its spread. COVID-19 is not something that happens to other people – it has happened to us all.

BOX 1.2 PRACTICE POINT

We acknowledge that the pandemic has been very difficult for many people, and you do not have to complete this activity if you do not wish to. Stop for a moment and reflect on your personal experience of the COVID-19 pandemic.

Have you been infected by COVID-19? What was that experience like for you, and the people around you? How long did it take you to recover? What impact did it have on your work and/or social life? Have you ever had personal experience of an illness, condition, or disability that one of your patients' lives with? Did that have any impact on how you worked with them?

The authors' experience of the early days of the pandemic included redeployment to front-line duties, the first of six community lockdowns and homeschooling our children. We calculated and juggled the risks of front line working with protecting ourselves, our loved ones, and our community. We spoke to colleagues in tears at the thought of catching COVID-19, traumatised by what they had witnessed in the wards and corridors of our hospitals. We became vigilant for every sneeze or scratchy throat and worried for our families. Like everyone else, we did our best to look after ourselves and each other during the most extraordinary and uncertain time of our lives.

As the Australian winter began to ease and the weather got warmer, we all started to wonder if the worst was finally behind us, relieved that Australia had seemingly dodged the widespread devastation we witnessed in other countries. Everyone celebrated the lifting of an extended community lockdown, but unbeknownst to many, a new and less obvious wave had reached our shores. Each subsequent wave brought further lockdowns and public health measures, with our home city, Melbourne, eventually spending over 250 days in lockdown in under 2 years.

Over time, the community attitude towards COVID-19 shifted from fear to acceptance in response to government messaging about moving to "COVID normal." The cognitive dissonance between the lived experience of people with Long COVID and general community attitudes regarding the risks of infection only grew as time went on. People with Long COVID experienced a profound shift. The focus moved away from collective safety measures towards personal responsibility for avoiding transmission and infection. To stay safe, people with Long COVID often withdrew from public life, as many spaces lacked protections like masking. In this new reality, people with Long COVID found themselves redefined as vulnerable, disabled, and marginalised. The combination of debilitating illness and societal exclusion created a double burden. Beyond the physical and emotional toll of being very unwell, the world itself was full of barriers to participation and connection.

People with lived experience of Long COVID were the first to recognise that not everyone was recovering from their acute infection. They began connecting online, forming peer support groups, organising grassroots awareness campaigns, and leading research.[7] In lieu of a formal name, the term "Long COVID" was rapidly adopted into both every day and professional language. By July 2020, it had appeared in WHO communications and the *British Medical Journal*.[8] While people with lived experience are increasingly included in health education, practice, and research, they were the ones who led the identification and initial exploration of Long COVID.[9] They were the first experts in Long COVID and continue to play a fundamental role in shaping our understanding and practices.

1.1.1 A Significant and Growing Public Health Issue

There are approximately 65 million people around the world (around 1 in 125) who meet the case description for Long COVID.[10] However, a lack of formal testing and consistent data collection makes it difficult to get an accurate picture of the magnitude of this public health problem. Its prevalence varies widely across studies (7.3–53%)[11] and the lack of diagnostic criteria means definitions differ across research. Prevalence rates also vary between groups and are generally higher for people hospitalised during their acute infection, females, older people, and those living with comorbidities.[11–13]

Many people find their Long COVID symptoms improve over time, with a minority reporting complete recovery after one year.[14] However, this still leaves the majority of people living with long-term problems, and many infected in early 2020 are entering their fifth year of illness and isolation. Every COVID-19 infection carries the risk of Long COVID, or relapse and exacerbation for people already living with this condition.[15,16] Long COVID is an increasingly common condition and will continue to affect millions of people worldwide as COVID-19 cases accumulate and new variants emerge.

1.2 ABOUT THIS BOOK

1.2.1 Overall Aim

Given its high prevalence, health professionals could see people with Long COVID in any service setting or healthcare sector. The aim of this book is to provide a comprehensive resource for health professionals working with people experiencing Long COVID. This may include physiotherapists, exercise physiologists, occupational therapists, speech pathologists, clinical psychologists, neuropsychologists, dietitians, social workers, nurses, physicians, and many others.

This book aims to enhance professional understanding of this condition and improve patient outcomes by offering detailed insights into interdisciplinary approaches, intervention strategies, and models of care. This book also seeks to explore the varying needs of distinctive community groups (such as culturally and linguistically diverse communities and women), emerging trends in the field, and ways to enable healthcare professionals to deliver effective, evidence-informed, and person-centred care. In doing so, we seek to answer a key question for health professionals – What can we do to help our patients with Long COVID?

1.2.2 Guiding Principles and Frameworks

A key characteristic of Long COVID is its diversity, both in clinical presentation and in its impact on daily life. The following principles and framework support a holistic perspective of Long COVID rehabilitation and provide readers with the context needed to practice effectively in their discipline or field.

The International Classification of Functioning, Disability, and Health (ICF),[17] developed by the WHO, is a framework for categorising health and disability. It considers physical, psychological, and social factors that impact a person's health and wellbeing. By providing a common language, the ICF enables healthcare professionals, policymakers, researchers, and others to communicate more effectively about health and disability, facilitating a clearer understanding of complex health issues.[18]

The ICF consists of two parts: Functioning and Disability (which includes body functions and structures, activities, and participation) and Contextual Factors (which include environmental and personal factors). The sections and chapters of this book touch upon all areas of the framework, with Figure 1.1 summarising how the ICF is embedded throughout.

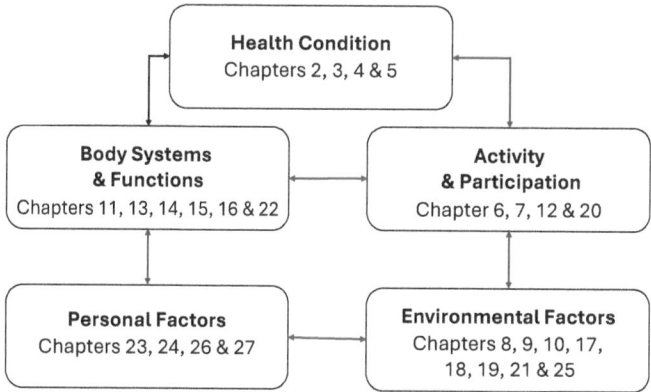

Figure 1.1 The presence of the International Classification of Functioning, Disability and Health (ICF) in this book.

1.3 KEY PRINCIPLES FOR LONG COVID REHABILITATION

Our perspective of Long COVID rehabilitation is informed by academic, professional, and lived experience. The key principles (Table 1.1) have driven the development of this book and are intended to give guidance on how to provide interventions that align with the principles of high-quality care. These principles also serve as a benchmark for evaluating practice, supporting both transparency and accountability. However, they are flexible enough to allow readers to adapt them to their local context while maintaining their core intent.

1.4 A WORD ABOUT LANGUAGE

We acknowledge that the language around Long COVID is diverse and rapidly changing, and we have advised our authors to use their preferred terms. However, we are choosing to use the term "Long COVID" rather than terminology recommended by the WHO and other institutions (e.g., Post-Acute COVID Condition). Long COVID is patient-named condition (see Chapter 4), and we acknowledge and respect the advocacy and hard-won lived experience behind it by using this as our preferred term.

Fundamentally, rehabilitation clinicians should take the lead from their patients about preferred terms for Long COVID symptoms and problems in daily life. Not all people with Long COVID experience their journey as "recovery," and opinions vary around whether Long COVID is a "condition," "syndrome," "disease," or "disability." Referring to symptoms as "normal" or "typical" may upset some patients and our

Table 1.1 Key Principles for Long COVID Rehabilitation

Principles	
Holistic Rehabilitation	Evaluate and understand the impact of Long COVID on all aspects of daily life to provide person-centred care.
Comprehensive Assessment	Ensure all potential explanations for symptoms or functional problems are explored to inform decision-making.
Responsive Rehabilitation	Early access to rehabilitation and tracking recovery over time to adjust rehabilitation interventions accordingly.
Integrated Care	Enable people with Long COVID to access and navigate the services they need as soon as possible.
Social Inclusion	Support people with Long COVID to remain connected with their family, friends and community.
Evidence Informed Care	Remain up to date on research findings and other emerging evidence to inform high-quality care.
Therapeutic Alliance	Supportive and respectful therapeutic relationships are central to Long COVID rehabilitation.
Managing Uncertainty	Realistic goal setting to enable people with Long COVID manage unpredictable symptoms and setbacks.
Equitable, Safe, and Accessible Care	Providing accessible and high-quality care to all people with Long COVID regardless of presentation, in a COVID-safe environment (i.e., with masking).

understanding of the natural history of Long COVID is still in its infancy. Words matter, and it is incumbent on all health professionals to reflect on their use when we partner with patients.

As in many areas of rehabilitation, reflective practice is crucial to building respectful therapeutic relationships. During the writing of this book, we learned that the term "biopsychosocial" has a very negative meaning for some people with Long COVID. It has become associated with neoliberal policies that downplay social and structural influences on health while attributing blame to individuals and emphasising personal responsibility.[19] As health professionals, we perceive "biopsychosocial" as a positive term that promotes engagement with the complex interplay between physical, psychological, and social factors that can influence health and wellbeing. Unfortunately, for many people living with Long COVID, the biopsychosocial model has become synonymous with misattributing causality to the social and psychological impacts of Long COVID and minimising patient experience.[20] Learning about this alternative meaning has prompted personal reflection on what we take for granted about health-related terminology, and we encourage readers to maintain a critically reflective perspective on the contents of this book.

1.5 STRUCTURE OF THIS TEXTBOOK

In accordance with these principles, every chapter of this book has been co-written with lived experience experts. While these contributions vary in form, all are acknowledged by co-authorship.

The seven sections of this book provide a comprehensive overview of the clinical and contextual landscape of Long COVID. The first section gives an overview of Long COVID as a syndrome and its emergence as a major public health issue. Chapter 2 provides an overview of the symptoms, epidemiology, and biological basis of Long COVID. Chapter 3 describes the relationship of Long COVID to other Post-Acute Infection Syndromes, with a particular focus on Myalgic Encephalitis/ Chronic Fatigue Syndrome. Chapter 4 recounts the role of people with Long COVID in recognising the condition and ongoing advocacy.

The second section of this book addresses the assessment phase of rehabilitation as the initial step to offering evidence-informed and effective support for people with Long COVID. Chapter 5 discusses tools for identifying Long COVID, addressing the challenges posed by an absence of diagnostic criteria and the application of big data to determine the magnitude of this issue at the population level. Chapter 6 explores the tools available to establish baseline health and track rehabilitation outcomes, emphasising the need to utilise clinician ratings, patient-reported outcomes, and patient experience measures for a comprehensive approach. Chapter 7 examines goal-setting practices to guide recovery and enable shared decision-making.

In Section Three, our authors describe the members of the multidisciplinary teams who work with people with Long COVID. Chapter 8 details the roles of various medical specialists, while Chapter 9 describes the contribution of diverse allied health professions and includes referral guidelines intended to ensure that people with Long COVID receive the right care at the right time. Chapter 10 discusses the integrated approaches to care recommended for people with Long

COVID, including a case study of a model of care co-produced with people with lived experience.

The fourth section of this book details evidence-informed rehabilitation and management strategies that address the issues faced by people with Long COVID. Chapter 11 outlines assessments and interventions to manage Post-Exertional Malaise and other physical symptoms, while Chapter 12 discusses strategies to support participation in daily life including pacing. Chapter 13 provides an overview of cognitive techniques, and Chapter 14 describes a range of psychosocial support strategies and interventions. Chapter 15 discusses nutritional approaches for Long COVID management, and Chapter 16 reviews treatment methods for Postural Orthostatic Tachycardia Syndrome associated with Long COVID.

In Section Five, the diverse models of care available to support people with Long COVID are reviewed and discussed within the broader contexts affecting care delivery. Chapter 17 explains the role of hospital-based services, while Chapter 18 provides an overview of allied health Long COVID clinics including a case study describing a hospital-based allied health-led service. Chapter 19 details general practitioner-led services in primary care, with case studies of face-to-face and telehealth models of care. Chapter 20 surveys self-management approaches, including those available online to people with Long COVID. From the broader perspective, Chapter 21 reviews economic factors impacting upon Long COVID care and resource allocation.

The sixth section of this book highlights and critiques the characteristics of specific groups of people with Long COVID, and the distinctive challenges they may face. Chapter 22 looks at the unique needs of Intensive Care Unit survivors, while Chapter 23 describes the care and support required by children and young people. Chapter 24 highlights the health equity issues faced by people from culturally and linguistically diverse communities, and best practice for working with these populations. Chapter 25 discusses the experiences and needs of people living in regional, rural, and remote communities, including case studies from Rural Australia and Canada. Chapter 26 explores the impact of gender for people with Long COVID, with a particular focus on women and the often highly gendered role of caregiving. Placing these chapters into context, Chapter 27 critiques the social issues related to the COVID-19 pandemic and their impact on the community experience of Long COVID.

The final chapter of the book looks to the future and poses the question "where to from here?" The field of Long COVID is rapidly evolving and we will end this book with an optimistic view of future opportunities.

NOTE

1 Sections of this chapter are adapted from "Enabling and Optimising Recovery from COVID-19: A handbook for health professionals and other caregivers of people with Long COVID" by Danielle Hitch, Genevieve Pepin, Kelli Nicola-Richmond, and Valerie Watchorn, used under CC BY 4.0.

REFERENCES

1 Allam Z. The first 50 days of COVID-19: a detailed chronological timeline and extensive review of literature documenting the pandemic. In: Allam Z, editor. Surveying the COVID-19 Pandemic and Its Implications. 1st ed. Amsterdam: Elsevier; 2020. p. 1–7. doi:10.1016/B978-0-12-824313-8.00001-2.

2 Bowles J. How Canadian AI start-up BlueDot spotted coronavirus before anyone else had a clue. *Diginomica*; 2020 Jan 27 [cited 2025 Feb 7]. Available from: https://diginomica.com/how-canadian-ai-start-bluedot-spotted-coronavirus-anyone-else-had-clue.

3 World Health Organization (WHO). Naming the coronavirus disease (COVID-19) and the virus that causes it [Internet]. Geneva: WHO; 2020 [cited 2025 Feb 7]. Available from: https://www.who.int/emergencies/diseases/novel-coronavirus-2019/technical-guidance/naming-the-coronavirus-disease-(covid-2019)-and-the-virus-that-causes-it.

4 World Health Organization (WHO). WHO Director-General's opening remarks at the media briefing on COVID-19 – 11 March 2020 [Internet]. Geneva: WHO; 2020 Mar 11 [cited 2025 Feb 7]. Available from: https://www.who.int/director-general/speeches/detail/who-director-general-s-opening-remarks-at-the-media-briefing-on-covid-19---11-march-2020.

5 Lee K, et al. Estimation of world seroprevalence of SARS-CoV-2 antibodies. J Appl Stat. 2024;51(15):3039–58. doi:10.1080/02664763.2024.2335569.

6 Leong DP, et al. Risk factors for recognized and unrecognized SARS-CoV-2 infection: a sero-epidemiologic analysis of the Prospective Urban Rural Epidemiology (PURE) study. Microbiol Spectr. 2024;12(2):e0149223. doi:10.1128/spectrum.01492-23.

7 McCorkell L, et al. Patient-Led research collaborative: embedding patients in the Long COVID narrative. PAIN Rep. 2021;6(1):e913. doi:10.1097/PR9.0000000000000913.

8 Mahase E. COVID-19: What do we know about "long covid"? Br Med J. 2020;370:m2815. doi:10.1136/bmj.m2815.

9 Callard F, et al. How and why patients made Long COVID. Soc Sci Med. 2021;268:113426. doi:10.1016/j.socscimed.2020.113426.

10 The Lancet. Long COVID: 3 years in. Lancet. 2023 Mar 11;401(10379):795. doi:10.1016/S0140-6736(23)00493-2.

11 Nittas V, et al. Long COVID through a public health lens: an umbrella review. Public Health Rev. 2022;43:1604501. doi:10.3389/phrs.2022.1604501.

12 Chen C, et al. Global prevalence of post-coronavirus disease 2019 (COVID-19) condition or Long COVID: a meta-analysis and systematic review. J Infect Dis. 2022;226(9):1593–1607. doi:10.1093/infdis/jiac136.

13 Muthuka JK, et al. Prevalence and predictors of Long COVID-19 and the average time to diagnosis in the general population: a systematic review, meta-analysis and meta-regression. COVID. 2024;4(7):968–81. doi:10.3390/covid4070067.

14 Mudgal SK, et al. Pooled prevalence of Long COVID-19 symptoms at 12 months and above follow-up period: a systematic review and meta-analysis. Cureus. 2023;15(3):e36325. doi:10.7759/cureus.36325.

15 Bosworth ML, et al. Risk of new-onset Long COVID following reinfection with severe acute respiratory syndrome coronavirus 2: a community-based cohort study. Open Forum Infect Dis. 2023;10(11):ofad493. doi:10.1093/ofid/ofad493.

16 Boufidou F, et al. SARS-CoV-2 reinfections and Long COVID in the post-Omicron phase of the pandemic. Int J Mol Sci. 2023;24(16):12962. doi:10.3390/ijms241612962.

17 World Health Organization (WHO). International classification of functioning, disability, and health: ICF. Geneva: World Health Organization; 2001.

18 World Health Organization (WHO). ICF beginner's guide: towards a common language for functioning, disability and health. Geneva: World Health Organization; 2002.

19 Hunt J. Holistic or harmful? Examining socio-structural factors in the biopsychosocial model of chronic illness, medically unexplained symptoms, and disability. Disabil Soc. 2024;39(4):1032–61. doi:10.1080/09687599.2022.2099250.

20 Cornish et al. Concerns regarding a suggested Long COVID paradigm. Lan Res Med. 2023; 11(4): e35. doi:10.1016/S2213-2600(23)00095-4.

SECTION ONE
UNDERSTANDING LONG COVID

Chapter 2

What Is Long COVID?

Erica Crome, Darcie Cooper, Catherine M. Bennett, and Danielle Hitch

---

BOX 2.1   LEARNING OBJECTIVES

By the end of this chapter, readers should be able to:

- Describe the key features of Long COVID and its relationship to common comorbidities.
- Outline the biological mechanisms underlying Long COVID.
- Evaluate the impact of inconsistent definitions on Long COVID research, clinical practice, and patient care.
- Identify strategies to apply evolving definitions and descriptions of Long COVID to rehabilitation practice while validating and integrating patient lived experience.

2.1 INTRODUCTION

Long COVID refers to ongoing symptoms persisting for weeks, months, or even years after the initial four weeks (or "acute" phase) of COVID-19 infection. These symptoms significantly impact daily life, health, and overall wellbeing. However, its varied symptoms, diverse presentations, overlap with other conditions, lack of biomarkers, and fluctuating course make it difficult to define. Patients, carers, health professionals, and researchers may prioritise different physical, psychological, or social aspects based on their perspectives. Symptoms may also overlay pre-existing health conditions and can present as a worsening of symptoms. Reconciling these views into a consistent description is a complex challenge.

DOI: 10.4324/9781003528104-3

Disagreements about Long COVID extend to what it should be called. Given its impact on general health, should it be described objectively as a "condition"? Can it be a "disease" given the biological causes remain unclear? Is it best described as an "illness" or "disability" to reflect subjective experience? Or does "syndrome" better capture the symptom patterns and phenotypes? We acknowledge the diversity of terms used around Long COVID, and Chapter 4 provides a detailed discussion of the various names proposed for this condition. We encourage health professionals to take a reflective approach to using language and terminology in practice.

BOX 2.2   PRACTICE POINT

What do you know about Long COVID? Jot down your understanding and one or two topics you want to learn more about.

2.2 DESCRIPTIONS AND DEFINITIONS OF LONG COVID

Several definitions and descriptions of Long COVID were developed in the initial years of the COVID-19 pandemic.[1-5] Some were created with contributions by patients, carers, and the public[1-2], while consortiums of academic or clinical experts formulated others.[3-5] They are broadly consistent. However, there are subtle differences regarding onset and duration and the need for COVID-19 infection confirmation and/or symptom patterns (Figure 2.1).

The WHO case description is widely adopted in research (particularly in clinical trials). However, in our opinion, the more recently published definition by the National Academies of Sciences, Engineering and Medicine (NASEM)[6] from the United States provides the most comprehensive description of Long COVID to date. Multiple strategies were used to develop this definition, including an extensive literature review, consultation with multidisciplinary experts and collaboration with patients, advocacy groups, and other stakeholders. This approach to developing a definition aims to enhance consensus, recognise the complex, systemic nature of Long COVID, and acknowledge its significant impact on daily life for the patient, their family, and their community. The key features of the NASEM definition are available in a one-page summary and an infographic (Figure 2.2).

The definition is designed to evolve as understanding and sociopolitical contexts change and highlights several important features of Long COVID (Box 2.3).

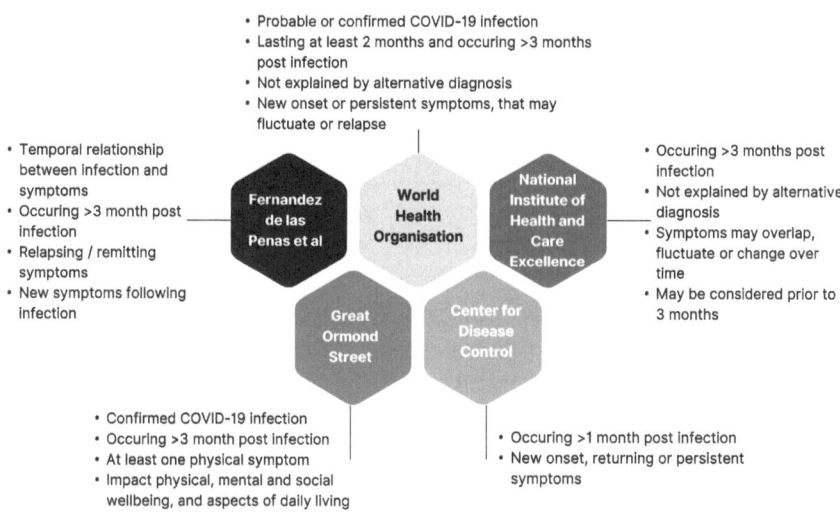

- Temporal relationship between infection and symptoms
- Occuring >3 month post infection
- Relapsing / remitting symptoms
- New symptoms following infection

- Probable or confirmed COVID-19 infection
- Lasting at least 2 months and occuring >3 months post infection
- Not explained by alternative diagnosis
- New onset or persistent symptoms, that may fluctuate or relapse

Fernandez de las Penas et al

World Health Organisation

National Institute of Health and Care Excellence

- Occuring >3 months post infection
- Not explained by alternative diagnosis
- Symptoms may overlap, fluctuate or change over time
- May be considered prior to 3 months

Great Ormond Street

Center for Disease Control

- Confirmed COVID-19 infection
- Occuring >3 month post infection
- At least one physical symptom
- Impact physical, mental and social wellbeing, and aspects of daily living

- Occuring >1 month post infection
- New onset, returning or persistent symptoms

Figure 2.1 Definitions and descriptions of Long COVID.[1–5]

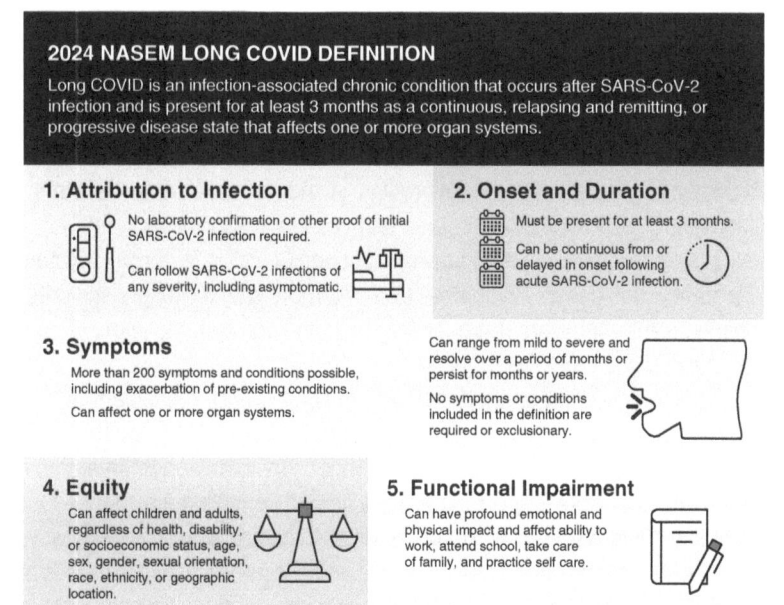

2024 NASEM LONG COVID DEFINITION

Long COVID is an infection-associated chronic condition that occurs after SARS-CoV-2 infection and is present for at least 3 months as a continuous, relapsing and remitting, or progressive disease state that affects one or more organ systems.

1. Attribution to Infection

No laboratory confirmation or other proof of initial SARS-CoV-2 infection required.

Can follow SARS-CoV-2 infections of any severity, including asymptomatic.

2. Onset and Duration

Must be present for at least 3 months.

Can be continuous from or delayed in onset following acute SARS-CoV-2 infection.

3. Symptoms

More than 200 symptoms and conditions possible, including exacerbation of pre-existing conditions.

Can affect one or more organ systems.

Can range from mild to severe and resolve over a period of months or persist for months or years.

No symptoms or conditions included in the definition are required or exclusionary.

4. Equity

Can affect children and adults, regardless of health, disability, or socioeconomic status, age, sex, gender, sexual orientation, race, ethnicity, or geographic location.

5. Functional Impairment

Can have profound emotional and physical impact and affect ability to work, attend school, take care of family, and practice self care.

Figure 2.2 Key features of the NASEM description of Long COVID.[6]

Note: Infographic: Elements of the 2024 Long COVID Definition. Used with permission of The National Academies Press, from *A Long COVID Definition: A Chronic, Systemic Disease State with Profound Consequences*, 2024; permission conveyed through Copyright Clearance Center, Inc.

BOX 2.3   KEY FEATURES OF LONG COVID

Long COVID can ....

- Follow asymptomatic, mild, moderate, or severe COVID-19 infections, which may or may not be formally diagnosed.
- Cause symptoms ranging from mild to severe that continue from the original infection or emerge several months after initial recovery. These symptoms may be new or exacerbate existing conditions.
- Affects anyone, regardless of their personal characteristics or location.
- Resolve over time or persist for years.
- Be diagnosed from clinical presentation, as no clinical biomarkers currently exist.
- Significantly impair a person's participation in daily life, including activities related to self-care, domestic, social, or community activities. These impairments take a severe toll on people with Long COVID, their families, caregivers, and communities.

The NASEM definition seeks to balance the vast individual variation in presentations while providing consistency to guide research, public policy, and funding decisions. It recognises that people with Long COVID present individually distinctive symptoms and functional profiles, including related diagnosable conditions (such as Postural Orthostatic Tachycardia Syndrome or Mast Cell Activation Syndrome). While recognising that Long COVID is "a chronic, systemic disease state,"[6] this description differs from the more specific diagnostic criteria that health professionals are more familiar with and comfortable with.

It is essential to describe the characteristics of Long COVID to enable the identification of a highly heterogeneous condition.[7] A lack of consistency in definitions or descriptions severely limits comparisons between interventions and outcomes and, therefore, opportunities to build and consolidate evidence.[8] A lack of consensus could also lead to inconsistencies in clinical practice and policy, potentially exacerbating inequities in access and outcomes.[9] Health professionals use these descriptions to plan assessments and interventions for specific symptoms. A definition helps them hypothesise what might work for their patient and provides a framework for organising their approach to care and collaboration with other disciplines.

A lack of consistent definition or description also impacts people with Long COVID's ability to obtain support, avoid stigma, and have their experiences validated.[10] It creates a shared explanation and language for symptoms and increases awareness of potential comorbid concerns or symptom trajectories. Definitions and descriptions may also provide eligibility criteria for some services, welfare supports, and insurance benefits.

BOX 2.4 PRACTICE POINT

What impact does the NASEM or other Long COVID definitions and descriptions have on your work as a health professional? From your perspective, do they facilitate your work with Long COVID? If not, what barriers do they pose for your patients? How do they compare with other definitions or diagnostic criteria for different conditions?

2.3 LONG COVID SYMPTOMS

While COVID-19 infection is primarily a respiratory illness, Long COVID is a multisystem condition, and its symptom profile can be highly variable depending on which body systems and structures are impacted. Over 200 symptoms are associated with Long COVID, although none are unique to this post-acute infection syndrome[6] (see Chapter 3). Some present more commonly than others.[11] The most commonly reported symptoms include Post-Exertional Malaise, fatigue, brain fog, dizziness or light-headedness, gastrointestinal complaints, and palpitations.[11] Other commonly identified symptoms are illustrated in Figure 2.3.

The symptoms of Long COVID overlap with many other syndromes, and Chapter 3 contains a detailed description of its relationship to other post-acute infection syndromes. People with Long COVID may also present with other diagnosable conditions (Figure 2.4).[6] It is unclear whether these conditions commonly co-exist with Long COVID due to shared causal mechanisms, direct precipitation by the COVID-19 virus, or their potential to increase the risk of developing Long COVID. There may also be a cascading impact across body systems, with symptoms in some systems leading to problems in other body systems.

Each experience of Long COVID (and other conditions they may live with) is as unique as the person living with it. Health professionals must be alert to the possibility of other commonly associated conditions and may need further training and education about any unfamiliar. Comorbid conditions may need monitoring and/or add complexity to shared decision-making and collaborative care planning.

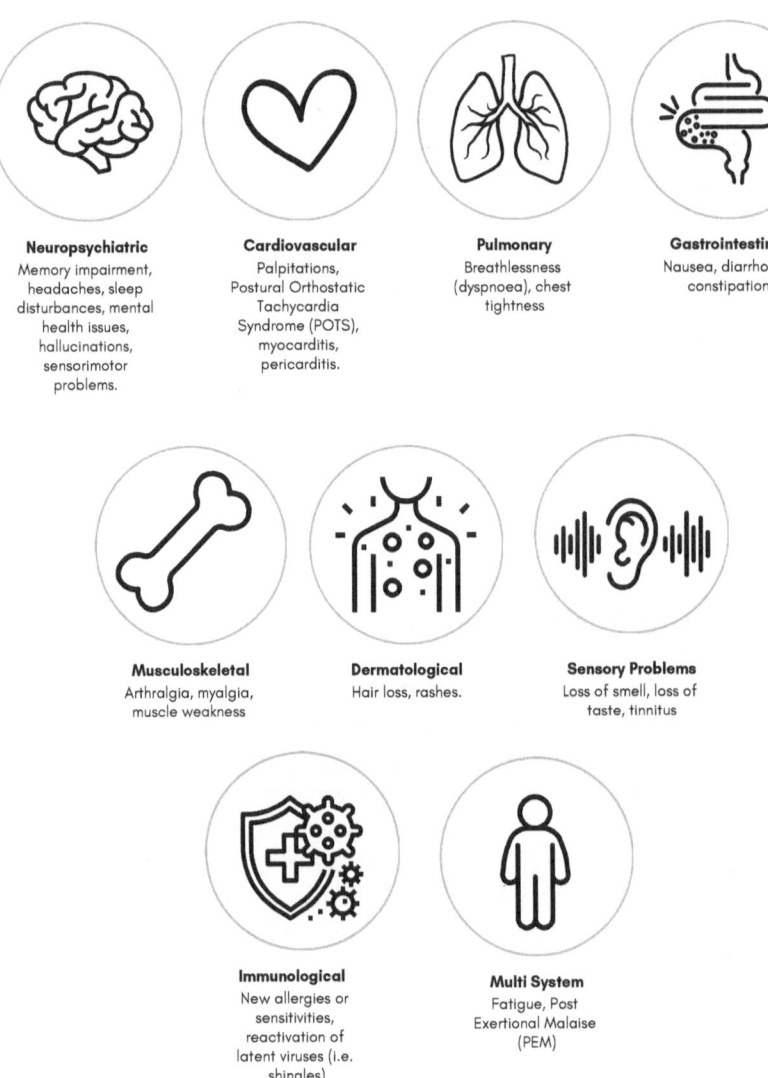

Neuropsychiatric
Memory impairment, headaches, sleep disturbances, mental health issues, hallucinations, sensorimotor problems.

Cardiovascular
Palpitations, Postural Orthostatic Tachycardia Syndrome (POTS), myocarditis, pericarditis.

Pulmonary
Breathlessness (dyspnoea), chest tightness

Gastrointestinal
Nausea, diarrhoea, constipation

Musculoskeletal
Arthralgia, myalgia, muscle weakness

Dermatological
Hair loss, rashes.

Sensory Problems
Loss of smell, loss of taste, tinnitus

Immunological
New allergies or sensitivities, reactivation of latent viruses (i.e. shingles)

Multi System
Fatigue, Post Exertional Malaise (PEM)

Figure 2.3 Commonly reported symptoms of Long COVID.[13]

Identifying Long COVID should not overshadow the need for comprehensive assessments or a willingness to adjust the diagnostic lens as new information comes to light.

As knowledge of Long COVID has grown, some researchers have sought to identify sub-types (phenotypes) based on symptom profiles. Several sub-types have been proposed, including between 3 and 33 symptoms clustered by body

Cardiovascular
- Arrhythmias, Postural Orthostatic Tachycardia Syndrome (POTS), dysautonomia, blood clots, hyperlipidemia.

Neurological
- Cognitive impairment, mood disorders, anxiety, migraine, stroke, Myalgic Encephalomyelitis / Chronic Fatigue Syndrome (ME/CFS).

Immunological
- Mast Cell Activation Syndrome (MCAS), lupus, rheumatoid arthritis, Sjogren's syndrome.

Respiratory
- Interstitial lung disease, hypoxemia.

Musculoskeletal
- Fibromyalgia, connective tissue diseases.

Renal
- Chronic kidney disease.

Endocrine
- Diabetes.

Figure 2.4 Conditions commonly associated with Long COVID.[6]

system (i.e., respiratory, cardiovascular). Other sub-types are organised around the number of symptoms experienced, with more symptoms associated with more severe Long COVID.[12–15] However, the clusters of symptoms identified often overlap and symptom profiles may change over time with the emergence of new issues or changes in severity. People with Long COVID may also experience significant day-to-day variation in symptoms, with activities that were easy one day feeling impossible the next. Sub-types may, therefore, have limited clinical usefulness due to the dynamic nature of Long COVID.

Being identified or diagnosed with Long COVID is not the end of the journey for many people; it's the start of a new phase in their relationship with health services. People with Long COVID and health professionals must remain open to the evolving nature of the condition and our understanding of it. New symptoms or complications may arise for individuals, and longer-term sequelae of COVID-19 infection may not yet be evident. The value of these Long COVID definitions and descriptions for health professionals, therefore, lies in their ability to both guide immediate treatment and shape dynamic and responsive approaches to rehabilitation into the future. Their value to people with Long COVID is their ability to help explain their experience of developing numerous, seemingly unrelated health conditions over a short time.

2.4 THE BIOLOGY OF LONG COVID

The biology underlying Long COVID involves a complex interplay of immune dysregulation, viral persistence, mitochondrial dysfunction, and organ-specific damage. Current research suggests that immune-mediated mechanisms, including chronic inflammation, autoimmune responses, and T-cell dysfunction, play a critical role in helping us understand the symptoms of Long COVID. Viral persistence and the resulting ongoing immune activation may also contribute to the persistence of symptoms. This is further complicated by dysregulation of the autonomic nervous system (ANS) and direct organ damage. The following four key focus areas are under investigation in Long COVID research.

2.4.1 Immune Dysregulation

Research confirms that some people with Long COVID have abnormal immune responses. Studies specifically looking at immune dysregulation have shown alternations to T cells,[16] which are white blood cells known as lymphocytes responsible for fighting off pathogens (like viruses) and cancerous cells. High levels of exhausted T cells have been found[17,18] in studies of people with Long COVID. This dysfunction is also found in other chronic infections, which means that the T cells can no longer perform their role in the immune response.

B cells are the lymphocytes that produce antibodies that allow your body to remember the pathogens you've encountered. Studies have shown an increase in double-negative B cells in people with Long COVID, which are cells that lack specific immune markers. These cells behave in different ways depending on the disease. For example, in Human Immunodeficiency Virus and malaria, they become exhausted and are no longer able to function correctly. However, in the autoimmune disease lupus, they secrete antibodies that contribute to flare-ups.[19] The COVID-19 virus can also reactivate underlying pathogens like Epstein-Barr virus (EBV),[20] with one study suggesting recent EBV reactivation is strongly associated with the fatigue experienced by people with Long COVID.[21]

2.4.2 Viral Reservoirs

Viral reservoirs are areas in the human body where viruses can persist, evading detection by the immune system and treatments and potentially reactivating to cause persistent symptoms. Particles and nucleic acids in the COVID-19 virus have been detected in numerous tissues up to 4 months post-recovery from mild infections, including the gastrointestinal tract, lung, thyroid, blood vessels, skin, breast, and brain.[22] They contribute to a prolonged immune response by becoming superantigens that activate a non-specific response in T cells, leading to immune overstimulation, hypersecretion of proteins that regulate and communicate immune responses (known as cytokines) and chronic inflammation.[23]

The discovery of SARS-CoV-2 (COVID-19) particles in gut tissue led researchers to link this systemic inflammation with potential changes in the gut microbiome of people with Long COVID. A study by Yeoh et al.[24] showed the effects of COVID-19 infection on bacteria, which modulates the immune response proportionate to disease severity and persists after the initial infection period. In a separate study, one year after initial infection, participants were found to have lower bacterial diversity and depleted short-chain fatty acids, which are key immunological components in both the gut lining mucosa and systemically.[25,26]

Persistent low-grade inflammation and cell damage from viral persistence can trigger a phenomenon called Damage-Associated Molecular Patterns (DAMPs).[27] These are molecules released by damaged or dying cells that trigger inflammation, often in response to injuries or stress. Studies have shown elevated levels of pro-inflammatory cytokines such as interleukin-6, tumour necrosis factor-alpha, and interleukin-1 beta in patients with Long COVID, which may lead to symptoms like fatigue, muscle pain, and general malaise.[17,28,29]

2.4.3 Mitochondrial Dysfunction

Mitochondria are colloquially known as "the powerhouse of the cell," so when the SARS-CoV-2 virus hijacks their energy-making capabilities, they can no longer function as part of innate immunity. Innate immunity is the body's first line of defence against viruses, providing a rapid and non-specific response to infections and injuries. SARS-CoV-2 uses parts of the mitochondria to replicate, increasing the Reactive Oxygen Species (ROS).[30,31] ROS are molecules our bodies produce as a byproduct of normal functions, like mitochondria producing energy. However, excessive ROS can cause significant damage to cells. Even after clearing the initial viral infection, mitochondrial function in tissues like the heart, liver, and lymph nodes remains impaired,[31] which can manifest as fatigue, muscle weakness, and poor stamina.

2.4.4 Autonomic Nervous System

Many people with Long COVID experience symptoms of dysautonomia, a disorder of the ANS that regulates involuntary functions such as heart rate, blood pressure, and digestion. POTS is an example of these disorders and is characterised by an abnormally high heart rate when standing up, leading to dizziness, light-headedness, and fatigue. Chapter 16 contains a comprehensive discussion of POTS and the impact of dysautonomia.

As our biological understanding of Long COVID evolves, ongoing research should focus on identifying biomarkers for diagnosis and potential therapeutic targets to treat the underlying mechanisms and pathways identified.

BOX 2.5   PRACTICE POINT

How might understanding the biological mechanisms of Long COVID help you validate patients' experiences and reduce stigma in clinical interactions? What additional training or resources might you seek to deepen your understanding of the biological basis of Long COVID?

2.5 THE EPIDEMIOLOGY OF LONG COVID

Epidemiology studies Long COVID patterns, causes, and distribution in populations to identify risks, track occurrence, and guide community-level public health interventions. Substantial research has been completed on the epidemiology of Long COVID; however, key aspects remain uncertain due to the complex causes and presentations of this systemic condition and challenges related to using real-world public health data (as discussed in Chapter 5). The evolution of the COVID-19 virus itself is also changing the epidemiology of Long COVID.

As discussed, the array and clustering of symptoms in Long COVID overlap with other conditions, and few have definitive features like biomarkers, making symptom-based diagnosis challenging. Some progress has been made towards identifying biomarkers that may support prognosis, diagnosis, and epidemiology in the future, but these may not be reliable for all forms of Long COVID.[32] Despite this, we continue to build our understanding of risk factors and our ability to identify particularly vulnerable populations.

Jeffrey et al.[33] conducted a national study of the Scottish electronic medical records of 4,676,390 people, and 1.7% were identified as having Long COVID. People with Long COVID were more likely to be female (65.1% versus 50.4%), aged 38–67 (63.7% versus 48.9%), overweight or obese (45.7% versus 29.4%), have one or more comorbidities (52.7% versus 36.0%), be immunosuppressed (6.9% versus 3.2%), shielding from infection (7.9% versus 3.4%), hospitalised within 28 days of testing positive (8.8% versus 3.3%%), and tested positive before Omicron (44.9% versus 35.9%). Vaccination with three doses before infection has also been associated with reduced incidence of Long COVID.[34]

While these findings on risk factors are consistent across many cohort studies, Long COVID prevalence estimates vary dramatically depending on study design, case definition, study population, and the timing of data collection. The highest estimates are reported for early variants and the lowest for Omicron infections that also occurred in the context of the added protection provided by natural immunity and vaccination. A systematic review[35] of 130 papers estimating the prevalence of Long COVID found results ranged from 0% to 93%, and most studies had a medium to high risk of bias.

Summarising what is known about Long COVID epidemiology highlights the challenges of working with complex real-world data. Determining prevalence and risk factors depends on reliable estimates of prevalence to compare relative risks across population subgroups. In the case of Long COVID, this is plagued by two epidemiological challenges: poor measurement of exposure with many undocumented infections and, as time has gone on, ubiquitous exposure. Long COVID incidence will be underestimated if symptoms are attributed to other causes, mainly if a COVID-19 infection was not recorded or suspected in the patient. However, its prevalence may also be overestimated if other conditions causing similar symptoms are misclassified as Long COVID. The likelihood of misdiagnosis also changes as testing practices change. Rapid Antigen Tests (RATs) have become less affordable, and the results of both Polymerase Chain Reaction and RATs have not been reported. Underlying reduction in the risk of severe COVID-19 disease, a Long-COVID risk factor linked to viral evolution and maturing immunity across the population, may also increase the chances of underdiagnosis as the index of suspicion decreases.

There is some evidence that experiencing repeat infections raises the overall risk of Long COVID, especially for older males.[36] It should be noted that the risk factors for repeat infection overlap those predisposing someone to severe acute disease, the development of Long COVID, and other conditions that may exacerbate Long COVID duration and severity.[37] The likelihood that a patient will be tested and confirmed as a COVID-19 case may also be related to the same risk factors for severe infection and Long COVID. For example, someone at higher risk of severe Long COVID due to an underlying condition is more likely to be tested and followed up by a doctor or hospital, which increases their chances of being identified as having both a COVID-19 infection and Long COVID.

Participants in hospital-based studies of Long COVID generally report higher Long COVID prevalence estimates than studies with people living in the community.[35] This suggests that prevalence estimates may not be generalisable to the broader population. In contrast, Woodrow et al.[35] also reported studies based on routine healthcare records generally reported lower prevalence estimates (13.6%) than studies based on self-report (43.9%), perhaps because those unwell from other conditions are shielding. Understanding the populations being studied, where very different prevalence estimates are generated, is essential because formally diagnosed and documented cases represent only a portion of genuine cases.

Controlled studies are an essential design, especially when the symptoms of the condition of interest are not unique. Controls reveal background rates of Long COVID-like symptoms that can be considered in Long COVID prevalence estimates. Hoeg et al.[38] note that the lack of Long COVID studies with control groups likely led to a risk distortion. Controlled studies can report the risk difference for symptoms between people with a history of COVID-19 infection and controls, providing an attributable risk estimate, a more meaningful estimate of the burden of Long COVID.[39] Few Long COVID studies are community-based with controls, showing relative risks from 1.0 to 51.4 and absolute risk differences from −1% to 35%.[37] Studies with low bias report a pooled relative risk of 1.33 and absolute differences of 1%–9%, highlighting that higher-quality studies show moderate relative risks and smaller, consistent absolute differences.[35]

BOX 2.6   EPIDEMIOLOGICAL TERMINOLOGY

Attributable risk estimates measure how much of a health condition is directly caused by a specific factor, such as infection or behaviour. These estimates identify the amount of risk that will be reduced if this factor is eliminated.

Pooled relative risks combine the findings of several studies to measure how much more likely an outcome is in one group compared to another on average.

While the true prevalence of Long COVID remains elusive, within cohort trends indicate it has decreased over time, with fewer new diagnoses and the recovery of existing cases. An Australian biomarker study of 62 people with COVID-19 infections from 2020 found significant improvements by 24 months. By 24 months, most people with Long COVID had similar biomarker levels to a control group of the same age and gender, with 62% of patients self-reporting improvement in their health-related quality of life.[32] This study followed people over time, identifying new onset and reinfections. However, improvement in biomarkers does not always translate into symptom relief. The risk of Long COVID has also been shown to differ by variant; for example, a US health worker study reported the prevalence to be 42% for the ancestral strain, 36% for the alpha variant, and 16% for the delta or omicron variants.[40]

The epidemiology of Long COVID is complex and evolving and influenced by study design, case definitions, and population characteristics. While substantial progress has been made in identifying risk factors, significant challenges remain. Also, the risk of new-onset long COVID after a second SARS-CoV-2 infection has been reported as being lower than after a first infection in those aged ≥16 years, but the risk is not zero.[36–37] While some evidence suggests Long COVID prevalence is decreasing over time, high-quality community-based research continues to have a crucial role in accurately assessing the burden of Long COVID, incidence of new Long COVID cases (whether new-onset or repeat diagnosis), and case relapse, to inform effective public health responses.

BOX 2.7 PRACTICE POINT

What steps can you take to identify and address risk factors for Long COVID in the populations you serve? Do you discuss risk factors with your patients? How can you incorporate your understanding of risk factors into your practice with people with Long COVID?

2.6 CONCLUSION

In summary, this chapter has shown that Long COVID is a complex and multifaceted condition characterised by persistent symptoms that significantly affect daily life, often long after the acute phase of COVID-19. Its varied presentations overlap with other conditions, and the lack of specific biomarkers makes diagnosis challenging. The biology of Long COVID involves immune dysregulation, viral persistence, mitochondrial dysfunction, and ANS disruptions, which contribute to its systemic and prolonged impact. While substantial research has shed light on risk factors, vulnerable populations, and the evolving epidemiology of Long COVID, estimating its true prevalence remains challenging due to methodological inconsistencies and biases. Continued high-quality research is essential to refine definitions, improve diagnosis, and guide effective public health and clinical responses to Long COVID.

REFERENCES

1 National Institute for Health and Care Excellence (NICE), et al. COVID-19 rapid guideline: Managing the long-term effects of COVID-19. Version 1.14. London: NICE, SIGN, RCGP; 2022.

2 Stephenson T, et al. Long COVID (post-COVID-19 condition) in children: A modified Delphi process. Arch Dis Child. 2022;107(7):674–80. doi:10.1136/archdischild-2021-323624

3 Centers for Disease Control and Prevention (CDC). Long-term effects of COVID-19 [Internet]. Atlanta: CDC; [updated 2023; cited 2025 Feb 7]. Available from: https://www.cdc.gov/covid/long-term-effects/.

4 World Health Organisation (WHO). A clinical case definition of post-COVID-19 condition by a Delphi consensus. Geneva: WHO; 2021.

5 Fernández-de-las-Peñas C, et al. Defining post-COVID symptoms (post-acute COVID, Long COVID, persistent post-COVID): An integrative classification. Int J Environ Res Public Health. 2021;18:2621. doi:10.3390/ijerph18052621.

6 National Academies of Sciences, Engineering, and Medicine (NASEM). A Long COVID definition: A chronic, systemic disease state with profound consequences. Washington, DC: The National Academies Press; 2024. doi:10.17226/27768.

7 Malone LA, et al. Multidisciplinary collaborative consensus guidance statement on the assessment and treatment of postacute sequelae of SARS-CoV-2 infection (PASC) in children and adolescents. PM R. 2022;14(10):1241–69. doi:10.1002/pmrj.12890.

8 Chaichana U, et al. Definition of post–COVID-19 condition among published research studies. JAMA Netw Open. 2023;6(4):e235856. doi:10.1001/jamanetworkopen.2023.5856.

9 Al-Aly Z, et al. Long COVID: Long-term health outcomes and implications for policy and research. Nat Rev Nephrol. 2023;19:1–2. doi:10.1038/s41581-022-00652-2.

10 Au L, et al. Long COVID and medical gaslighting: Dismissal, delayed diagnosis, and deferred treatment. SSM Qual Res Health. 2022;2:100167. doi:10.1016/j.ssmqr.2022.100167.

11 Davis HE, et al. Characterising Long COVID in an international cohort: 7 months of symptoms and their impact. EClinicalMedicine. 2021;38:101019. doi:10.1016/j.eclinm.2021.101019.

12 Kenny G, et al. Identification of distinct Long COVID clinical phenotypes through cluster analysis of self-reported symptoms. Open Forum Infect Dis. 2022;9(4):ofac060. doi: 10.1093/ofid/ofac060.

13 Zhang H, et al. Data-driven identification of post-acute SARS-CoV-2 infection subphenotypes. Nat Med. 2023;29(1):226–35. doi: 10.1038/s41591-022-02116-3.

14 Frontera JA, et al. Post-acute sequelae of COVID-19 symptom phenotypes and therapeutic strategies: A prospective, observational study. PLoS One. 2022;17(9):e0275274. doi:10.1371/journal.pone.0275274.

15 Reese J, et al. Generalisable Long COVID subtypes: Findings from the NIH N3C and RECOVER programmes. EBioMedicine. 2023;87:104413. doi: 10.1101/2022.05.24.22275398.

16 Glynne P, et al. Long COVID following Mild SARS-CoV-2 Infection: Characteristic T Cell Alterations and Response to Antihistamines. J Investig Med. 2022;70:61–67. doi:10.1136/jim-2021-002051.

17 Phetsouphanh C, et al. Immunological dysfunction persists for 8 months following initial mild-to-moderate SARS-CoV-2 infection. Nat Immunol. 2022;23:210–16. doi:10.1038/s41590-021-01113-x.

18 Klein J, et al. Distinguishing features of Long COVID identified through immune profiling. Nature. 2023;623:139–48. doi:10.1038/s41586-023-06651-y.

19 Sachinidis A, et al. Double Negative (DN) B cells: A connecting bridge between rheumatic diseases and COVID-19? Mediterr J Rheumatol. 2021;32:192–99. doi:10.31138/mjr.32.3.192.

20 Gold JE, et al. Investigation of Long COVID Prevalence and its relationship to Epstein-Barr Virus reactivation. Pathogens. 2021;10:763. doi: 10.3390/pathogens10060763.

21 Peluso MJ, et al. Chronic viral coinfections differentially affect the likelihood of developing Long COVID. J Clin Invest. 2023;133. doi:10.1172/JCI163669.

22 Zuo W, et al. The persistence of SARS-CoV-2 in tissues and its association with Long COVID symptoms: A cross-sectional cohort study in China. Lancet Infect Dis. 2024;24:845–55. doi:10.1016/S1473-3099(24)00171-3.

23 Cheng MH, et al. Superantigenic character of an insert unique to SARS-CoV-2 spike supported by skewed TCR repertoire in patients with hyperinflammation. Proc Natl Acad Sci U S A. 2020;117:25254–62. doi:10.1073/pnas.2010722117.

24 Yeoh YK, et al. Gut microbiota composition reflects disease severity and dysfunctional immune responses in patients with COVID-19. Gut. 2021;70:698–706. doi:10.1136/gutjnl-2020-323020.

25 Zhang D, et al. Gut microbiota dysbiosis correlates with Long COVID-19 at one-year after discharge. J Korean Med Sci. 2023;38:e120. doi:10.3346/jkms.2023.38.e120.

26 Mann ER, et al. Short-chain fatty acids: Linking diet, the microbiome and immunity. Nat Rev Immunol. 2024;24:577–95. doi:10.1038/s41577-024-01014-8.

27 Maamar M, et al. Post-COVID-19 syndrome, low-grade inflammation and inflammatory markers: A cross-sectional study. Curr Med Res Opin. 2022;38:901–9. doi:10.1080/03007995.2022.2042991.

28 Schulthei C, et al. The IL-1ß, IL-6, and TNF cytokine triad is associated with post-acute sequelae of COVID-19. Cell Rep Med. 2022;3. doi:10.1016/j.xcrm.2022.100663.

29 Peluso MJ, et al. Markers of immune activation and inflammation in individuals with post-acute sequelae of severe acute respiratory syndrome coronavirus 2 infection. J Infect Dis. 2021;224:1839–48. doi:10.1093/infdis/jiab490.

30 Saleh J, et al. Mitochondria and microbiota dysfunction in COVID-19 pathogenesis. Mitochondrion. 2020;54:1–7. doi:10.1016/j.mito.2020.06.008.

31 Guarnieri JW, et al. Core mitochondrial genes are down-regulated during SARS-CoV-2 infection of rodent and human hosts. Sci Transl Med. 2023;15:eabq1533. doi:10.1126/scitranslmed.abq1533.

32 Phetsouphanh C, et al. Improvement of immune dysregulation in individuals with Long COVID at 24-months following SARS-CoV-2 infection. Nat Commun. 2024;15:3315. doi:10.1038/s41467-024-47720-8.

33 Jeffrey K, et al. Prevalence and risk factors for Long COVID among adults in Scotland using electronic health records: A national, retrospective, observational cohort study. EClinicalMedicine. 2024;71. doi:10.1016/j.eclinm.2024.102590.

34 Slawson DC. Likelihood of Long COVID varies by variant, sex, and vaccination status. Am Fam Physician. 2023;107:199.

35 Woodrow M, et al. Systematic review of the prevalence of Long COVID. Open Forum Infect Dis. 2023;10. doi:10.1093/ofid/ofad233.

36 Bowe B, et al. Acute and postacute sequelae associated with SARS-CoV-2 reinfection. Nat Med. 2022;28:2398–405. doi:10.1038/s41591-022-02051-3.

37 Boufidou F, et al. SARS-CoV-2 reinfections and Long COVID in the post-omicron phase of the pandemic. Int J Mol Sci. 2023;24. doi:10.3390/ijms241612962.

38 Høeg TB, et al. How methodological pitfalls have created widespread misunderstanding about long COVID. BMJ Evid Based Med. 2024;29:142–46. doi:10.1136/bmjebm-2023-112338.

39 Xuereb RA, et al. Long COVID syndrome: A case-control study. Am J Med. 2023. doi:10.1016/j.amjmed.2023.04.022.

40 Azzolini E, et al. Association between BNT162b2 vaccination and Long COVID after infections not requiring hospitalisationhospitalisation in health care workers. JAMA. 2022;328(7): 676–78. doi:10.1001/jama.2022.11691.

Chapter 3

Long COVID, ME/CFS, and Other Post-Acute Infection Syndromes

Raeya Bognar, Julie Hughes, and Danielle Hitch

BOX 3.1   LEARNING OBJECTIVES

By the end of this chapter, readers should be able to:

- Understand the similarities and differences between Long COVID and other PAIS and their implications for accurate diagnosis and effective care.
- Apply the Weerasekera 5P's model to identify and analyse the predisposing, precipitating, perpetuating, and protective factors shaping Long COVID and other PAIS.
- Develop practical management strategies for Long COVID in collaboration with patients, drawing on the lived experiences of people with ME/CFS to support recovery and resilience.
- Advocate for person-centred and equitable care for individuals with PAIS, emphasising empathy, respect, validation, and collaboration in therapeutic relationships.

3.1 INTRODUCTION

Viruses have been infecting humans for millennia, influencing our evolutionary and immunological development as a species.[1] Post-Acute Infection Syndromes (PAIS) have long been recognised by healthcare providers, with the first reports dating back to the second half of the 19th century.[2] Long COVID is the latest in a long line of PAIS, which have a range of similar and distinctive symptoms. This chapter explores where Long COVID sits within the broader landscape of PAIS and what this means for rehabilitation.

DOI: 10.4324/9781003528104-4

3.1.1 Post-Acute Viral Syndromes

Many, but not all, PAIS are caused by viruses. A virus is a microscopic infectious agent that can only replicate inside the living cells of an organism. They are composed of DNA or RNA enclosed in a protein envelope. Viruses can evolve (or mutate) rapidly, which may allow them to outpace immune responses and develop resistance to treatment.

BOX 3.2   DID YOU KNOW?

Viruses are the most common biological things on the planet. There are approximately one decillion (1,000,000,000,000,000,000,000,000,000,000,000) known to science.[3]

Most PAIS share a core set of similar symptoms, but each also has distinctive aspects in their presentation (see Figure 3.1).

Each PAIS is also associated with one or more distinctive symptoms, reflecting the unique characteristics of their causative virus. These include joint swelling and stiffness (Chikungunya); extensive joint involvement (Ross River Fever); liver

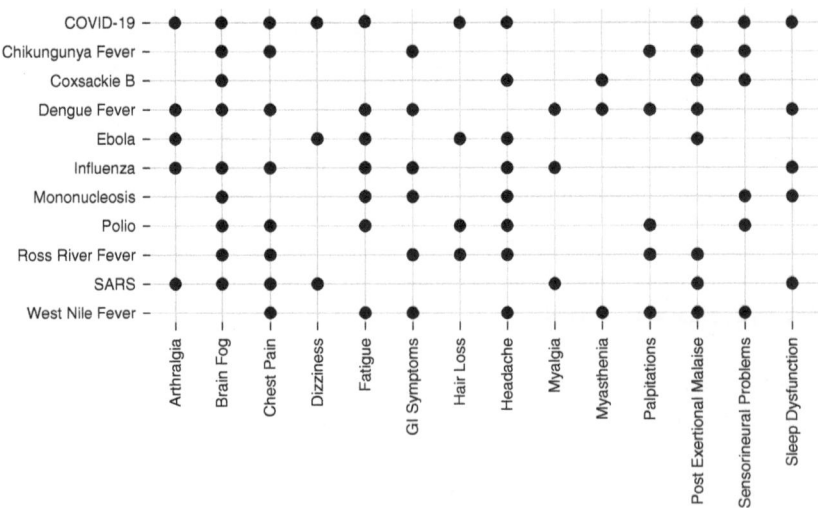

Figure 3.1 Examples of shared and distinctive features of Post Acute Infection Syndromes (PAIS).

Note: The Epstein-Barr virus causes mononucleosis (also known as Glandular Fever).

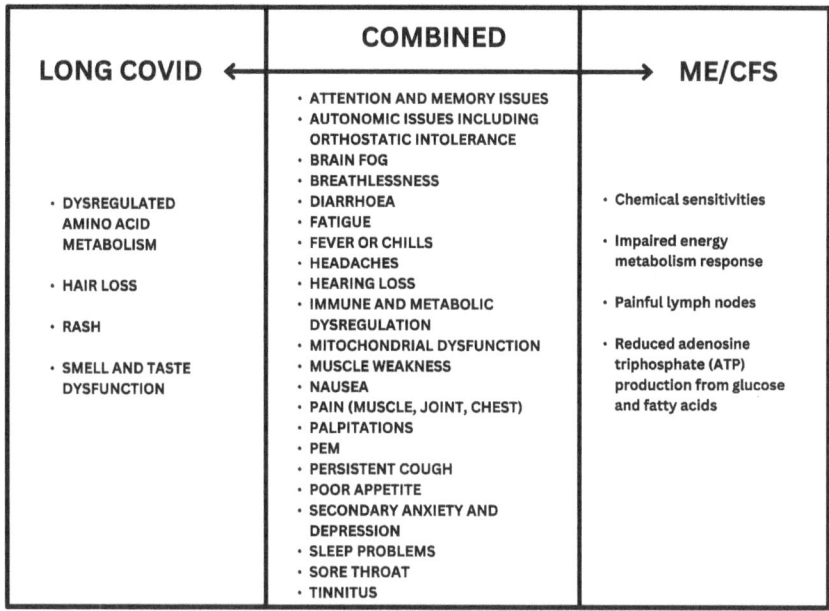

LONG COVID	COMBINED	ME/CFS
• DYSREGULATED AMINO ACID METABOLISM • HAIR LOSS • RASH • SMELL AND TASTE DYSFUNCTION	• ATTENTION AND MEMORY ISSUES • AUTONOMIC ISSUES INCLUDING ORTHOSTATIC INTOLERANCE • BRAIN FOG • BREATHLESSNESS • DIARRHOEA • FATIGUE • FEVER OR CHILLS • HEADACHES • HEARING LOSS • IMMUNE AND METABOLIC DYSREGULATION • MITOCHONDRIAL DYSFUNCTION • MUSCLE WEAKNESS • NAUSEA • PAIN (MUSCLE, JOINT, CHEST) • PALPITATIONS • PEM • PERSISTENT COUGH • POOR APPETITE • SECONDARY ANXIETY AND DEPRESSION • SLEEP PROBLEMS • SORE THROAT • TINNITUS	• Chemical sensitivities • Impaired energy metabolism response • Painful lymph nodes • Reduced adenosine triphosphate (ATP) production from glucose and fatty acids

Figure 3.2 Shared and distinctive features of ME/CFS and Long COVID.

dysfunction, rash, fever, and swollen glands (Mononucleosis/Glandular Fever); paraesthesia (Coxsackie B), menstrual cessation (Ebola), motor incoordination (West Nile), and progressive muscle weakness (Post-Polio Syndrome).

Myalgic Encephalomyelitis/Chronic Fatigue Syndrome (ME/CFS) is one of the most widely known PAIS and provides a standard benchmark for comparison with Long COVID. No specific viral cause has been identified for ME/CFS, with Epstein-Barr, Cytomegalovirus, Enteroviruses, Borna disease virus, and Parvovirus all implicated.[4–6] The relationship between ME/CFS and Long COVID will be explored in detail throughout this chapter, but Figure 3.2 provides an evidence-based overview of shared and distinctive symptoms.[7–10] It is important to note that while ME/CFS has several established diagnostic criteria, Long COVID does not at the time of writing.

BOX 3.3 PRACTICE POINT

From your perspective, are ME/CFS and Long COVID the same, or are they distinctive syndromes? There is no right or wrong answer to this question, but consider how your perspective might influence your work with patients.

Understanding PAIS's overlapping and unique aspects is essential for both the person and healthcare professionals. Recognising their similarities helps to highlight the shared challenges people face and fosters opportunities for peer support. For some, Long COVID may be their first encounter with PAIS, but others may have had lived experiences of other viral infections. On the other hand, recognising the distinct characteristics of these conditions allows for more personalised interventions and approaches that better address the specific needs of each person impacted. Seeing both sides of the PAIS coin can support a holistic approach that leverages existing knowledge and enables person-centred care.

3.1.2 PAIS Can Cause Invisible Disabilities

Invisible disability (or hidden disability) is a broad term describing impairments that are not immediately obvious when looking at someone but which nevertheless cause significant symptoms like chronic pain and exhaustion and daily challenges such as social isolation.[11] These disabilities are caused by a wide range of physical and mental conditions and have a significant impact on participation in daily life.[12] These conditions are not rare, with approximately 90% of Australians living with a disability having an invisible condition.[13] Inexperience or misunderstandings from others about the impact of these disabilities can result in stigma and discrimination within society,[11] which in turn has a significant impact on the person's mental health and wellbeing.

Not "looking disabled" or "looking well" can lead to an underestimation of challenges and limitations, particularly when clinicians lack knowledge or experience about the causative condition. Inaccurate professional judgements and expectations by health professionals can contribute to this problem, and comprehensive assessment must be founded on information gathered from multiple formal and informal sources.[14] Asking open and curious questions, along with a commitment to learning from the lived experiences of patients, allows clinicians to enact person-centred practice and more effectively addresses the impact of invisible disabilities for people with Long COVID.

3.2 THE 5P'S OF PAIS

Given that most PAIS fit the definition and experience of an invisible disability, the Weerasekera 5P's model of formulation[15] provides a helpful structure for health professionals to consider their impact on health and wellbeing (see Figure 3.3).

While sufficient evidence exists about the presenting, predisposing, and precipitating factors for Long COVID, ME/CFS provides the most examples of

The 5P's

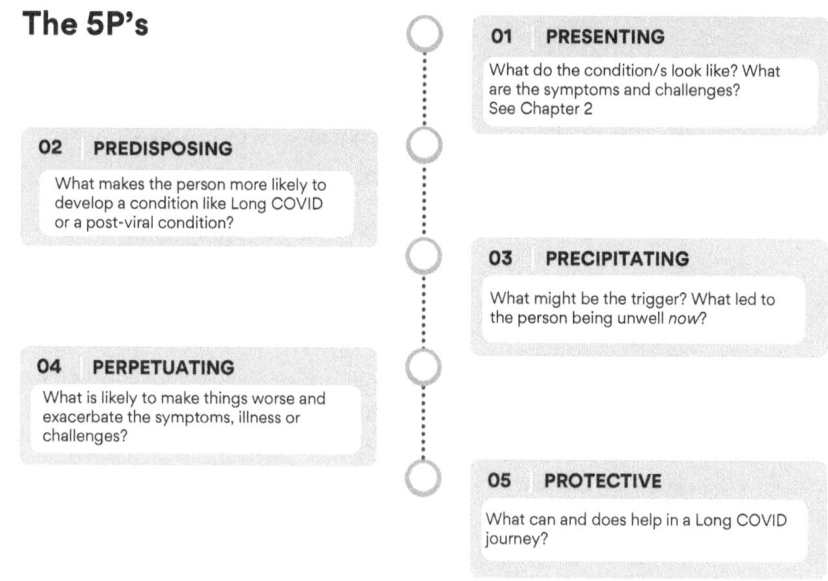

01   PRESENTING

What do the condition/s look like? What are the symptoms and challenges? See Chapter 2

02   PREDISPOSING

What makes the person more likely to develop a condition like Long COVID or a post-viral condition?

03   PRECIPITATING

What might be the trigger? What led to the person being unwell *now*?

04   PERPETUATING

What is likely to make things worse and exacerbate the symptoms, illness or challenges?

05   PROTECTIVE

What can and does help in a Long COVID journey?

Figure 3.3 5P's formulation applied to PAIS.

perpetuating and protective factors due to its more prolonged presence in the research literature. The controversies surrounding ME/CFS are also relevant to understanding Long COVID, given their many similarities, illustrating collective learning about what to do and what not to do.

3.2.1 Presenting

Briefly, Long COVID manifests as a range of persistent symptoms that affect individuals for weeks or months after acute SARS-CoV-2 infection.[16–17] Common symptoms include fatigue, shortness of breath, cognitive dysfunction (often called "brain fog"), headaches, sleep disturbances, and chest pain. Long COVID can impact multiple organ systems, potentially exacerbating pre-existing conditions or introducing new health issues. Symptoms can fluctuate, and some patients experience relapses, which are both distressing and disruptive to recovery.

The symptoms of Long COVID significantly impact function and participation in daily life, leading to difficulties in self-care, domestic and community activities, as well as education and work. The impact of this syndrome, therefore, extends beyond physical health, affecting emotional wellbeing and resulting in social and economic problems for people with Long COVID, as well as their families and carers. For more detailed information about presentations of Long COVID, please see Chapter 2.

BOX 3.4 PRACTICE POINT

Do you have any assumptions about who will likely develop Long COVID? Are you assumptions the same or different from the risk factors associated with COVID-19 infection?

3.2.2 Predisposing Factors

Viruses infect people of any age, and people accumulate multiple viral infections over their lifetimes. So, what predisposes or makes a person more likely to develop Long COVID? Many patients ask the question, "Why did my symptoms not go away? Why did I get Long COVID?" It is important to say they are not at fault – Long COVID can affect anyone, regardless of the precautions they take or their general health or wellbeing. However, several factors are known to increase the risk of developing a PAIS, which may support people with Long COVID to make sense of their experience.

Hereditary factors (including genetics and epigenetics) may predispose some people to developing Long COVID and other PAIS. People assigned female at birth are more likely to be diagnosed with these conditions, as are those with pre-existing autonomic or cardiovascular issues (including blood pressure issues and heart rate abnormalities) and iron deficiency.[18–20] Hypermobility disorders causing excessive flexibility are also associated with Long COVID, potentially due to connective tissue dysfunction.[21] These factors highlight the complex interplay of biological and physiological mechanisms underlying susceptibility to Long COVID.

Psychological factors may also predispose people to develop Long COVID by influencing the body's stress response and overall resilience to illness. A history of trauma, including adverse childhood events, plays a critical role in shaping the nervous system[22]. This can lead to dysregulation in how the body processes and reacts to stressors, increasing susceptibility to Long COVID.[23] Personality traits, including emotional sensitivity (also known as neuroticism), perfectionism, and Type D personality (negative emotions with social inhibition), are thought to influence how people experience and cope with the challenges of conditions like Long COVID and ME/CFS,[24–26] reflecting the complex interplay between personality, stress, and anxiety. Pre-existing anxiety also adds an additional layer of stress to the nervous and immune systems, which may contribute to the development of Long COVID.[27] While Long COVID is not a psychosomatic disorder, there are many links between the physical, psychological, and cognitive aspects of this syndrome.

Physical health factors also significantly predispose individuals to Long COVID due to their demands on the immune system and overall physiological resilience. Pre-existing Mast Cell Activation Syndrome (MCAS) leads to inappropriate stimulation of mast cells, a type of white cell that protects against pathogens, promotes wound healing, and mediates allergic responses. Pre-existing MCAS could increase the likelihood of hyperinflammation, which has, in turn, been implicated in the development of Long COVID symptoms.[28] While some evidence is emerging about potential roles for pre-existing sleep disorders and allergies in increasing Long COVID risk, research findings are mixed.[29–31] Finally, the presence of other chronic health issues also increases risk by compromising recovery from acute COVID-19, including obesity and Human Immunodeficiency Virus.[32–33]

Finally, socioeconomic factors may also predispose people to developing Long COVID. People from Culturally and Linguistically Diverse and disadvantaged communities are more vulnerable to acute COVID-19 infection, experience more severe outcomes and have higher rates of Long COVID.[34,35] Their outcomes reflect the compounded impact of social determinants of health, including poverty, poor quality housing, low educational attainment, unemployment, migration status, and social isolation.[36] An intersectional perspective, which recognises that patients may belong to one or many of these risk groups, is essential when working with people with PAIS to understand their unique experiences and circumstances fully.

3.2.3 Precipitating Factors

As shown in Figure 3.4, one or more events may trigger the development of Long COVID. Infection with COVID-19 is the common precipitating factor for all cases of Long COVID, but severe and multi-symptom illness during the acute phase is a well-established risk factor.[37] Recent infection with other viruses, such as Epstein-Barr,[32] and severe or sustained stress[38] may also encourage the development of Long COVID.

3.2.4 Perpetuating Factors

Perpetuating factors can exacerbate the symptoms and functional problems of Long COVID and may extend its duration. Although each person with Long COVID has their own risk factors, people with ME/CFS have more experience with the perpetuating and protective factors that have accompanied this condition, many of which are also relevant to Long COVID and other PAIS. The history of ME/CFS has much to teach us about both beneficial and harmful approaches to supporting these patients.

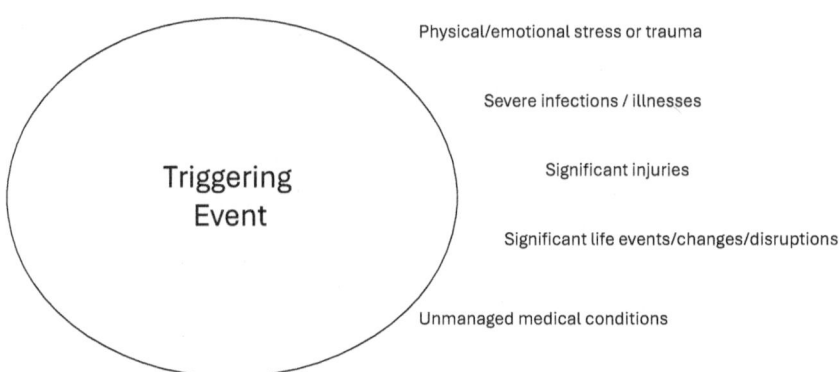

Physical/emotional stress or trauma

Severe infections / illnesses

Significant injuries

Significant life events/changes/disruptions

Unmanaged medical conditions

Figure 3.4 Precipitating factors for Long COVID.

Note: People with Long COVID may have experienced one or more of these events.

Myalgic encephalomyelitis (ME), also known as chronic fatigue syndrome (CFS), is an acquired neurological disease-causing complex dysfunction in the nervous, immune, and endocrine systems.[39] A cardinal feature is the exacerbation of fatigue and other symptoms following minimal exertion,[40] but symptom severity and functional impairments vary widely between people. Severe ME/CFS may lead to decades-long illness with limited recovery.[41]

Historic misconceptions about ME/CFS resulted in inaccurate prevalence estimates, inaccurate diagnostic criteria, flawed theories of aetiology, inappropriate treatments, and insufficient research. Prevalence is hard to estimate due to over 20 case definitions worldwide.[42] However, Emerge Australia[43] estimates that 75–80% of patients identify as female, 0.4–1% of Australians are affected, and 25% experience severe symptoms leaving them housebound or bedbound.

Historically, patients waited over five years for diagnosis and had to make persistent efforts to receive it once they had lived with symptoms for at least six months.[41,44] Broad diagnostic criteria and the lack of definitive biomarkers led to frequent misses and misdiagnoses.[39,41] Many clinicians did not have the skills to recognise or did not believe in the existence of the condition,[41] leaving patients untreated and unsupported. Without a diagnosis, people were left to cope with their condition alone.

Despite decades of misunderstanding and misdirection, research has only recently begun to uncover underlying pathological processes. Until recently, people with ME/CFS were viewed by health professionals through a chronic pain or health psychology lens. These theories and practices were prioritised over lived experience and provided a foundation for treatments like graded exercise therapy and cognitive behavioural therapy.[45] The methodological quality of research on these interventions is contested[46]; they have limited or negative patient-reported impact on health[47] and may contribute to the danger of "psychologising" ME/CFS.[48]

The ME/CFS community became self-taught experts[41] challenging flawed research, which likely included people without ME/CFS due to broad diagnostic criteria and therefore wasted scarce funding.[41,49] This united consumer voice has reframed ME/CFS history as a case of "medical gaslighting," where patient perspectives were dismissed and symptoms attributed primarily to psychological causes.[48,49] Sadly, history appears to have repeated itself for Long COVID, with the downplaying of symptoms and viewing the condition as largely psychosomatic, a common theme in the international literature.[50]

As a result, many people with ME/CFS experience stigma, discrimination, and neglect from their families, health professionals, and the broader community. ME/CFS has been found to reduce a person's quality of life[51] significantly and causes long-standing disruption to work and other meaningful activities and leisure roles, social isolation, poorer mental health, and relationship breakdowns.[41,52] People with severe ME/CFS are rarely seen by health professionals and remain underrepresented in research due to access difficulties and reluctance resulting from negative past interactions with health professionals[41]. Globally, there remains little in the way of support for people with ME/CFS and eligibility criteria related to "permanence" often prevent these patients from accessing disability and welfare supports.[52,53]

The history of ME/CFS offers critical insights into the challenges inherited by people with Long COVID. These systemic failures highlight the importance of early intervention and validation of people's experiences, prioritising research that centres on patient-reported outcomes, and creating integrated healthcare pathways. Learning from past mistakes means avoiding the marginalising of Long COVID patients by framing their symptoms as psychosomatic, delaying care, or neglecting tailored rehabilitation. Transparent, evidence-based, multidisciplinary rehabilitation approaches that prioritise equity with other conditions could ensure Long COVID patients do not have to fight the same protracted battles faced by the ME/CFS community. Their hard-earned lived experience should teach us the necessity of systemic accountability and proactive measures to build trust, improve outcomes, and dismantle inequities.

3.2.5 Protective Factors

Research has primarily focused on predisposing and perpetuating factors, but limited studies on protective factors for ME/CFS, Long COVID, and other PAIS highlight avenues for further exploration. Being of an older age and having shorter diagnostic delays are linked to better outcomes for ME/CFS,[54] while blood types O and B may play a protective role in Long COVID.[55]

The quality of care provided by rehabilitation health professionals is a key protective factor against poor outcomes for people with PAIS. Clear diagnostic criteria for some PAIS, like Glandular Fever, enable timely diagnosis and early intervention to reduce symptom severity and functional challenges. Without diagnostic criteria for Long COVID, rehabilitation health professionals should refer to the National Academies of Science, Engineering, and Medicine working definition or the World Health Organization case description for guidance.[16,17]

Most importantly, people with Long COVID need health professionals who actively listen to them and do not ignore or negate their experience. They need support from people who accept and acknowledge their lived experience, even though the underlying pathology is not entirely understood. Access to compassionate and evidence-informed advice and support can and does help people with Long COVID, despite the current absence of evidence about effective treatments or recovery expectations.

A careful assessment of symptoms, functional capacity, and the impact of Long COVID on personal quality of life by healthcare professionals is vital. Healthcare professionals working with people experiencing Long COVID have a wide range of interventions at their disposal, including evaluating time use via activity diaries,[56] assessments of functional capacity,[57] assistive equipment or home modifications, as well as pacing and energy conservation.[41–45] Informal (family, friends, and Long COVID peers) and formal supports (like health and disability services) also provide essential protection against relapse. In summary, rehabilitation health professionals already have a toolbox complete of strategies to help protect people with Long COVID from poor outcomes and promote sustained recovery.

3.3 RAEYA'S STORY

At 14 years old, Raeya was highly academic, very sporty, slightly hypermobile, and prone to viruses, with a family history of low blood pressure. When she developed Glandular Fever (EBV), she thought it was just a cold. So, she "pushed through" and continued attending school and Netball tournaments. Instead of recovering, she became extremely unwell.

After 12 months of ill health and seeing nine different Doctors, she was finally diagnosed with CFS. Between the ages of 14 and 16 years, her health steadily declined, and she was only able to attend school 40% of the time. She spent most of her time at home and/or in bed. At the age of 16, Raeya was finally offered an evidence-based treatment for her CFS. However, she continued to struggle with everyday life and school expectations, entering a cycle of "pushing through" despite her symptoms and then crashing. As a result, she couldn't finish school and was regularly "gaslit" by teachers, peers, and even health professionals into thinking her CFS wasn't real because it was "rare" and someone "so young" was unlikely to have the condition.

By the age of 19 years, Raeya found some helpful support and returned to study, followed by part-time work and slowly increasing her return to a regular life. However, it wasn't until she was 25 that she was diagnosed with Orthostatic Intolerance and hypermobility. She can only wonder how her life could have been different if she had received this information and some informed support early in her experience with CFS. Now, at 30 years old, she has a family, works full-time as a health professional, and runs a successful business with people with invisible conditions. She can finally say that she is living without health challenges and limitations.

Looking back on her illness journey as a health professional, Raeya understands she had many of the predisposing factors that increased her likelihood of developing CFS, along with several precipitating and perpetuating factors outlined in this chapter. She eventually found and focused on protective factors, all of which allowed her to regain her current level of health. Knowing the perpetuating and protective factors enabled Raeya to self-manage and shorten her COVID journey, even though she experienced fatigue, orthostatic intolerance (again), loss of smell and taste, and a daily headache for 4 months. As a result, she was able to return to her previous normal. She believes her previous CFS journey and health professional knowledge prepared and helped her to avoid developing Long COVID.

BOX 3.5   PRACTICE POINT

Compare Raeya's experience of CFS with what you know about the experience of people with Long COVID. What is similar and what is different? What (if anything) do you ask patients about prior experiences of PAIS?

3.4 CONCLUSION

The comparison of Long COVID with other PAIS, such as ME/CFS, highlights a critical opportunity to learn from the challenges and successes of these conditions. ME/CFS offers a cautionary example of how health professionals should – and should not – approach Long COVID. Early diagnosis, patient validation, and person-centred care models are essential to addressing systemic inequities within PAIS. Clinicians and researchers must leverage lessons from other PAIS, recognising patients as experts in their own experiences. While its relative recency has led some health professionals to see Long COVID as an unknown condition, there is a plethora of relevant and transferable knowledge and skills available within their existing practice.

Frameworks for Long COVID care should integrate lived experiences into inclusive, evidence-based, and unbiased care systems. This approach will improve outcomes for Long COVID and strengthen care for all PAIS. Our advice to readers is to go slowly - look, listen, and learn from the person about the impact of Long COVID on their lives and what they need to improve their situation. Health professionals must listen, collaborate, and support patients, taking thorough histories to understand how symptoms affect daily life and capacity over time. Please keep in mind that many peoples' journey with ME/CFS and now Long COVID can be very tumultuous and is not linear. It changes daily, year by year, and from illness to illness. Many with pre-existing ME/CFS may now be worse since having Long COVID, which is extremely challenging on many fronts. Professional expertise is crucial, but the lived experience of patients is equally vital, especially as research continues to fill gaps in PAIS knowledge.

REFERENCES

1 Sharp PM, et al. Evaluating the evidence for virus/host co-evolution. Curr Opin Virol. 2011;1(5):436–41. doi:10.1016/j.coviro.2011.10.018.

2 Stefano GB. Historical insight into infections and disorders associated with neurological and psychiatric sequelae similar to Long COVID. Med Sci Monit. 2021;27:e931447. doi:10.12659/MSM.931447.

3 Tajouri L. What is a virus? How do they spread? How do they make us sick? [Internet]. The Conversation. 2020 Mar 10 [cited 2025 Feb 7]. Available from: https://theconversation.com/what-is-a-virus-how-do-they-spread-how-do-they-make-us-sick-133437.

4 Ariza ME. Myalgic encephalomyelitis/chronic fatigue syndrome: The human herpesviruses are back! Biomolecules. 2021;11:1–12. doi:10.3390/biom11020185.

5 Lerner AM, et al. A paradigm linking herpesvirus immediate-early gene expression apoptosis and myalgic encephalomyelitis/chronic fatigue syndrome. Virus Adapt Treat. 2011; 3:19–24. doi:10.2147/VAAT.S15105

6 O'Neal AJ, et al. The enterovirus theory of disease etiology in myalgic encephalomyelitis/chronic fatigue syndrome: A critical review. Front Med. 2021. doi:10.3389/fmed.2021.688486.

7 Falfán-Valencia R, et al. ME/CFS and Long COVID share similar symptoms and biological abnormalities: Road map to the literature. Front Med. 2023;10:1–15. doi:10.3389/fmed.2023.1187163.

8 Li GH, et al. Systems modeling reveals shared metabolic dysregulation and novel therapeutic treatments in ME/CFS and Long COVID. bioRxiv. 2024. doi: doi:10.1101/2024.06.17.599450.

9 Shankar V, et al. Oxidative stress is a shared characteristic of ME/CFS and Long COVID. bioRxiv. 2024. doi:10.1101/2024.05.04.592477.

10 Wong TL, et al. Long COVID and myalgic encephalomyelitis/chronic fatigue syndrome (ME/CFS)—A systemic review and comparison of clinical presentation and symptomatology. Medicina. 2021;57:1–12. doi:10.3390/medicina57050418.

11 UK Government Disability Unit. Living with non-visible disabilities [Internet]. London: UK Government; 2020 Dec 17 [cited 2025 Feb 7]. Available from: https://disabilityunit.blog.gov.uk/2020/12/17/living-with-non-visible-disabilities/

12 Invisible Disabilities Association. What is an invisible disability? [Internet]. Parker, CO: Invisible Disabilities Association; [cited 2025 Feb 7]. Available from: https://invisibledisabilities.org/what-is-an-invisible-disability/

13 Leedon C. Tackling the invisible: The hidden world of 'invisible illness' [Internet]. Australian National University; [cited 2025 Feb 7]. Available from: https://studylib.net/doc/8911040/the-hidden-world-of--invisible-illness-#google_vignette

14 Prince MJ. Drawing hidden figures of disability: Youth and adults with disabilities in Canada. Evid Policy. 2021. doi:10.1332/174426421X16146827140135.

15 Weerasekera P. Multiperspective case formulation: A step towards treatment integration. Malabar, FL: Krieger; 1996.

16 National Academies of Sciences, Engineering, and Medicine. A Long COVID definition: A chronic, systemic disease state with profound consequences. Washington, DC: National Academies Press; 2024. doi:10.17226/27768.

17 World Health Organization. A clinical case definition of post-COVID-19 condition by a Delphi consensus. Geneva: WHO; 2021.

18 Sylvester SV, et al. Sex differences in sequelae from COVID-19 infection and in Long COVID syndrome: A review. Curr Med Res Opin. 2022;38:1391–99. doi:10.1080/03007995.2022.2081454.

19 Itua B, et al. Long COVID and its effects on the cardiovascular system: A literature review. Int J Res Med Sci. 2023;21:211–18. doi:10.1080/14779072.2023.2184800.

20 Lenehan PJ, et al. Longitudinal lab test analysis confirms pre-existing anemia as a severe risk factor for post-viral clearance hospitalisation in COVID-19 patients. medRxiv. 2020. doi:10.1101/2020.12.02.20242958.

21 Logarbo B, et al. Long COVID and the diagnosis of underlying hypermobile Ehlers-Danlos syndrome and hypermobility spectrum disorders. PM R. 2024;16(8): 935–37. doi:10.1002/pmrj.13120.

22 Hurk AW, et al. Childhood trauma exposure increases Long COVID risk. medRxiv. 2020. doi:10.1101/2022.02.18.22271191.

23 Amsterdam D, et al. Long COVID-19 enigma: Unmasking the role of distinctive personality profiles as risk factors. J Clin Med. 2024;13. doi.org/10.3390/jcm13102886.

24 Delgado-Alonso C, et al. Personality traits in post-COVID syndrome. 2021. doi:10.21203/rs.3.rs-1099432/v1.

25 Wright A, et al. Perfectionism, depression and anxiety in chronic fatigue syndrome: A systematic review. J Psychosom Res. 2021;140:110322. doi:10.1016/j.jpsychores.2020.110322.

26 Paul E, et al. Does pre-infection stress increase the risk of Long COVID? medRxiv. 2022. doi: 10.1101/2022.04.06.22273444.

27 Afrin LB, et al. COVID-19 hyperinflammation and post-COVID-19 illness may be rooted in mast cell activation syndrome. Int J Infect Dis. 2020;100:327–32. doi:10.1016/j.ijid.2020.09.016.

28 Arun S, et al. Mast cell activation syndrome and the link with Long COVID. Br J Hosp Med. 2022;83(7):1–10. doi:10.12968/hmed.2022.0123.

29 Schilling C, et al. Pre-existing sleep problems as a predictor of post-acute sequelae of COVID-19. J Sleep Res. 2023;33:e13949. doi:10.1111/jsr.13949

30 Goldstein CA, et al. The prevalence and impact of pre-existing sleep disorder diagnoses and objective sleep parameters in patients hospitalised for COVID-19. J Clin Sleep Med. 2021;17(5):1039–50. doi:10.5664/jcsm.9132.

31 Wolff D, et al. Allergic diseases as risk factors for long-COVID symptoms: Systematic review of prospective cohort studies. Clin Exp Allergy. 2023;53:1162–76. doi:10.1111/cea.14391.

32 Peluso MJ, et al. Long COVID in people living with HIV. Curr Opin HIV AIDS. 2023;18:126–34. doi:10.1097/COH.0000000000000789.

33 Loosen SH, et al. Obesity and lipid metabolism disorders determine the risk for development of Long COVID syndrome. Infect. 2022;50:1165–70. doi:10.1007/s15010-022-01784-0.

34 Subramanian A, et al. Symptoms and risk factors for Long COVID in non-hospitalised adults. Nat Med. 2022;28:1706–14. doi:10.1038/s41591-022-01909-w.

35 de Leeuw E, et al. Long COVID: Sustained and multiplied disadvantage. Med J Aust. 2022;216:222–24. doi:10.5694/mja2.51435.

36 Hitch D, et al. Beyond the case numbers: Social determinants and contextual factors in patient narratives of recovery from COVID-19. Aust N Z J Public Health. 2023;47(1):100002. doi:10.1016/j.anzjph.2022.100002.

37 Fernández-de-las-Peñas C, et al. Symptoms experienced at the acute phase of SARS-CoV-2 infection as risk factor of long-term post-COVID symptoms. Int J Infect Dis. 2022;116:241–44. doi:10.1016/j.ijid.2022.01.007.

38 Yavropoulou MP, et al. Protracted stress-induced hypocortisolemia may account for the clinical and immune manifestations of Long COVID. Clin Immunol. 2022;245:109133. doi:10.1016/j.clim.2022.109133.

39 Carruthers BM, et al. Myalgic encephalomyelitis: International consensus criteria. J Intern Med. 2011;270(4):327–38. doi:10.1111/j.1365-2796.2011.02428.x.

40 Goudsmit E, et al. Bias, misleading information and lack of respect for alternative views have distorted perceptions of myalgic encephalomyelitis/chronic fatigue syndrome and its treatment. J Health Psychol. 2017;22(9):1159–67. doi:10.1177/1359105317707216.

41 Montoya JG, et al. Caring for the patient with severe or very severe myalgic encephalomyelitis/chronic fatigue syndrome. Healthcare. 2021;9:1331. doi:10.3390/healthcare9101.

42 Lim EJ, et al. Review of case definitions for myalgic encephalomyelitis/chronic fatigue syndrome (ME/CFS). J Transl Med. 2020;18:289. doi:10.1186/s12967-020-02455-0.

43 Emerge Australia. Emerge Australia: Advocacy, education & support for ME/CFS [Internet]. Melbourne: Emerge Australia; [cited 2025 Feb 7]. Available from: https://www.emerge.org.au.

44 Cairns R. A systematic review describing the prognosis of chronic fatigue syndrome. Occup Med. 2005;55:20–31. doi:10.1093/occmed/kqi013.

45 Goudsmit EM, et al. Pacing as a strategy to improve energy management in myalgic encephalomyelitis/chronic fatigue syndrome: A consensus document. Disabil Rehabil. 2012;34(13):1140–47. doi:10.3109/09638288.2011.635746.

46 Ahmed SK, et al. Assessment of the scientific rigour of randomised controlled trials on the effectiveness of cognitive behavioural therapy and graded exercise therapy for patients with myalgic encephalomyelitis/chronic fatigue syndrome: A systematic review. J Health Psychol. 2020;25:240–55. doi:10.1177/1359105319847261.

47 Geraghty KJ, et al. Myalgic encephalomyelitis/chronic fatigue syndrome patients' reports of symptom changes following cognitive behavioural therapy, graded exercise therapy and pacing treatments: Analysis of a primary survey compared with secondary surveys. J Health Psychol. 2019;24:1318–33. doi:10.1177/1359105317726152.

48 Greenhalgh T, et al. Long COVID: A clinical update. Lancet. 2024;404(10453):707–24. doi:10.1016/S0140-6736(24)01136-X.

49 Smith ME, et al. Treatment of myalgic encephalomyelitis/chronic fatigue syndrome: A systematic review for a National Institutes of Health pathways to prevention workshop. Ann Intern Med. 2015;162:841–50. doi:10.7326/M15–0114.

50 Owen R, et al. Long COVID quality of life and healthcare experiences in the UK: A mixed-method online survey. Qual Life Res. 2023;33:133–43. doi:10.1007/s11136-023-03513-y.

51 Eaton-Fitch N, et al. Health-related quality of life in patients with myalgic encephalomyelitis/chronic fatigue syndrome: An Australian cross-sectional study. Qual Life Res. 2020;29: 1521–31. doi:10.1007/s11136-019-02411-6.

52 Bartlett C, et al. Living with myalgic encephalomyelitis/chronic fatigue syndrome: Experiences of occupational disruption for adults in Australia. Br J Occup Ther. 2022;85(4): 241–50. doi:10.1177/03080226211020656.

53 Strand EB, et al. Myalgic encephalomyelitis/chronic fatigue syndrome (ME/CFS): Investigating care practices pointed out to disparities in diagnosis and treatment across the European Union. PLoS One. 2019;14:e0216792. doi:10.1371/journal.pone.0225995.

54 Ghali A, et al. Factors influencing the prognosis of patients with myalgic encephalomyelitis/chronic fatigue syndrome. Diagnostics. 2022;12:2540. doi:10.3390/diagnostics12102540.

55 Tamayo-Velasco Á, et al. ABO blood system and COVID-19 susceptibility: Anti-A and Anti-B antibodies are the key points. Front Med. 2022;9:882477. doi:10.3389/fmed.2022.882477.

56 Roxburgh R, et al. Using time diaries to inform occupational therapy practice for people with myalgic encephalomyelitis/chronic fatigue syndrome: An exploratory study. Br J Occup Ther. 2024;87(9):583–92. doi:10.1177/03080226241249279.

57 Sommerfelt K, et al. Assessing functional capacity in myalgic encephalopathy/chronic fatigue syndrome: A patient-informed questionnaire. J Clin Med. 2024;13:3486. doi:10.3390/jcm13123486.

Chapter 4

Long COVID as a Patient Identified Disease Entity

*Elisa Perego, Elyse McInerney, Julie Taylor,
Tara Barton, Ali Harrington, and Danielle Hitch*

BOX 4.1 LEARNING OBJECTIVES

By the end of this chapter, readers should be able to:

- Describe how people living with Long COVID contributed to identifying and naming the condition.
- Analyse how patient-led advocacy has shaped research, healthcare policies, and public awareness about Long COVID.
- Critically discuss the socio-political challenges of recognising and naming Long COVID and consider their implications for rehabilitation practice.
- Reflect on how patient narratives and grassroots efforts have informed and validated scientific understandings and challenged traditional hierarchies in knowledge production.

4.1 INTRODUCTION

Reports began emerging of an illness similar to Severe Acute Respiratory Syndrome (SARS) from Wuhan, China, in late 2019.[1] It was soon recognised the illness was caused by a novel SARS coronavirus (SARS-CoV-2) and was initially named 2019-nCov before the World Health Organization (WHO) settled on the name Coronavirus Disease 2019 (COVID-19).[2] In the early days and weeks of 2020, people around the globe started becoming ill as COVID-19 spread through globalised travel.[3] Many turned to social media to seek answers about this poorly understood new illness as the world collectively struggled to come to terms with its rapid spread and impact on society.

DOI: 10.4324/9781003528104-5

Due to widespread fear and uncertainty about what we were facing, people began to take proactive control of their health in March 2020 by masking, wearing protective shields or eyeglasses, or removing their children from school long before mandates or lockdowns.[4] At the same time, hospitals in China began "proning" to manage acute COVID-19 infections and judge when patients needed to go to Intensive Care Units.[5]

BOX 4.2   PRONING

Proning involves moving a person from lying on their back (supine position) to lying face-down on their front (prone position).[4] This position improves oxygenation and reduces the need for mechanical ventilation.

Social media played a crucial role in spreading accessible information about COVID-19, particularly to and from global hotspots in Asia (China and South Korea), the Middle East (Iran), Europe (Italy, France, Germany, Spain, and Switzerland), and the United States of America (US).[6,7] By mid-2020, numerous stories about the lived experiences of people affected by COVID-19 were circulating, and it became clear that the disease had prolonged effects on many people. Others appeared to recover initially but were hit with delayed health effects.

The personal stories of lived experience collectively highlighted the emergence of a new post-viral illness. This condition exhibited distinctive multi-system features beyond those expected from a disease (COVID-19) initially described as a respiratory illness. People with severe acute COVID-19 described long and difficult recoveries, persistent symptoms, and prolonged disease. However, ongoing issues were also reported by people with mild to moderate symptoms who had received no acute care from overwhelmed hospital systems.[8] People who were older, living with a disability or chronic illness or with socioeconomic disadvantage tended to have poorer outcomes.[9] However, there were also many testimonials from younger people who were previously in good health. Everyone was potentially at risk from this new illness, and citizen science on an unprecedented scale was building a global collection of case reports.[10]

> I was in the early hotspot of Lombardy, and people who weren't recovering were middle age and elderly, and some had preexisting conditions. I was myself chronically ill before Covid. It crosscut age, gender and prior health status although certain demographics were more likely to join discussions on media platforms (younger, Internet literate).
>
> Elisa[21]

In this chapter, we will explore the evolving role of patients in shaping our understanding of Long COVID. We will delve into how people with lived experience formed online communities that identified the illness and drove critical advocacy and research efforts. We will also discuss the ongoing challenges related to formal recognition of Long COVID, from initial reluctance to acknowledge its existence to efforts by the scientific and policymaking community to give the illness a different name, sanctioned within conventional medicine's framework. This chapter provides you with a deeper appreciation of the fundamental role patient-led initiatives have played, and continue to play, in shaping healthcare responses and public awareness of Long COVID. All but one of the authors of this chapter live with Long COVID, and we draw upon those experiences.

4.2 IDENTIFYING AND NAMING LONG COVID

In the words of Callard and Perego, "Long COVID has a strong claim to be the first illness created through patients finding one another on Twitter."[10][p4] Patient advocacy is recognised in other health fields, but uniquely, it was Long COVID patients who named and defined the disease before the medical community. Along with their lived experience, people with prolonged symptoms after COVID-19 infections were using social media to connect with others living through similar experiences, pushing back the boundaries of knowledge-building in unprecedented ways.[11] The novelty of COVID-19 meant the world was "flying the plane while building it," and at the time, patients held the most comprehensive understanding of how the virus could impact daily life. Without proven treatments, they also applied their lived experience to problem-solve the issues they encountered and shared those solutions with their peers. In other words, patients were (and still are) leading experts in Long COVID.

As the number of these lived experience experts grew, the broadly consistent symptoms and sequelae they described needed a name. Naming these symptoms and sequelae was key to bringing the world's attention to this rapidly growing problem and the potential for its impact to eclipse that of acute COVID-19. Naming their experience could support an open approach to possible aetiology without providing a prior explanation for all symptoms and, therefore, avoid premature predictions or prognoses about diverse disease pathways.[12,13] It would also give this growing community a plain language, easily understandable name.

In the US, Amy Watson used the term Long Haul COVID and "long hauler" after the trucking cap she wore the day she was tested for COVID. In Europe, Elisa Perego coined the term "Long COVID" and used it on Twitter to address her own experience of the disease and emerging knowledge.[14] Both terms resonated with the community because they reflected the long-term nature of the illness. Due to public health messaging at the time, most had expected their symptoms would quickly resolve because they had shaken off other infectious illnesses easily, and COVID-19 was described as lasting at most two to six weeks. This felt very different; it was unusual to be sick for so long, and it was difficult to know how much their health would decline or how long they would be disabled. However, people with lived experience were beginning to sound the alarm about potentially severe and enduring illness and disability.

> *I recall being in complete shock that I couldn't do the simplest things. I trusted my body to recover and be strong. I tried to walk 100m up the street and collapsed. Making myself a tea led to half a day in bed. I had to fully revise how I thought of myself and my functionality which was incredibly frightening.*
>
> Karen

BOX 4.3   PRACTICE POINT

Reflect on the ongoing uncertainty people with Long COVID live with. How does this affect the advice and information you provide as a health professional? What approach do you adopt to illnesses with uncertain prognoses or natural histories? How do you acknowledge and validate the lived experience of your patients to build genuine therapeutic partnerships?

It was the "first wavers" who began trying to alert the public, policymakers and health officials about the serious problems they were experiencing, all while being seriously unwell themselves. Many people were infected before the WHO declared the pandemic. In early 2020, these patients had no chance or option to mask, vaccinate (with vaccines unavailable until 2021), obtain Polymerase Chain Reaction, or benefit from subsequent pandemic risk mitigations. A key motivation for naming this illness was to warn others and mobilise action from leaders.

Experiences vary, but those infected in later waves of the pandemic still face many of the same issues. While the WHO case description of Long COVID in 2021[15] was a turning point for recognising the condition, general awareness of the condition remained low in some contexts, and many patients had to campaign to access the few existing services.

> *Having a GP who never had a 'long covid' patient, I had to be my own advocate to at least be considered for an (Australian) Long COVID clinic, which*

at least existed by this stage. I had to fight to get access to services, especially if you weren't an 'in patient' of the facility support the Long Covid Clinic.

Julie.

The naming of Long COVID also acted as a catalyst for people to share their lived experiences online. As more and more people joined this global conversation, they collectively identified patterns of symptoms and other problems that were commonly experienced by people with prolonged illness following COVID-19.[16] As the problems caused by Long COVID became increasingly evident, the lived experience community urged leaders to collect data, which could be done, for example, under the clinical code "Post-COVID Condition."Patients have been advocating for improved data collection since 2020, for instance, under the hashtag #countlongcovid, to understand better the disability and chronic illness emerging from the pandemic.[16] In response to a TikTok about the long-term effects of COVID-19 infection, disability advocate Imani Barbarin commented in late 2020, "I can't stress this to you all enough, but COVID-19 is a mass disabling event. People are becoming disabled because of COVID-19. This society, America in particular, is not prepared for it—at all."[17]

Starting in April 2020, the first online groups to support affected patients were created, such as Slack and Facebook support groups like "Long Haul COVID Fighters" created by Amy Watson in the US, "Long COVID Support" created by Claire Hastie in the United Kingdom (UK),[16] and the "Australian Long COVID Community." Body Politic emerged as a global network of COVID-19 patients and allies that developed from a pre-pandemic queer feminist collective focused on the relationship between wellness, politics, and personal identity.[18] While some (like Survivor Corps[19]) have disbanded, many have grown in membership and influence as more people developed Long COVID. For example, the "Long COVID for Endurance Athletes" support group now includes over 2000 members and supports this underrepresented cohort of patients. These groups have played a pivotal role in raising awareness about Long COVID, mainly in the absence of public health information campaigns. They also influence research and policy by producing patient-led research, sharing compelling testimonials, and collaborating with medical and academic institutions.

In many ways, Long COVID became a grassroots movement that rapidly moved from local to global. As described by Ryan Prior,

Many had no medical degree or academic specialisation in infectious disease or immunology. What they had was a suffering human body, the consciousness to describe it, and the technological tools to form a global collective of citizen scientists called to action.[20] [p41–42]

The first wavers are now in their fifth year of advocacy, asking health and political leaders to address the multifaceted health, social, and other impacts of Long COVID. International efforts are accelerating to collect the epidemiological and biomedical data needed to rigorously assess prevalence and pathophysiology more thoroughly to improve and formulate appropriate health responses, including treatments and trials. National inquiries into pandemic responses and Long COVID have been held in Australia[21] and the UK.[22] Progress is happening, with different trajectories in different countries, but it cannot come soon enough for people with Long COVID.

4.3 WHY USE THE TERM LONG COVID?

Despite the identification of Long COVID by people with lived experience, a debate has continued around the name given to sustained symptoms and sequelae following COVID-19 infection. There has been resistance to adopting Long COVID as standard terminology from medical and academic institutions, who have proposed several other terms.

Health professionals, healthcare bodies, and officials proposed "Post-Acute Sequelae of SARS-CoV-2 infection" and Post-COVID Syndrome to describe the condition in clinical and academic contexts in late 2020. The WHO formalised the term "Post COVID-19 Condition" in October 2021[15] to promote more consistent definitions as a basis for diagnostic criteria while capturing the complexity of symptoms. Others utilise the term "Chronic Post COVID Syndrome,"[23] which is closer to the traditional medical perspective on acute and chronic stages of illness.

Long COVID has also been challenged in debates around its boundaries with Myalgic Encephalitis/Chronic Fatigue Syndrome (ME/CFS). In late 2020, some health professionals and ME/CFS community members began questioning whether Long COVID and ME/CFS were distinct conditions. These queries raised concerns that the stigma and controversy surrounding other post-acute infection syndromes (see Chapter 3) might become associated with Long COVID.[24] Some people also interpret the term Long COVID as an extended period of acute infection rather than the sustained and chronic symptoms experienced by people with Long COVID.

Resistance to using the term "Long COVID" reflects broader socio-political issues related to subjective evidence, illness identity, epistemic authority, and medical knowledge.[25-27] Health professionals and academics prefer disease names that fit within their existing taxonomies because these are reputed to support accurate and consistent diagnosis of disease states.[28] This reflects assumptions by many health professionals and researchers around the relative value of subjective or anecdotal patient experiences versus "scientific" clinical evidence, preferably produced in the context of extensive studies.

This reflects a very narrow and erroneous view of what counts as "scientific." Science is the process of building knowledge from isolated facts into coherent and comprehensive understanding. The name Long COVID emerged from individual patient stories, rich in contextual detail about diverse symptoms, signs, sequelae, and recovery trajectories – generating multiple hypotheses and data for future exploration. Many of the early hypotheses proposed by the patient community have since been proven correct by biomedical studies.[29] As citizens and sometimes professional scientists, people with lived experience of Long COVID are leaders in the field and continue to conduct innovative and inclusive studies of the issues that matter most to their community.[30]

The fact that Long COVID was also quickly adopted in the scientific literature demonstrates its accessibility and capacity to drive rigorous research and guide effective practice. International governments, research institutions, and healthcare professionals use Long COVID in their documentation and discussions.[30] However, it often remains an alternative term added to medical terminology in brackets or parentheses. Therefore, its acceptance is incomplete; however, its widespread adoption remains a significant achievement in validating lived experience, amplifying patient voices, and recognising the importance of different forms of expertise.

BOX 4.4 PRACTICE POINT

Use the following prompts to consider whose voices are heard in the Long COVID patient community. What might this mean for your practice as a rehabilitation clinician?

1 Which patients tend to have their voices heard in healthcare advocacy and research?
   - *Consider factors like education, access to resources, severity of symptoms and social privilege.*
2 What does it mean for people with Long COVID to be experts in their condition in the current healthcare system?
   - *Consider requirements for diagnoses to be validated by evidence from medical professionals and levels of health professional acceptance of the value of lived experience.*

3   How does the level of recognition of the term "Long COVID" in your location impact people's access to healthcare and other supports?
   • *Consider the evidence required to meet service eligibility criteria.*

4   What are the benefits of having well-educated and resourceful patients leading healthcare advocacy?
   • *Consider how their contributions shape policies, practices, and access to care.*

5   How do you feel about the following quote from a doctor with Long COVID?
   "There's a certain responsibility to put down our experiences so they [patients who are not medical professionals] can be opened up to other people who don't have the language and the access that we potentially have to communicate it to primary healthcare to access the services that need to be put in place for them (Doctor)."[31]
   • *Consider the role and responsibility of patient advocates and what is expected of them.*

6   What are the implications of privileging certain voices in Long COVID advocacy?
   • *Consider the impact on the evidence base, policies, and practices.*

7   How can the voices of patients with less presence in the Long COVID community be heard?
   • *Consider the needs of specific groups and communities and potential engagement strategies, such as adaptations required for people with severe Long COVID who cannot leave their homes or are bed-bound.*

8   How can you ensure the lived experiences of diverse people with Long COVID inform your practice?
   • *Identify one or two actions based on your responses to the questions and prompts above.*

4.4 SUPPORTING PATIENT ADVOCACY AND ACTION

While they may or may not have lived experience of this condition, rehabilitation health professionals can be essential allies for people with Long COVID. Patient action at the policy level may also have a widespread impact, leading to better funding and resourcing for everyone in the Long COVID community. However, enabling individual patients to advocate for their unique needs is equally important. The following story reflects the lived experience of just one person with Long COVID, but every person's journey is unique.

BOX 4.5   ALI'S STORY

"My symptoms were misunderstood and overlooked. It was a constant struggle to continually repeat myself – over and over – while experiencing debilitating and ongoing fatigue. I felt unheard and invisible. Not only was I forging the path of my illness and having to guide the doctors, but I was also fighting my employers who could not understand the severity of my condition. Every day feels like a fight, and this has felt like a fight for over two years for me personally, with no real end in sight. I have had to constantly advocate for myself, and it is tiring and depressing.

Fifteen-minute doctors' consults do not allow time for new illnesses, especially one that only started a few years prior. Doctors are too busy in their day-to-day, so it had to be me pushing for help to get anywhere, all while I was barely able to get out of bed, let alone have the energy to advocate. I had to diagnose myself then convince my doctor to send me to a Long COVID clinic. The forms themselves were exhausting, and it was clear no one really knew how to fill them out. I had already tried a multitude of supplements and sought different opinions, but there was no one clear direction to heal. It was extremely isolating.

Adding to my struggle, the clinic forms were not accepted, but no one told me, and months later I was forced to do the whole process all over again. This put me months behind on the waiting list. I had to re-do the multitude of forms and make the fatigue-inducing trip to my doctor once again. All I could do in the meantime was continue research myself on what could help this debilitating fatigue.

For me, contracting Long COVID in 2023 at least meant there were Facebook support groups already established, but the lack of knowledge even at that stage from doctors was overwhelming. It felt like no one believed me even though I was begging for other tests to uncover some kind of direction to heal. Now, over two years into my Long COVID journey, endless hours at exhausting appointments, tons of tests, a multitude of medications and supplements, and thousands of dollars out of pocket, I am still suffering from debilitating fatigue.

As part of the online Long COVID community, I had plenty of support and understanding from those who were suffering like me. It is a lifeline for many sufferers – what alternative did we have? The same sentiment is throughout our posts – we often feel invisible and in disbelief that there is no clear treatment to heal. Trying to explain to family, friends and employers how unwell you feel is difficult especially when you feel scared. Doctors do not know what to do, so it is little wonder that hope feels lost for many. It is evident within the support groups there were many jobs lost, dreams shattered and countless lives still in turmoil.

*Having Long COVID means most of us feel worse after attempting even the smallest of tasks and outings, let alone the energy it takes to logistically organise an appointment. Simple allowances like telehealth consults could help. When we see health professionals, we want to feel heard and supported, with clear directions about what to do next. **Please help us advocate for our health, instead of leaving us to struggle behind closed doors. Work with us. You don't need to have all the answers – please acknowledge our condition and help us look for a way forward."***

BOX 4.6   PRACTICE POINT

Imagine Ali has been referred to your rehabilitation service. How might the symptoms of Long COVID impact Ali's ability to advocate for her needs? Identify two to three ways you could support her in advocating for her needs.

4.5 ONGOING RESEARCH AND ADVOCACY BY THE LONG COVID COMMUNITY

The Long COVID community has organised and produced significant research and advocacy over time. Patient-driven collaboration or groups, like the Patient-Led Research Collaborative originating from the Body Politic Slack support group, have published extensively, independently, and with other researchers. The work of patient-driven collectives has provided foundational data on diverse topics, including suspected physiological mechanisms and the critical role of patient advocacy,[12,14] symptom profiling,[30] and experiences of under-represented groups like people with disabilities.[31]

Many of these studies were groundbreaking, establishing key knowledge for future research. Early in the pandemic, brief tweets often contained insights ahead of current medical knowledge. Simple polls began consolidating this knowledge despite many facing severe illness and experiencing brain fog, which was then poorly understood. Inclusive research practices remain crucial to ensure those with Long COVID can contribute as researchers and participants, with internet platforms, digital technologies, and social media all providing accessibility options.[32]

The foundations of Long COVID research are still evolving, with significant gaps remaining. Many people with Long COVID who have engaged in research and advocacy were infected early in the pandemic, yet most global infections have occurred since Omicron's emergence. The experiences of more recent Long COVID people are under-represented in the evidence base. Systematic epidemiological data on COVID-19 morbidity related to all variants needs improvement,[33] and discrepancies between patient self-reports and clinical coding[34] further obscure the impact of newer variants.

Activism by people with Long COVID was recognised by WHO only three months after the term was coined and continues to gain international traction (see Figure 4.1). For example, the first International Long COVID Awareness Day, on 15 March 2023, featured the theme #ConfrontLongCOVID. Tracey Thompson

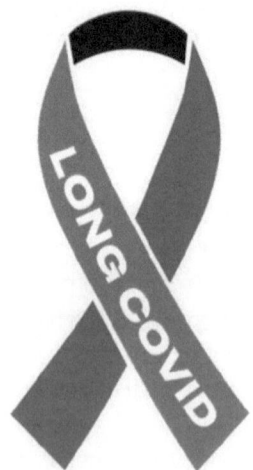

Figure 4.1 Symbol of International Long COVID Awareness Day. "LCAEnglish.white" by Long COVID Awareness is licensed under CC0 1.0 Universal (https://creativecommons. org/publicdomain/zero/1.0/).

created the original International Long COVID Awareness Ribbon in the US (Figure 4.1). The grey in the ribbon represents loss and sadness due to the pandemic, the teal represents hope and support, and the black represents the loneliness and rest that comes with Long Covid. Members of the LC global community selected the colours in January 2023.

In 2024, the US grassroots group LC/DC held a live-streamed demonstration advocating for awareness, change, action, and transparency. In Australia and Canada, public buildings were illuminated in teal to symbolise hope and support, while the UK launched an online tool offering tailored support. These actions increased awareness, offered solidarity, and highlighted the need for research and support. In Melbourne, Australia, a small group lay on the steps of state parliament surrounded by 200 pillowcases with stories of those too ill to attend (Figure 4.2).

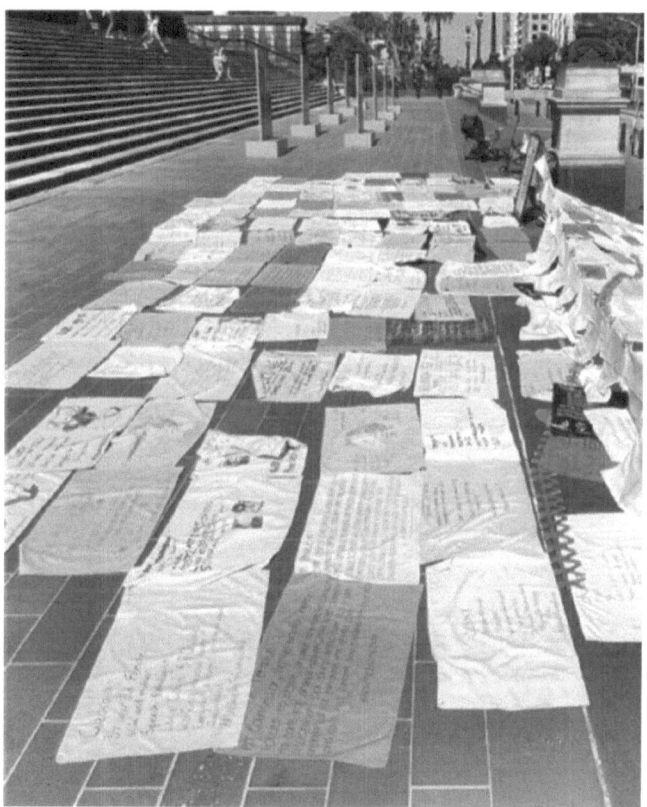

Figure 4.2 Representation of people too unwell to attend Long COVID Awareness Day event in Melbourne, Australia. © 2024 Alicia Newham and Miquette Abercrombie, Long COVID Support Australia.

Advocacy and research fuel each other. For example, the US Long COVID Action Project advocates for non-partisan support for investigating biomarkers and treatments.[35] Similarly, the Long COVID Moonshot campaign[36] seeks $1 billion annually from the US government for sustainable research. The US National Institutes of Health (NIH) has also founded the "RECOVER" collaborative, which includes health professionals, clinicians, scientists, caregivers, community members, and people with Long COVID in an adaptive research network.[37] Globally, people with Long COVID are urging local representatives to act.

4.6 CONCLUSION

Long COVID exemplifies a transformative, patient-identified disease entity. A grassroots movement of lived experience experts named the condition, shaped its understanding, and advocated for recognition in healthcare systems and policies. This effort demonstrates the critical role of lived experience in expanding medical knowledge, especially during a global health crisis when science lags behind patients' realities. Using social media, online communities, and advocacy, people with Long COVID modelled citizen science, influencing both research and public health priorities.

Despite progress, challenges persist. Tensions between patient narratives and medical frameworks hinder full recognition, and systemic inequities limit representation in advocacy and research. Integrating diverse lived experiences into healthcare responses is essential to drive equitable and inclusive practices. By valuing patient-led initiatives and fostering collaboration between patients, researchers, and policymakers, there is hope for a future where lived experience is acknowledged and deeply embedded in the fabric of healthcare innovation.

REFERENCES

1 Whitworth J. COVID-19: a fast evolving pandemic. Trans R Soc Trop Med Hyg. 2020;114: 241–48. doi:10.1093/trstmh/traa025.
2 Sun P, et al. Understanding of COVID-19 based on current evidence. J Med Virol. 2020;92: 548–51. doi:10.1002/jmv.25722.
3 Huang C, et al. Clinical features of patients infected with 2019 novel coronavirus in Wuhan, China. Lancet. 2020:395(10223):497–506. doi:10.1016/S0140-6736(20)30183-5.
4 Forman R, et al. 12 Lessons learned from the management of the coronavirus pandemic. Health Policy. 2020;124(6):577–80. doi:10.1016/j.healthpol.2020.05.008.
5 Prasad M, et al. Should I prone non-ventilated awake patients with COVID-19? Cleve Clin J Med. 2020;92(6):548–51. doi:10.1002/jmv.257222572225722.
6 Jamshidi B, et al. Mathematical modeling the epicenters of coronavirus disease-2019 (COVID-19) pandemic. Epidemiol Methods. 2020;9(S1):20200009. doi:10.1515/em-2020.0009.

7 Gottlieb M, et al. Information and disinformation: social media in the COVID-19 crisis. Acad Emerg Med. 2020;27:640–41. doi:10.1111/acem.14036.

8 Moynihan R, et al. Impact of COVID-19 pandemic on utilisation of healthcare services: a systematic review. BMJ Open. 2021; 11(3):e045343. doi:10.1136/bmjopen-2020-045343045343045343.

9 de Leeuw E, et al. Long COVID: sustained and multiplied disadvantage. Med J Aust. 2022; 216:222–24. doi10.5694/mja2.51435

10 Perego E, et al. How and why patients made Long COVID. Soc Sci Med. 2021;268:113426. doi:10.1016/j.socscimed.2020.113426.

11 Russell D, et al. Support amid uncertainty: Long COVID illness experiences and the role of online communities. SSM Qual Res Health. 2022;2:100177. doi:10.1016/j.ssmqr.2022.100177.

12 Perego E, et al. Why the patient-made term 'Long COVID' is needed. Wellcome Open Research. 2020;5:224. doi:10.12688/wellcomeopenres.16307.1.

13 Burdick CE. Naming chronic illness: Diagnosis and disability. Incl Dis. 2022;(2):101–14. doi:10.51357/id.vi2.193.

14 Turner M, et al. The #longcovid revolution: A reflexive thematic analysis. Soc Sci Med. 2023;333:116130. doi:10.1016/j.socscimed.2023.116130

15 World Health Organization (WHO). A clinical case definition of post COVID-19 condition by a Delphi consensus. Geneva: WHO; 2021.

16 McClymont GC. The role of patients and patient activism in the development of Long COVID policy. Camb J Sci Policy. 2021;2(1):1–12. doi:10.17863/CAM.75505.

17 Crutches and Spice. Disabled people aren't your justification for not following Covid-19 rules [Internet]. TikTok; 2021 Jan 1 [cited 2025 Feb 7]. Available from: https://www.tiktok.com/@crutches_and_spice/video/6905830183601769733.

18 Body Politic. Body Politic: A grassroots health justice organization [Internet]. [place unknown]: Body Politic; [cited 2025 Feb 7]. Available from: https://www.wearebodypolitic.com/.

19 Survivor Corps. Advocacy [Internet]. [place unknown]: Survivor Corps; [cited 2025 Feb 7]. Available from: https://www.survivorcorps.com/advocacy.

20 Prior R. The Long Haul: How Long COVID survivors are revolutionising healthcare. Cambridge: MIT Press; 2024.

21 Parliament of Australia. Sick and tired: Casting a long shadow. Canberra: Standing Committee on Health, Aged Care and Sport; 2023.

22 UK COVID-19 Inquiry. UK COVID-19 public inquiry [Internet]. London: UK COVID-19 Inquiry; [cited 2025 Feb 7]. Available from: https://covid19.public-inquiry.uk/.

23 Halpin S, et al. Long COVID and chronic COVID syndromes. J Med Virol. 2021;93(3):1242–43. doi:10.1002/jmv.26587.

24 Byrne EA. Understanding Long COVID: Nosology, social attitudes and stigma. Brain Behav Immun. 2021;99:17–24. doi:10.1016/j.bbi.2021.09.012.

25 Roth PH, et al. The contested meaning of "Long COVID" – Patients, doctors, and the politics of subjective evidence. Soc Sci Med. 2022;292:114619. doi:10.1016/j.socscimed.2021.114619.

26 Hitch D. Why we must keep using the term 'Long COVID' [Internet]. InSight+; 2024 Apr 8 [cited 2025 Feb 7]. Available from: https://insightplus.mja.com.au/2024/13/why-we-must-keep-using-the-term-long-covid/.

27 Harada Y, et al. Diagnostic errors in uncommon conditions: a systematic review of case reports of diagnostic errors. Diagnosis. 2023;10:329–36. doi:10.1515/dx-2023-0030.

28 Puhan MA. Literature report on Long COVID [Internet]. Bern: FOPH; 2023 Jan 24 [cited 2025 Feb 7]. Available from: https://www.bag.admin.ch/dam/bag/en/dokumente/mt/k-und-i/ aktuelle-ausbrueche-pandemien/2019-nCoV/Literaturrecherchen/literaturrecherchen_ long_covid_20220608.pdf.download.pdf/FOPH_LitReport_Covid-19%20LongCOVID_ 20230124.pdf

29 Gorna R, et al. Long COVID guidelines need to reflect lived experience. Lancet. 2021 Feb 6;397(10273):455–57. doi:10.1016/S0140-6736(20)32705-7.

30 Davis H, et al. Characterising Long COVID in an international cohort: 7 months of symptoms and their impact. eClinical Med. 2021;38:101019. doi:10.1016/j.eclinm.2021.101019.

31 Hall JP, et al. Long COVID among people with preexisting disabilities. Am J Public Health. 2024;114:1261–64. doi:10.2105/AJPH.2024.307794.

32 Hitch D, et al. Occupational being during the COVID-19 pandemic. In: Kara H, Khoo S- M, editors. Researching in the Age of COVID-19. Vol 2: Care and Resilience. Bristol: Bristol University Press; 2020. p. 111–20.

33 Al-Aly Z, et al. Long COVID science, research and policy. Nat Med. 2024;30:2148–64. doi:10.1038/s41591-024-03173-6.

34 Knuppel A, et al. The Long COVID evidence gap: comparing self-reporting and clinical coding of Long COVID using longitudinal study data linked to healthcare records. medRxiv. 2023.02.10.23285717. doi:10.1101/2023.02.10.23285717.

35 Long COVID Action Project. Long COVID action project: Advocacy, research, and support [Internet]. [place unknown]: Long COVID Action Project; [cited 2025 Feb 7]. Available from: https://longcovidactionproject.com/.

36 United States Congress. Text – S.4964 – 118th Congress (2023-2024): Long COVID Moonshot Act [Internet]. [Washington, US]: US Congress; [cited 2025 May 9]. Available from: https:// congress.gov/bill/118th-congress/senate-bill/4964/text/is.

37 National Institutes of Health (NIH). RECOVER: Researching COVID to enhance recovery [Internet]. [Bethesda, Maryland, US: NIH; [cited 2025 May 9]. Available from: https:// recovercovid.org/.

SECTION TWO
LONG COVID IDENTIFICATION AND PLANNING

Chapter 5

The Importance of Screening for and Identifying Long COVID in Individuals, Communities, and Populations

Michael Muleme, Angela Crombie, Danielle Hitch, Andrew Georgiou, Judith Thomas, Kylie Ovenden, Kevin Masman, Darcie Cooper, Sophie Julian, James Boyd, and Sarah Annesley

---

BOX 5.1 LEARNING OBJECTIVES

By the end of this chapter, readers should be able to:

- Understand the importance of a patient-centred approach in identifying Long COVID.
- Appreciate health professionals' role in assessing, reporting, and identifying Long COVID.
- Be aware of the role that big health datasets can have in assessing risks, prevalence, and usage of health services – and how this can be used to improve outcomes for Long COVID patients.

5.1 INTRODUCTION

Long COVID was first introduced into our vocabulary in May 2020 when Dr Elisa Perego took to Twitter to describe her experience after her initial COVID-19 infection. The hashtag and the term Long COVID hit the literature in October of that year, and patients, doctors, and researchers have been discussing it since. One of the main challenges is a lack of consensus across these groups about

DOI: 10.4324/9781003528104-7

what Long COVID is and how it can be diagnosed. Some existing definitions, like the World Health Organisation Long COVID definition,[1] are broad and may not be easily operationalised in scenarios of limited diagnostic resources and concurrent infections. It is also unclear whether Long COVID includes people with long-term functional impact from the acute illness (e.g., post-ICU syndrome, stroke, hypoxic brain injuries). The pathophysiology of these sequelae is known and is part of the rehabilitation pathways.

Taking a collaborative approach to understanding Long COVID, where patients, researchers, and clinicians work together, utilises the strength of each of these parties. This was the approach taken by the National Academy of Sciences, Engineering and Medicine (NASEM) to come up with their definition of Long COVID.[2] Their definition states: "Long COVID is an infection-associated chronic condition that occurs after SARS-CoV-2 infection and is present for at least 3 months as a continuous, relapsing and remitting, or progressive disease state that affects one or more organ systems."[2] An essential feature of this definition is that the acute infection does not need to be confirmed, allowing patients who did not keep a copy of their rapid antigen test or had an asymptomatic infection, for example, also to be diagnosed. The definition also states that a Long COVID diagnosis is made on clinical grounds, as no diagnostic biomarkers are available.

Diagnosing Long COVID is a challenge, particularly with over 200 reported symptoms. A study by the Patient-Led Research Collaborative using a large (3,500+) international cohort highlighted many symptoms that weren't commonly mentioned in other Long COVID studies.[3] This emphasises the need for a personalised approach in diagnosing and managing Long COVID patients.

Long COVID can affect anyone, but certain people may be more at risk, including females, those with an increased Body Mass Index, those over the age of 40 years, those who experienced a severe acute infection, or those with a preexisting condition such as type 2 diabetes, inflammatory bowel disease, or cardiovascular disease (CVD).[4] It is crucial to accurately identify these risks so appropriate precautions and health management plans can be made. The importance of big data in the search for new or repurposed therapeutics and risk stratification of Long COVID is imperative. For example, a review of US Department of Veterans Affairs healthcare databases highlighted the risks and burdens of long-term cardiovascular events post-COVID-19 infection.[5] In this chapter, we outline screening processes for Long COVID from general practice and allied health perspectives and how big data can help address the issue of identifying Long COVID.

5.2 GETTING STARTED: IDENTIFYING LONG COVID AS A CLINICAL PROBLEM

> ### BOX 5.2   THE JOURNEY TO DIAGNOSIS, A PATIENT'S PERSPECTIVE
>
> *"I caught COVID in 2022. A few months later, the fatigue and brain fog were still significantly impacting my ability to work, so I went to my GP. She didn't have any treatment pathway for me, but I was extremely fortunate that she was aware of a local doctor who had Long COVID himself and became a self-taught expert in the condition. I was able to get in and see him (lucky again, as not long after, he was so overbooked he stopped accepting new Long COVID patients). This doctor had collected research data from all over the world and collated it into potential treatment options. They were all supplements so were a fairly safe option to try and gain some functionality back. Sadly, I was still struggling to get through the day. I managed to get a referral to a General Physician but it took three attempts to find one who would be willing to take on a potential Long COVID patient.*
>
> *This doctor tested me for one hundred and fourteen other things before confirming a diagnosis of Post Viral Syndrome from Covid (i.e. Long COVID). He provided a variety of prescriptions for me to try so that I could find one that worked for me. Nearly three years since the original infection, I have found medication that keeps me working part time. I have been referred to Exercise Physiologists and Physiotherapists to assist with symptom management. I consider myself one of the lucky patients as I had doctors that were able to help me to a diagnosis relatively quickly (approximately a year). Many others that I've spoken to are on waiting lists for years to see a doctor, and as there is so much variety in symptoms, there is also a wide variety of possible treatments – many of which are off label. It's very difficult (and expensive!) as a patient to know what to do, where to go, or who to see when you need help getting through the day or getting back to some form of normal life."* Sophie.

BOX 5.3   PRACTICE POINT

Pause and reflect on your own beliefs about Long COVID. From your perspective, what causes Long COVID? What sort of disease or condition is it? What roles do physical, mental health, and social factors play in its development?

People experiencing Long COVID may present in any clinical setting, given the variety of symptoms and functional problems caused by this condition.[2] However, they may not realise they have Long COVID due to generally poor awareness of the condition in the community or incorrect information from healthcare providers or others. International research indicates both patients and healthcare providers have variable, at best, and poor, at worst, knowledge about Long COVID.[6-9] Like other chronic and unexplained conditions, some providers have also been reluctant to acknowledge its distinct features in comparison to other Post-Acute Infection Syndromes or attribute purely psychiatric causes for its symptoms.[10] This lack of consistent knowledge and awareness hinders accurate diagnosis, timely intervention, and appropriate care for these patients. It harms their health and wellbeing due to the impact of being dismissed and disbelieved.

So, where could a rehabilitation provider start with David? Only doctors are qualified to diagnose Long COVID, but all health professionals have a contribution to make to the identification of potential cases of Long COVID. The following recommendations are within the scope of practice of most rehabilitation disciplines and provide a foundation for further investigation to ensure he receives the best possible care and achieves his rehabilitation goals.

5.2.1 Collect a Detailed Health and Social History

Comprehensively document David's COVID-19 history, including dates of infections and the symptoms he experienced during and after each episode. This helps to establish the timeline of symptom emergence and may also provide additional information about characteristic symptoms related to some variants (such as olfactory dysfunction from earlier variants). From a biopsychosocial perspective, understanding his social circumstances (i.e., employment, housing, family members) is vital for identifying both opportunities and potential barriers to treatment and support. Therefore, this history provides a foundation for patient-centred care tailored to David's needs.

BOX 5.4   DAVID'S STORY

David is a 42-year-old small business owner who self-referred to a multidisciplinary allied health clinic in his local community. His medical history is unremarkable overall, but he does have obesity and reports he has had COVID "three or four times" since the end of 2021. David runs a contract hire agency for the construction industry, a role that involves both physical site visits and managing administrative tasks from his home office. Over the past few months, he has struggled with persistent fatigue, which isn't improving. David also experiences muscle aches and joint pain, particularly after long hours of work or periods of physical exertion. These symptoms have become increasingly difficult to manage, making it challenging for him to keep up with the demands of his business. He feels like he is "running on empty" and is worried about how this might affect his business's future. David has researched online and believes exercise and diet changes could help him improve. His wife is a former clinic patient who suggested it due to her good experience with their service.

5.2.2 Comprehensively Assess Current Symptoms and Functional Impact to Establish a Baseline

Explore the onset, duration, and variability of his fatigue, muscle aches, and joint pain. Asking David to describe how these symptoms affect his daily life and his ability to fulfil his life roles will help to understand their impact on his overall functioning and quality of life. This assessment may also help identify effective self-management strategies the patient already uses, which can be enabled while exploring other treatment options.

5.2.3 Screen for Common Long COVID Symptoms

While no validated screening tools for long COVID are currently available, a range of existing outcome measures allows for high-quality assessment of individual symptoms (see Chapter 6). Depending on your scope of practice, these may include evaluations of cognitive symptoms, sleep disturbances, cardiovascular symptoms, respiratory difficulties, and mental health concerns. Information about baseline symptom characteristics, as well as their causes and relievers, can also be extended where indicated. Given David's experience of fatigue, an assessment of his energy levels, both at rest and after exertion, is indicated to identify potential

Post-Exertional Malaise. All symptoms should be fully assessed, given the wide variety of ways in which Long COVID can present.

5.2.4 Consider Differential Diagnoses

Whether diagnosis is within a professional's scope of practice or not, keeping an open mind about differential diagnoses is essential to ensure a thorough approach. Assessment findings may also indicate the presence of other conditions, such as Myalgic Encephalomyelitis/Chronic Fatigue Syndrome or fibromyalgia, which may influence your advice and recommendations for next steps. People with Long COVID report their symptoms are often attributed to preexisting conditions, even when they are significantly exacerbated or presenting differently. While some health professionals see Long COVID as a diagnosis of exclusion,[11] it can and does exist alongside other conditions (see Chapter 2).

5.2.5 Assess Long COVID Awareness and Understanding

Initiating a conversation with David about Long COVID will identify his current awareness of the condition and its symptoms. If appropriate, provide transparent, current, and credible information about potential causes, common symptoms, and the possibility that his persistent symptoms could be related. Inviting David to describe any previous interactions with health professionals about Long COVID also sets the scene for ongoing discussion. An essential part of this process is acknowledging the limits of our current understanding to manage expectations, forming respectful therapeutic relationships, and building shared knowledge.

5.2.6 Shared Decision-Making Regarding Next Steps

David may or may not pursue further advice or assessment around his potential Long COVID diagnosis. If he does, adopt a shared decision-making approach to ensure his preferences and values are integrated into all care plans. This transparency also helps David make an informed choice that aligns with his needs and priorities based on his lived experience and priorities. A plan can then be co-created that balances his recovery aspirations with realistic goals for his personal and professional life. Regularly revisit the shared decision-making process to allow for adjustment as David's needs change, new priorities evolve, or new information about best practices for long-term COVID emerges.

This plan may include referral for further assessments or to other providers, following a discussion about who may be best placed to help him achieve his recovery goals (see Chapters 8 and 9). David might also work on his symptoms and their functional impact without obtaining a formal diagnosis. However, patients with suspected long COVID should always be encouraged to visit their general practitioner (GP) for a confirmatory diagnosis and access to a range of primary care services and support.

5.3 DIAGNOSING LONG COVID IN GENERAL PRACTICE

General practice is often the first point of call for patients experiencing continuing symptoms or health concerns following a COVID-19 infection. As such, GPs are key in diagnosing Long COVID and referring patients for further investigations, specialist consultation, and/or allied health treatment and support.

Until a universally agreed set of diagnostic investigations and treatment and management criteria for Long COVID is established, frontline practitioners are likely to face challenges in identifying the condition. Understanding these experiences was the subject of an Australian qualitative study[11] examining the difficulties faced by GPs in diagnosing Long COVID. The key challenges identified in the study reflect the complexity of many interrelated dimensions of clinical practice, including clinical (diagnosis, management, and referral), social (declines in rapid antigen and polymerase chain reaction testing), technical (reporting and documentation), and educational (patients and clinicians) factors.[11] These contribute to uncertainty as described by a study participant:

> And is this long COVID? Is (this) something else? … So, I think, really, the uncertainty for general practitioners is the most difficult thing, and you know, being able to be confident that that is the diagnosis. Particularly when there's a bit of a delay in that symptomatology coming forward.
>
> Participant 2[(1)11]

While the development of Long COVID is preceded by a COVID-19 infection, establishing when the causative infection occurred may not be straightforward, as Long COVID symptoms may present after an asymptomatic or mild infection.[12] A study of general practice data (n=1588 patients)[13] found that only 41.3% of patients diagnosed with Long COVID by their GP (based on Systemised Nomenclature of Medicine coding) had a previous COVID-19 diagnosis documented. The absence of documented COVID-19 infection (including date of infection) may not only exacerbate diagnostic uncertainty (given a timeframe of 12 or more weeks of symptoms before a Long COVID diagnosis)[14] but can also impede research into understanding Long COVID. Without rapid recognition of Long COVID, patients may not benefit from early interventions that can moderate the impact of their symptoms on daily life.[15] Improving clinical documentation of COVID-19 infections and detailing symptoms in patient records would enrich the quality of data and its meaningfulness and provide a greater understanding of Long COVID.

As a locus for coordinating multidisciplinary care for patients with post COVID-19 symptoms, general practice is well placed to record the diverse symptomatology and medical concerns experienced by patients with Long COVID. De-identified general practice clinical record data, therefore, holds the potential to provide meaningful insights and understanding into their temporal medical and healthcare experiences. General practice data can also provide crucial insights into the patient's journey from first encounter to diagnosis and treatment.

Moving forward, greater integration between general practice, medical specialists, and allied health is needed to ensure consistent messaging and continuity of care and support integrated diagnostic and care practices. While digital health can play a role in multidisciplinary care coordination and understanding the metrics of Long COVID, it requires high-quality de-identified data that is secure, timely, and accessible. When used appropriately by practitioners, researchers, and healthcare planners, such big data can contribute to the quality of coordinated care.

5.4 MONITORING LONG COVID TRENDS USING BIG DATA: CHALLENGES AND OPPORTUNITIES

BOX 5.5   "BIG DATA"

In the healthcare context, the term "big data" refers to data collected from mulitiple agencies, including healthcare services, research institutes, and governments. These form very large and complex dataset for analysis.

Integrating big data analytics into studying Long COVID trends represents a transformative approach to understanding and managing this complex condition. However, this approach is hindered by the absence of a standardised or widely accepted definition for Long COVID. It becomes difficult to compare across research and clinical settings if research and health organisations apply diverse symptom sets and durations. Some proposed definitions require symptoms to persist for a minimum of 12 weeks, while others use different thresholds.[1,2,16,17]

Other notable differences include the requirement of proof of acute infection or excluding other illnesses.

There is a risk that patients may struggle to receive appropriate care and support without a precise diagnosis. The ambiguity surrounding Long COVID can lead to delays in diagnosis, misdiagnosis, or the dismissal of symptoms, -affecting patient wellbeing and recovery and hindering access to specialised services and support networks designed for this patient group. This issue affects the establishment of dedicated clinics, rehabilitation programmes, and research funding specific to Long COVID.

5.4.1 Leveraging Big Data to Illuminate the Magnitude of the Long COVID Problem

The resources required to develop and maintain specialised supports for people with Long COVID must be founded on an accurate understanding of the magnitude of the problem. It is estimated that around 5–10% of COVID-19 cases in Australia result in symptoms persisting for more than ten months.[18] However, estimates vary significantly in international data, ranging from 9% to 81%.[18] This is mainly due to differences in the definitions of Long COVID, including the time points at which patients were monitored, the variant of COVID-19 that caused their infection and possibly the individual's vaccination status at the time of infection. Despite the varied estimates, the high numbers of SARS-CoV-2 infections indicate that Long COVID is a growing concern, and its impact on livelihoods is consistent.

A study by Murray et al.[19] used the International Classification of Disease, 10th Revision (ICD-10)-coded hospital admissions data from Victoria, Australia, during the pandemic period, 2020–2023, to identify admissions for COVID-19 and post-COVID-19 conditions. Post-COVID-19 admissions were identified using specific ICD-10 coding of episodes for which medical assessment of the patients determined the admission diagnosis was related to their previous COVID-19 illness.[19] The study identified 108,830 post-COVID-19 admissions, a figure 27% higher than acute COVID-19 admissions identified in the same study. This highlights the impacts post-acute COVID-19 may have on the hospital system.

This big data project also provides a more nuanced perspective on the relationship between COVID-19 infection, Long COVID, and preexisting chronic disease. Only 9% of post-COVID-19 admissions identified were among patients with a chronic condition, despite evidence from other studies indicating a higher burden of Long COVID within this population.[19,20] However, the prevalence of secondary infections was 3.5 times higher among those with post-COVID-19 conditions and chronic disease (18.1%) compared to admissions with post-COVID-19 conditions and no chronic conditions (5.2%). This may imply that chronic conditions predispose Long COVID patients to an increased risk of secondary infections, which prolong the duration and severity of illness.

Several other studies highlight the interplay between chronic diseases, COVID-19, and Long COVID, revealing key insights into disease severity, healthcare disruptions, and long-term impacts.[21–24] Some studies have pointed to the interruption of chronic disease management during the pandemic by hindering access to diagnosis, treatment, and follow-up care due to healthcare closures and service reductions. The authors suggest this disruption may explain the increased severity of COVID-19 outcomes and the higher risk of Long COVID among those with chronic conditions, compared to those without.[21,22] Other studies pointed to Long COVID impacting the clinical course of hypertension-related disorders, such as CVD, kidney diseases, and endocrine diseases, as well as older adults and women.[24] While these reports emphasise the need for strategies to prioritise the surveillance of Long COVID in these vulnerable populations, changes in the COVID-19 disease dynamics and management, including new variants, vaccinations, and treatments, as well shifts in societal behaviours, may have profound impacts on the risk of Long COVID.

Collectively, these studies identified more severe outcomes for post-COVID-19 patients with chronic conditions, although the long-term impacts of Long COVID on individuals go far beyond their hospital admission. More studies are required to assess the effects of Long COVID on other health services and the hospital system, including primary and community health. Assessment of the magnitude of these symptoms and health service usage patterns may help to inform Long COVID models of care and service delivery. A broad array of symptoms significantly impacts patient quality of life and needs to be captured in future studies.

> *Those of us who are fatigued - a non-life-threatening condition - are lost outside of the system. Studies exclude us so medical practitioners don't have the information on what to do with us.*
>
> Sophie

BOX 5.6   PRACTICE POINT

How might the findings of this study contribute to planning or resource allocation for Long COVID services? Do you see any potential for big data to contribute to service planning and resource allocation in your service setting? If so, what specific data would need to be extracted from existing data?

5.5 CASE STUDY: ANALYSING BIG DATA AT COVIDTHON

A substantial volume of healthcare data, including comprehensive COVID-19-related information, is being generated and archived at an accelerating pace. Despite this abundance of data, a standardised framework for converting this raw data into actionable insights to enhance healthcare quality and safety remains noticeably absent at international, national, state, regional, and individual healthcare service levels. Extensive healthcare datasets, particularly when integrated across multiple sources, can generate a highly accurate virtual representation of clinical practice, enabling in-depth analysis to optimise patient outcomes.[25] Big data interrogation requires a rigorous methodology and precise analysis, with statisticians and data scientists who are the best skilled in these areas. Transforming the data into useful health information that can be translated into policy and practice requires the expertise of senior clinicians and healthcare workers.

A health Datathon provides the ideal forum to facilitate collaborative exploration of large and linked formal collections of healthcare data to stimulate ongoing viable and meaningful research activity aimed at better health outcomes.[26] Bendigo Health, a large regional health service in Central Victoria, Australia, hosted a Datathon event called "COVIDthon." This brought together clinicians and health sector researchers to find preliminary answers to COVID-related variations in healthcare by teaming up data scientists, statisticians, epidemiologists, and performance reporting experts to interrogate the data using robust querying techniques.

Bendigo Health led the COVIDthon in close collaboration with the Victorian State Government Department of Health (DoH), Centre for Victorian Data Linkage (CVDL), and academic partners from across Australia. With the approval of the data custodians, nine disparate datasets were linked by CVDL. In this linking process, patients were anonymised according to set anonymisation rules applied to the data, for example, five-year age groups and SA2 level geographic data. The CVDL conducted the patient-based data linkage. The dataset was accessed via ten Virtual Machine instances hosted by the CVDL. Only data scientists with dual-key secure authentication were granted permission to query the data using commonly employed statistical software. Figure 5.1 provides an overview of the COVIDthon data schema.

Over the two-day event, five collaborative teams accessed the large, linked health datasets and were supported to explore priority research questions to gather

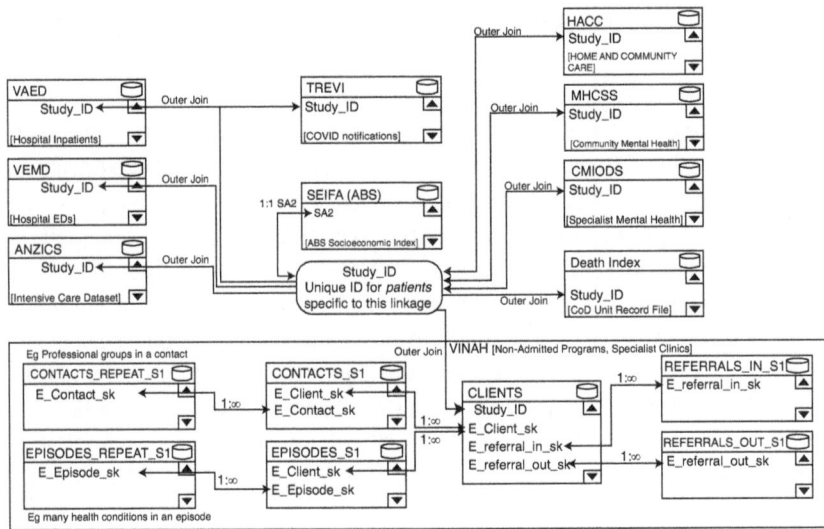

Figure 5.1 Bendigo Health COVIDTHON Schema shows the variety of person-level linked administrative datasets from Victoria, Australia, used during the datathon.

Note: All data sets were joined, and a Study ID was allocated for patients specific to this data linkages. The data sets included the Victorian Admitted Episode (VAED) dataset, Victorian Emergency Minimum (VEMD) dataset, Australian and New Zealand Intensive Care Society (ANZICS) database, Transmission and Response Epidemiology Victoria (TREVI) database, Home and Community Care (HACC) database, Mental Health Community Support Services (MHCSS) database, Client Management Interface/Operational Data Store (CMIODS), Victorian Integrated Non-Admitted Health (VINAH) dataset, Socio-Economic Indexes for Areas (SEIFA) dataset, and Death Index. The lower section of the figure shows an expanded view of the VINAH data linkage configuration, expanded because it is a slightly more complicated data structure than the other data sets.

evidence that could otherwise take years to accumulate from smaller disparate datasets. The event was unique as there have been very few occasions and opportunities for researchers to gain access to such extensive linked datasets. The event aimed to view the *whole* health service footprint of COVID-19 patients across multiple health collections.

Each team had clinicians, health researchers, allocated data scientist/s, student data scientists, and epidemiologists. This was coupled with a group of 19 support personnel with expertise to facilitate the event and interrogation of the data. The teams focused on exploring research questions from a diverse range of priority areas, including COVID impacts on CVD, elective surgery waiting lists, family violence (including physical and sexual assault hospitalisation rates), mental health, and Long COVID.

At the end of the event, each team "pitched" their findings to the expert judging panel, and the winning team was the team that explored the long-term sequelae of COVID-19. They interrogated the big data, finding initial answers to the questions:

- What are the service use patterns for people diagnosed three to six months after a COVID-19 diagnosis?
- What are the risk factors for seeking access to health services three to six months after their COVID-19 diagnosis?
- What severity outcomes are associated with Long COVID-19 (seeking access to health service three to six months after their COVID-19 diagnosis)?

The main goal of the COVIDthon was to facilitate and evaluate collaborative exploration of large and linked formal collections of healthcare data. The aim was to encourage sustained and impactful research, particularly to enhance health outcomes for individuals in rural and regional communities. A secondary aim was to subsequently establish a blueprint for the robust analysis of big data in healthcare that protects the privacy of individuals and complies with all ethical aspects of using individuals' health data, particularly those living in rural and regional areas where smaller population numbers can increase the risk of an individual's data being potentially identifiable. We believe that the COVIDthon achieved these aims.

The substantial volume and scale of healthcare data collected represent a significant untapped resource for enhancing population health and wellbeing. The failure to leverage this data effectively is a missed opportunity. As healthcare workers, we have an inherent responsibility to our community to ensure that this data is translated into meaningful information to inform healthcare policy and practice. Health Datathons like the COVIDthon can drive and accelerate value-based healthcare. The ability to responsibly apply analytics to "big data" has the potential to revolutionise evidence-based healthcare.[27] Events like the COVIDthon ensure the efficient and responsible use of the enormous reservoirs of available health data to improve our community's health and wellbeing outcomes in the future and build our nation's Digital Health capabilities.

Some remaining questions that big data events could help address include

- What patterns or correlations can be identified in large datasets that reveal the variability of Long COVID symptoms across different demographic groups (age, gender, ethnicity, and preexisting health conditions)?

- Can big data help establish clear, evidence-based diagnostic criteria for Long COVID by analysing the various manifestations of the condition across large populations?

5.6 CONCLUSION

Identifying and managing Long COVID presents a complex challenge for healthcare providers due to the multifaceted nature of the condition and the absence of universally agreed-upon criteria. GPs and other healthcare specialists are crucial in identifying symptoms, coordinating care, and making timely referrals to specialists, but the variability in diagnostic protocols can impede effective management and research. As Long COVID continues to affect a significant portion of the population, big data analytics holds immense potential for improving our understanding of the condition and optimising patient care. Data-driven insights can help reveal the true scope of Long COVID, refine diagnostic criteria, and support the development of tailored interventions. The COVIDthon initiative exemplifies how health data, when appropriately harnessed, can drive impactful research and improve healthcare outcomes, particularly for vulnerable populations affected by Long COVID. Moving forward, the strategic use of big data can enhance the quality of care for Long COVID patients and inform broader healthcare policies and resource allocation.

NOTE

1 Reproduced with permission from The Royal Australian College of General Practitioners from: Thomas J, Prgomet M, Weeding S, McGuire P, Goodger B, Joss N, Mackintosh CF, McLeod A, Georgiou A. A qualitative study of the general practice experience of diagnosing and managing long COVID: Challenges and practical recommendations. Aust J Gen Pract 2024;53(10):732–36.

REFERENCES

1 World Health Organization. COVID-19 clinical management: living guidance, 25 January 2021. Geneva: World Health Organization; 2021.

2 National Academies of Sciences, Engineering, and Medicine. A Long COVID definition: A chronic, systemic disease state with profound consequences. Washington, DC: The National Academies Press; 2024. doi:10.17226/27768.

3 Davis H, et al. Characterising long COVID in an international cohort: 7 months of symptoms and their impact. eClinicalMedicine. 2021;38:101019. doi:10.1016/j.eclinm.2021.101019.

4 Adhikari A, et al. Beyond acute infection: mechanisms underlying post-acute sequelae of COVID-19 (PASC). Med J Aust 2024;221(9): S40–48. doi:10.5694/mja2.52456.

5 Xie Y, et al. Long-term cardiovascular outcomes of COVID-19. Nat Med. 2022;28:583–90. doi:10.1038/s41591-022-01689-3.

6 Pfaff E, et al. Who has long-COVID? A big data approach. medRxiv. 2021;10.18.21265168. doi:10.1101/2021.10.18.21265168.

7 Cooper E, et al. Awareness and perceptions of long COVID among people in the REACT programme: Early insights from a pilot interview study. PLoS One. 2023;18. doi:10.1371/journal.pone.0280943.

8 Fisher KA, et al. Long COVID awareness and receipt of medical care: A survey among populations at risk for disparities. Front Public Health. 2024;12. doi:10.3389/fpubh.2024.1360341.

9 Ojha S, et al. A quantitative evaluation of knowledge, perception, awareness, and preparedness of "Long COVID" among healthcare professionals and students in India. J Radiol Nurs. 2023. doi:10.1016/j.jradnu.2023.10.005.

10 Little J, et al. Long COVID – Can we deny a diagnosis without denying a person's reality? Australas Psychiatry. 2024;32(1):44–46. doi:10.1177/10398562231222809.

11 Thomas J, et al. A qualitative study of the general practice experience of diagnosing and managing long COVID: Challenges and practical recommendations. Aust J Gen Pract. 2024;53(10):732–36. doi:10.31128/AJGP-10-23-6983.

12 Adler L, et al. Long-COVID in patients with a history of mild or asymptomatic SARS-CoV-2 infection: A Nationwide Cohort Study. Scan J Prim Health Care. 2022;40(3):342–49. doi:10.1080/02813432.2022.2139480.

13 Kamalakkannan A, et al. Factors associated with a general practitioner-led diagnosis of long COVID: An observational study using electronic general practice data from Victoria and New South Wales, Australia. Med J Aust. 2024; 221 Supp9:S18–22. doi:10.5694/mja2.52458.

14 National Clinical Evidence Taskforce. COVID-19 living guidelines Version 74.1 [Internet]. Melbourne: Living Evidence; [cited 2025 Feb 7]. Available from: https://livingevidence.org.au/living-guidelines/covid-19/.

15 Ghali A, et al. The relevance of pacing strategies in managing symptoms of post-COVID-19 syndrome. J Transl Med. 2023;21(1):375. doi:10.1186/s12967-023-04229-w.

16 National Institute for Health and Care Excellence (NICE), Scottish Intercollegiate Guidelines Network (SIGN), & Royal College of General Practitioners (RCGP). COVID-19 rapid guideline: Managing the long-term effects of COVID-19. Version 1.14. London: NICE, SIGN, RCGP; 2022.

17 Fernández-de-las-Peñas C, et al. Defining post-COVID symptoms (post-acute COVID, long COVID, persistent post-COVID): An integrative classification. Int J Environ Res Public Health. 2021;18:2621. doi: 10.3390/ijerph18052621.

18 Australian Institute of Health and Welfare. Long COVID in Australia: A review of the literature [Internet]. Canberra: AIHW; 2023 [cited 2025 Feb 7]. Available from: https://www.aihw.gov.au/reports/covid-19/long-covid-in-australia-a-review-of-the-literature/summary.

19 Murray H, et al. Prevalence, risk factors, and outcomes of secondary infections among hospitalised patients with COVID-19 or post-COVID-19 conditions in Victoria, 2020–2023. Int J Infect Dis. 2024;145:107078. doi:10.1016/j.ijid.2024.107078.

20 Song Z, et al. Demographic and clinical factors associated with Long COVID. Health Aff. 2023;42(3): 433–42. doi:10.1377/hlthaff.2022.00991.

21 Geng J, et al. Chronic diseases as a predictor for severity and mortality of COVID-19: A systematic review with cumulative meta-analysis. Front. Med. 2021;8:588013. doi:10.3389/fmed.2021.588013.

22 Fekadu G, et al. Impact of COVID-19 pandemic on chronic diseases care follow-up and current perspectives in low resource settings: a narrative review. Int J Physiol Pathophysiol Pharmacol. 2021 Jun 15;13(3):86–93.

23 Kendzerska T, et al. The effects of the health system response to the COVID-19 pandemic on chronic disease management: A narrative review. Risk Manag Healthcare Policy. 2021;14, 575–84. doi:10.2147/RMHP.S293471/.

24 Matsumoto C, et al. Long COVID and hypertension-related disorders: a report from the Japanese Society of Hypertension Project Team on COVID-19. Hypertens Res. 2023;46(3):601–19. doi:10.1038/s41440-022-01145-2.

25 Aboab J, et al. A "datathon" model to support cross-disciplinary collaboration. Sci Transl Med. 2016;8:333. doi:10.1126/scitranslmed.aad9072.

26 Silver JK, et al. Healthcare hackathons provide educational and innovation opportunities: A case study and best practice recommendations. J Med Syst. 2016;40:177. doi:10.1007/s10916-016-0532-3.

27 Roski J, et al. Creating value in health care through big data: Opportunities and policy implications. Health Aff. 2014;33(7):1115–22. doi:10.1377/hlthaff.2014.0147.

Chapter 6

Measuring What Matters in Long COVID

Outcome Measures and Monitoring

Miquette Abercrombie and Danielle Hitch

BOX 6.1   LEARNING OUTCOMES

By the end of this chapter, readers should be able to:

- Describe the role of outcome measures in Long COVID rehabilitation, including clinical measures, Patient-Rated Outcome Measures (PROMs), and Patient-Rated Experience Measures (PREMs).
- Apply a framework for selecting meaningful, high-quality outcome measures aligning with patient goals and organisational requirements.
- Critically evaluate outcome measures by assessing their psychometric properties, practicality, relevance and validity for people with Long COVID.
- Explore strategies to integrate patient goals and lived experience into implementing outcome measures.

6.1 INTRODUCTION

Measuring baseline health and treatment outcomes is vital to assess intervention impacts and personalise care. Outcome measures help monitor progress and address unexpected changes or setbacks for people with Long COVID. Hillier et al.[1][p511] state, "A basis of good clinical practice is to use valid and reliable outcome measurement tools that are also responsive to the interventions offered."

DOI: 10.4324/9781003528104-8

Many people with Long COVID find ways to track their progress, highlighting the importance of hope to the therapeutic process.

> *I deliberately left video journals on my Facebook so I could actually see what the difference is on my bad days. There are a lot of them that I do look back on when I'm feeling down and see that I have fought back to be better.*

In healthcare, "outcome" refers to results or changes observed after an intervention, whether or not they are directly linked to that treatment.[2] However, clinical measures are often used only during the initial rehabilitation assessment. A key feature of outcome measures is their ability to show change over time.[3] Thus, clinical measures in Long COVID rehabilitation must be administered at least twice to capture improvement and recovery.

BOX 6.2   REMEMBER

It's not an outcome measure if you only use it once.
Outcomes result from change over time.

Outcome measures are also vital to link the healthcare provided and the outcomes experienced by people with Long COVID.[3] This is often challenging due to the diversity of Long COVID presentations and multidisciplinary treatment approaches.[4] Evidence suggests some people may experience spontaneous recovery over time, with improvements reported even without access to rehabilitation in the early pandemic months.[5] Despite the challenges of capturing the relationship between the care provided and outcomes achieved, outcome measures are essential for evidence-based practice, personalised care, and advancing research on effective Long COVID treatments. Without outcome measures, people with Long COVID and health professionals may lose trust or motivation in rehabilitation, especially with slow or fluctuating recovery.[6]

This chapter aims to guide the selection of meaningful measures and their implementation into practice. It describes identifying meaningful outcomes for people with Long COVID and selecting and implementing appropriate measures that balance the needs of patients and services. Given the diversity of Long COVID presentations and practice settings, this chapter focuses on general principles and processes rather than specific outcome measures relevant to Long COVID.

6.2 MEASURING WHAT MATTERS

Outcome measures should reflect the rehabilitation goals of people with Long COVID, incorporating input from health professionals. Meaningful goals stem from the lived experience of the person with Long COVID, while realistic goals are informed by professional expertise. Health professionals also gather clinical data to support reasoning and meet organisational metrics. Some measures may not align with clients' priorities but are essential to the service response, serving multiple purposes and stakeholders' needs.

BOX 6.3   PRACTICE POINT

Reflect on the outcome measures you need to inform your clinical reasoning. How do you choose which one to use for each patient? Do you use some more frequently than others? Are there organisation wide outcome measures at your service?

The concept of "measuring what matters" is commonly associated with quality improvement in health services[7] and is embedded in policy frameworks like the Australian National Wellbeing Framework.[8] Identifying meaningful, actionable outcomes is crucial for the therapeutic relationship between people with Long COVID and health professionals. While priorities often overlap, prioritising the needs of health professionals or services over those of patients inevitably disrupts the therapeutic alliance.[9]

BOX 6.4   WHAT IS A PATIENT-RATED OUTCOME MEASURE?

These tools capture people's subjective perspectives on health outcomes. Patient-rated outcome measure (PROMs) enable health professionals to capture lived experiences, support patient-centred care, and collect data systematically for quality improvement.

Many PROMs have design features that limit their ability to measure what matters. Despite their name, most PROMs were developed without involving people with lived experience,[10] reflecting developers' priorities rather than what matters to patients. This threatens their content validity, compromising their ability to measure all essential aspects of an outcome. For example, the widely used Modified Medical Research Council (mMRC) Dyspnoea Scale[11] primarily evaluates breathlessness during physical exertion but fails to account for delayed and disproportionate symptom exacerbation resulting from Post-Exertional Malaise (PEM).

Outcome measures are structured and standardised to ensure consistent implementation and comparison of health outcomes between services and patient groups.[12] Few outcome measures have been validated specifically for people with Long COVID, and rehabilitation measures often prioritise participation in self-care activities.[13] There have also been calls to update options on long-established measures that no longer reflect activities in which people regularly participate.[14] However, goal attainment measures like the Goal Attainment Scale (GAS)[15] and Multidisciplinary Goal Attainment Measure (MGAM)[16] offer patient-centred alternatives to scales that focus on function or the performance of measuring their participation in specific activities.

In our experience, measuring what matters often means using outcome measures of function and participation in daily life. People with Long COVID have repeatedly told us that their symptoms are what Long COVID "is," but their impact on their daily life is what Long COVID "means."[16] Functional measures are valued by people with Long COVID and healthcare professionals; however, symptom measures play an equally important role in understanding people's lived experiences.

BOX 6.4   WHAT IS A CLINICAL MEASURE?

Clinical measures are objective tools or assessments (often observational) used by health professionals to evaluate a person's health status, function, or symptoms. In the context of Long COVID, they are frequently used to assess aspects like fatigue, breathlessness, or PEM.

Clinical measures, particularly symptom scales, are often prioritised by health professionals and services alongside Patient-Rated Experience Measures (PREMs). Symptom measures provide insights into specific symptoms' severity, frequency, and triggers that may otherwise go unreported. For example, tools that assess fatigue, breathlessness, or pain can capture subtle changes over time, enabling health professionals to adjust interventions proactively. Symptom measures can also help identify patterns, such as exacerbations triggered by exertion, to inform self-management strategies like pacing. Incorporating symptom measures alongside functional assessments ensures a comprehensive approach to outcome measurement, addressing what Long COVID "is" (symptom severity) and what it "means" (impact on daily life).

BOX 6.5   WHAT IS A PATIENT RATED EXPERIENCE MEASURE?

These tools capture the lived experience of accessing healthcare, covering communication, accessibility, coordination, and satisfaction. They assess care quality, enabling health professionals to improve systems, enhance safety, meet standards, and support health equity.

Quality of Life (QoL) measures are also commonly employed with people with Long COVID and are highly valued by those with Long COVID and healthcare professionals. QoL is often used as an umbrella term, encompassing a range of factors that might influence physical, functional, economic, spiritual, and psychosocial wellbeing.[17,18] Many QoL measures include items measuring both function and symptoms; however, there is no current consensus about how the concept is defined overall.[19]

BOX 6.6   PRACTICE POINT

Review these recommendations for measuring what matters for people with Long COVID. Do they reflect your current practice? If not, select one and consider how you could change your practice to improve outcome measurement.

- Ensure outcome measures reflect outcomes relevant to the person's goals and achievable through rehabilitation.
- Recognise each measure's purposes and ensure all stakeholders' needs are met.
- Understand the development process of chosen measures, including the degree of patient involvement in its formulation.
- Use goal-focused measures to evaluate whether rehabilitation supports personal goal achievement.

- Use standardised, structured measures to enhance data quality.
- Utilise both objective (i.e., clinical) and subjective (i.e., PROMs, PREMs) measures to access multiple perspectives across diverse formats (i.e., checklists, patient narratives, observational).

6.3 SELECTING MEANINGFUL AND HIGH-QUALITY OUTCOME MEASURES

Selecting outcome measures for people with Long COVID requires balancing personal goals with standardised clinical data. Coster[20] outlines a process for selecting outcome measures in research, which can also guide practice. Multidisciplinary teams should collaboratively identify primary and secondary measures. Primary measures focus on critical rehabilitation outcomes like symptom severity, function, and QoL. In contrast, secondary measures address broader and complementary factors such as mental health, patient experiences, and environmental or contextual outcomes. Consistent use of measures supports clinician information sharing and streamlines overlapping measures across disciplines. Health professionals can use these steps to align measures with their expertise or the specific goals of people with Long COVID.

6.3.1 Identify Rehabilitation Goals for the Person with Long COVID

As stated, clearly articulated rehabilitation goals are the foundation of outcome measurement selection. (see Chapter 7)

6.3.2 Identify Relevant Outcome Domains

The Core Outcome Measures in Effectiveness Trials (COMETs) initiative sought international consensus on a core outcome set for Long COVID research.[21] People with Long COVID and their carers participated in the process, which included a literature review, an online Delphi process with 1,535 participants, and a consensus meeting. Twelve core outcomes were identified: seven clinical outcomes (cardiovascular; nervous; respiratory; cognitive and mental systems; fatigue; pain; and post-exertion symptoms), two participation outcomes (physical functioning and work or study challenges), survival, and recovery. Research outcome measures are used to generate generalisable evidence, often prioritising standardisation and statistical validity. In contrast, clinical outcome measures are

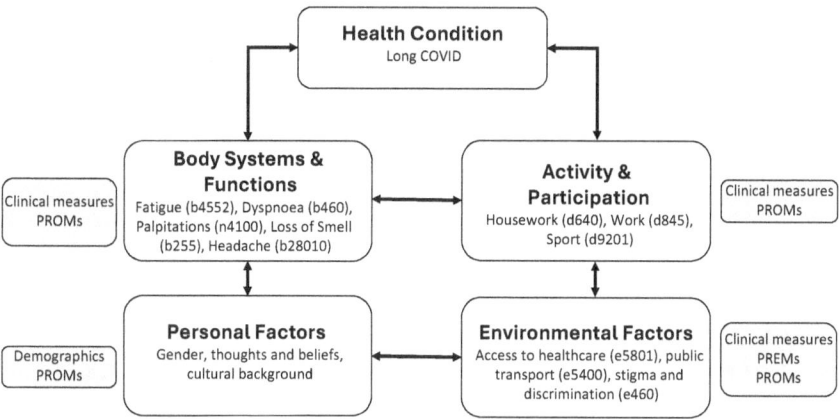

Figure 6.1 Identifying relevant outcome domains using the International Classification of Function.

used to improve health and functioning through rehabilitation. Clinical measures can be used in research, but they are applied for different purposes.

While these outcomes may apply broadly to people with Long COVID, a personalised approach to identifying meaningful outcomes is essential. The International Classification of Functioning (ICF)[22] offers a multidisciplinary framework to understand interactions between a person's health condition, personal factors, and environmental influences on their functioning and participation. It helps map meaningful health domains for people with Long COVID and identify potential relationships. Outcomes should always be interpreted within the context of all data collected for the patient, just as each component of the ICF cannot be considered in isolation (Figure 6.1).

Figure 6.1 maps common rehabilitation goals for people with Long COVID to their ICF classifications and relevant outcome measure categories. Although personal factors are included in the ICF, they remain unclassified due to their diversity and individual nature.[22]

6.3.3 Review Existing Measures

Long COVID research evolves rapidly, with around 300 new studies published monthly,[23] and no health professional can realistically read ten journal articles daily. Review articles synthesise current practice, reducing the need to read multiple articles. Consulting Long COVID-specific resources is another efficient way to find relevant measures. LitCovid,[23] a searchable database updated monthly, is currently the only Long COVID-specific database available.

While larger health services have the capacity to conduct systematic reviews, benchmarking exercises, and implement extensive outcome measures, sole practitioners often operate with limited resources and support. Curated resources (like LitCovid), professional guidelines, and communities of practice provide ready-made, practical alternatives. Networking with peers from larger services also offers opportunities for mutual learning and sharing tools and resources with less well-resourced health professionals. Health professionals generally cannot validate outcome measures for themselves but can partner with universities on studies that confirm or evaluate their psychometric properties.

Health professionals can also identify measures already used through benchmarking, which compares practice with other services working with people with Long COVID. It improves service quality by identifying best practices, fostering shared learning, and building professional networks.[24] Benchmarking also helps identify outcome measures feasible for everyday practice, not just those applicable to research. Finally, many more extensive health services have links to universities or hospital libraries that can assist with formalised systematic literature reviews.

6.3.4 Review Existing Measures for Psychometric Rigour and Practicality

Once potentially relevant outcome measures are identified, they must be thoroughly evaluated to ensure they measure what matters. Rehabilitation clinicians usually prefer to use familiar outcome measures, making this review process crucial when considering new ones. The following case study from a community rehabilitation service illustrates this process using the World Health Organization Disability Assessment Schedule 2.0 (WHODAS)[25] as an example of the review process. Not all services will have the resources to complete this process, but elements of it may be feasible.

BOX 6.7   CASE STUDY: REVIEWING THE SUITABILITY OF WHODAS FOR LONG COVID REHABILITATION

The review began with an overview of the outcome measure's characteristics and scoring to enhance clinician familiarity. The WHODAS is a generic tool for assessing health status and disability across cultures and settings linked to the Activity and Participation domain of the ICF.[26] It assesses disability across six domains: understanding and communicating, getting around, self-care, getting along with people, life activities (household, work, and/or school), and social participation.

There are two versions (12 and 36 items), and the measure can be self-administered or completed with an interviewer. The WHODAS is scored based on a person's self-reported difficulty performing activities over the past 30 days, using a 5-point scale from "no difficulty" to "extreme difficulty or unable to do." Three additional questions assess days of impaired activity engagement but do not contribute to the WHODAS score. Domain scores are summed to calculate the overall score.

The community-based rehabilitation team examined how the WHODAS was developed. This began with a review of over 300 measures and literature on disability, compiling a pool of items with associated psychometric properties. An international task force then led field testing across multiple countries, gathering feedback on psychometric qualities, redundancy, screener performance, and recall times. The public and people with physical, mental, and substance use disorders contributed through interviews, focus groups, field testing, and exploring the measure's cross-cultural relevance.[26]

The next phase of the review evaluated the psychometric properties of the outcome measures, ensuring reliability, validity, and responsiveness. The WHODAS has been validated with people with Long COVID,[27] though most evidence for its psychometric properties comes from studies with other patient groups. These properties were reviewed using the COnsensus-based Standards for the selection of health Measurement Instruments (COSMIN), and evidence quality was rated using the Grading of Recommendations, Assessment, Development, and Evaluations (GRADE) approach[28,29] (see Table 6.1).

The community-based rehabilitation team used a conservative approach, basing their evaluation on the lowest scores. As a result, the WHODAS was deemed to have adequate psychometric properties and moderate evidence quality.

Client-centred practice underpins integrated care[30] and is a key community rehabilitation approach. Guided by its principles,[31] the team considered these questions to assess the WHODAS against this core value (see Table 6.2).

Table 6.1 Psychometric Properties of the WHODAS

Psychometric Property	Rating	Evidence Quality
Measure Development	Very good	Very good
Content Validity	Very good	Good
Structural Validity	Very good	Good
Internal Consistency	Adequate	Moderate
Cross Cultural Validation	Adequate	Moderate
Reliability	Very good	Good
Measurement Error	Very good	Good
Criterion Validity	Adequate	Moderate
Construct Validity	Very good	Good
Responsiveness	Adequate	Moderate
Minimally Important Change	Adequate	Moderate

Table 6.2 WHODAS Alignment with Client-Centred Practice Principles

Client-Centred Practice Principle	WHODAS Evaluation
Getting to know the person beyond their diagnosis or functional impairment.	It covers diverse domains beyond impairment and encompasses all areas of daily life.
Sharing power and responsibility through meaningful partnerships between health professionals and clients in goal setting, care planning, and decision-making.	Self-rated by the person, providing predetermined information on specific items and guiding shared decision-making about function and participation.

Accessibility supports people's choices by providing timely, complete, accessible, and accurate information for decision-making.	Clear response categories written in everyday language.
Flexibility by eliciting and being sensitive to people's values, preferences, and expressed needs.	Applicable to various diagnoses, but response options are predetermined.
Enables teams to collaborate and coordinate, reducing duplication and supporting care continuity.	Designed to be multidisciplinary for use by various health professionals.
Understanding the person's physical, social, and cultural environment.	Includes items that explicitly address the environment.

The team considered the practicalities of using WHODAS with clients. The tool is quick to complete (36 items: 7–10 minutes, 12 items: 2–3 minutes) and not burdensome. No training or accreditation is required, and it is free to use with acknowledgment of the World Health Organization. WHODAS is available in multiple languages, including those common in their local community. It also has proven utility with people experiencing various disabilities, including cardiovascular and musculoskeletal conditions.[32,33]

BOX 6.8   PRACTICE POINT

Every service and community are unique, making context crucial. After reading this case example, would you use the WHODAS in your service with people with Long COVID? What factors would support or discourage its implementation in practice?

6.3.5 Pilot Testing of Outcome Measure in Practice

Pilot testing new outcome measures in context is essential before full implementation.[20] Testing with a small group of people with Long COVID provides opportunities to identify potential issues, adjust its use and gather feedback about the experience of completing the measure.[34] This groundwork prepares health professionals for implementation and potential impacts on practice.[34] A service may decide against finalising a tool if it proves infeasible or lacks impact on decision-making during testing.

6.3.6 Selection Finalisation and Roll Out

The final step in this process focuses on the sustainability of the chosen outcome measure. Barriers to consistent adoption can arise within the service context (e.g., competing demands), health professional engagement, and perceptions of benefits to patient outcomes,[35] which may not have been evident during pilot testing. Additional support may include training on practice use, data interpretation, and troubleshooting; infrastructure investment in data systems or administrative support; and addressing logistical issues around analysis and reporting.

Systems must ensure that outcome measures are completed at least twice to track change. These may be completed routinely for all people with Long COVID or during short but intense periods (i.e., two weeks) to reduce the burden during high demand. The latter reflects a service-driven approach but may be the only feasible option in some cases. Feedback loops should provide health professionals with data summaries showing the value of these measures. Routine data monitoring supports evidence-based service reforms that respond to the evolving needs of people with Long COVID.

6.4 MEASURING WHAT MATTERS AT THE INDIVIDUAL LEVEL

The foundation of outcome measurement is the personal goals of people with Long COVID; their primary purpose is to support recovery. Based on lived and practice experience, the following recommendations offer a guide to health professionals to use outcome measures respectfully and effectively.

6.4.1 Actively Listen During Every Appointment

Begin assessments by inviting people with Long COVID to share what brought them in. This allows them to voice key concerns without being influenced by clinician assumptions. Listen for repeated phrases and observe emotional responses to identify outcomes that matter to them. Initial appointments can be stressful due to the need to share information and build rapport, so offer additional chances to clarify priorities, "I ask so many questions as I don't like that I am perceived as loopy because I am on anti-depressants. I am so anxious when any new health professional sees my medication list, and all of a sudden, I am treated differently, especially being in a wheelchair as well."

Continuing this approach in every clinical encounter ensures you measure and address what matters. For example, it mattered to Miquette that her pain levels at home were accurately assessed.

> I begged the Paramedics not to treat my pain as I felt no one would believe I had it when we got to hospital. I was ignored and pain relief given. As a result, the Emergency Department doctor said that there was nothing wrong with me.

Active listening is essential for building a therapeutic alliance in rehabilitation. International experience shows that people with Long COVID often feel health professionals dismiss their symptoms. Poor listening risks missing crucial health information and undermines long-term treatment, "In a telehealth appointment with a Neurologist he was eating his lunch and preoccupied with maybe his phone."

6.4.2 Place Equal Value on Objective (Clinical) and Subjective (PROM or PREM) Outcome Measures

Many people with Long COVID have received normal test results that do not reflect their lived experience. Long COVID is often invisible, with key symptoms not readily observable. Health professionals are trained to prioritise objective over subjective data, yet validating lived experience is essential for high-quality outcome measurement. This emergency physician recognised the need to include all perspectives after developing Long COVID.

> My test results were normal … but I did not feel fine, and still do not. As a result, I have been reminded of the need to listen to the patient first, even in the absence of conclusive testing. The next time I care for someone with … any of the myriad conditions that are uncomfortable on the inside but look fine on the outside, I will remember that these symptoms are real and impactful for patients. There is a marked difference between tests being within normal limits and a patient being well.[36]

Objective outcome measures for depression and anxiety are particularly challenging to interpret for people with Long COVID. Due to symptom overlap, these measures may inadvertently pathologise physical symptoms as mental health issues. For example, a person with Long COVID may score highly on a depression scale due to fatigue or sleep disruption despite the absence of depressive symptoms. Health professionals must balance these objective measures with patient-reported experiences to validate and contextualise their lived experiences. Using Long COVID specific outcome measures can help bridge this gap and prevent the mischaracterisation of symptoms.

This chapter's comprehensive outcome measurement approach, using multiple instruments and perspectives, helps avoid dismissing or discharging people with Long COVID who remain unwell. While normal results may reassure in some cases, telling people they are fine when their body says otherwise will not change their minds.

6.4.3 Share Outcome Measurement Results with People with Long COVID

Many people (but not all) want to know the results of outcome measures to understand their condition or track recovery better. This data is co-constructed information about their health, wellbeing, and identity. Ethical practice requires transparency in data use, appropriate consent, and shared decision-making with people with Long COVID. Health professionals should provide outcome measure results and support people in interpreting them within their personal context.

To ensure accessibility, results should be presented and communicated in suitable formats. Visual aids or plain language summaries can address brain fog and improve accessibility for people from culturally and linguistically diverse backgrounds. Verbal explanations must be supported by written information, enabling patients to review and share results with other health providers, "Due to anxiety, lack of energy or spoons or just not being good cognitively on the day, I will retain ALL results for my own records or to read when I am better."

6.4.4 Think about What You Really Need to Measure

There are many things you could measure for people with Long COVID. Still, excessive outcome measures risk overwhelm and add to their already significant administrative burdens, "I have had weekly appointments for two years to keep up to date with all tests and specialists follow up – that's a minimum of 104 appointments just to keep on top of everything."

Adopting the "measuring what matters" principles helps health professionals streamline outcome measurement, with the selection process identifying measures that cover multiple outcome domains. This avoids the need for people with Long COVID to tell their story repeatedly, which contributes to feeling they are not being heard. Regular check-ins with people with Long COVID, through PREMs or informally, can reveal if they feel overwhelmed by outcome measure completion or feedback, "Biweekly my health professional calls to check in to see if I am OK if appointments have overwhelmed or upset me."

6.5 CONCLUSION

In conclusion, this chapter emphasises the critical role of outcome measures in delivering and evaluating effective, person-centred rehabilitation for people with Long COVID. Healthcare professionals must select and use measures that capture clinical and patient-reported outcomes to reflect the condition's complexity and impact on daily life. Aligning these measures with people's personal goals supports recovery, strengthens the therapeutic alliance, fosters trust, and builds motivation throughout rehabilitation.

Health professionals are encouraged to evaluate their measures critically, balancing service-level metrics with the needs and priorities of people with Long COVID. Embedding routine outcome measures into practice requires thoughtful selection, reflection, patient involvement, and adaptability. These strategies help rehabilitation professionals meet clinical standards while respecting the lived experiences of people with Long COVID.

REFERENCES

1 Hillier S, et al. Development of a participatory process to address fragmented application of outcome measurement for rehabilitation in community settings. Disabil Rehabil. 2010 Jan;32(6):511–20. doi:10.3109/09638280903171519.
2 Boyce NW, et al. Quality and outcome indicators for acute healthcare services: A research project for the National Hospital Outcomes Program (NHOP) Health Service Outcomes Branch. Canberra: Australian Government Publishing Service; 1997.
3 Unsworth C. Measuring the outcome of occupational therapy: Tools and resources. Aust Occup Ther J. 2000 Dec;47(4):147–58. doi:10.1046/j.1440-1630.2000.00239.x.
4 Haroon S, et al. Therapies for Long COVID in non-hospitalised individuals: From symptoms, patient-reported outcomes and immunology to targeted therapies (The TLC Study). BMJ Open. 2022;12(4):e060413. doi:10.1136/bmjopen-2021-060413.
5 Hitch D, et al. Beyond the case numbers: Social determinants and contextual factors in patient narratives of recovery from COVID-19. Aust N Z J Public Health. 2023 Feb;47(1):100002. doi:10.1016/j.anzjph.2022.100002.
6 Servier C, et al. Trajectories of the evolution of post-COVID-19 condition, up to two years after symptoms onset. Int J Infect Dis. 2023;133:67–74. doi:10.1016/j.ijid.2023.05.007.

7 Vyas A, et al. Measuring what matters: A proposal for reframing how we evaluate and improve experience in healthcare. Patient Exp J. 2022;9(1):5–11. doi:10.35680/2372-0247.1696.

8 Australian Government. Measuring what matters [Internet]. Canberra: Australian Government; 2023 [cited 2025 Feb 7]. Available at: https://treasury.gov.au/policy-topics/measuring-what-matters.

9 Barnett A, et al. Patients' experiences with rehabilitation care: A qualitative study to inform patient-centred outcomes. Disabil Rehabil. 2023;45(8):1307–14. doi:10.1080/09638288.2022.2057597.

10 Wiering B, et al. Asking what matters: The relevance and use of patient-reported outcome measures that were developed without patient involvement. Health Expect. 2017 Dec;20(6):1330–41. doi:10.1111/hex.12573.

11 Sunjaya A, et al. Qualitative validation of the modified Medical Research Council (mMRC) dyspnoea scale as a patient-reported measure of breathlessness severity. Respir Med. 2022;203:106984. doi:10.1016/j.rmed.2022.106984Liao Z, et al.

12 Li Z, et al. Challenges to global standardisation of outcome measures [Internet]. In: AMA Virtual Summit 2021; 2021 [cited 2025 Feb 7]. Available at: https://scholar.harvard.edu/files/yuriquintana/files/amia_virtualsummit2021_paper_zl-yq_revision.pdf.

13 Romli MH, et al. Overview of reviews of standardised occupation-based instruments for use in occupational therapy practice. Aust Occup Ther J. 2019;66(4):428. doi:10.1111/1440-1630.12572.

14 Fessler EB, et al. Rebooting instrumental activities of daily living for the 21st century. Ann Intern Med. 2021;175:278–79. doi:10.7326/M21-3065.

15 Kiresuk T, et al. Goal attainment scaling: A general method of evaluating comprehensive mental health programmes. Community Ment Health J. 1968;4:443–53. doi:10.1007/BF01530764.

16 Kendall M, et al. Measuring goal attainment within a community-based multidisciplinary rehabilitation setting for people with spinal cord injury. Edorium J Disabil Rehabil. 2016;2:43–52. doi:10.5348/D05-2016-10-OA-6.

17 Fayers P, et al. Quality of life. 3rd ed. West Sussex: Wiley; 2016.

18 Liddle J, et al. Quality of life: An overview of issues for use in occupational therapy outcome measurement. Aust Occup Ther J. 2000;47(2):77–85. doi:10.1046/j.1440-1630.2000.00217.x.

19 Lombardi M, et al. The concept of quality of life as framework for implementing the UNCRPD. J Policy Pract Intellect Disabil. 2019;16(3):180–90. doi:10.1111/jppi.12279.

20 Coster WJ. Making the best match: Selecting outcome measures for clinical trials and outcome studies. Am J Occup Ther. 2013 Mar-Apr;67(2):162–70. doi:10.5014/ajot.2013.006015.

21 Munblit D, et al. PC-COS project steering committee. A core outcome set for post-COVID-19 condition in adults for use in clinical practice and research: An international Delphi consensus study. Lancet Respir Med. 2022 Jul;10(7):715–24. doi:10.1016/S2213-2600(22)00169-2.

22 World Health Organization. International classification of functioning, disability and health (ICF). Geneva: World Health Organization; 2001.

23 National Center for Biotechnology Information (NCBI). Coronavirus research database: Long COVID [Internet]. Bethesda, MD: U.S. National Library of Medicine; [cited 2025 Feb 7]. Available from: https://www.ncbi.nlm.nih.gov/research/coronavirus/docsum?filters=e_condition.LongCovid.

24 Willmington C, et al. The contribution of benchmarking to quality improvement in healthcare. A systematic literature review. BMC Health Serv Res. 2022;22. doi: 10.1186/s12913-022-07467-8

25 Ustun T, et al. Measuring health and disability: Manual for WHO disability assessment schedule (WHODAS 2.0). Geneva: World Health Organization; 2010.

26 Ustün TB, et al. Developing the World Health Organization disability assessment schedule 2.0. Bull World Health Organ. 2010 Nov;88(11):815–23. doi:10.2471/BLT.09.067231.

27 Hitch D, et al. Validation of the WHODAS 2.0 (36-item) in people recovering from COVID-19 infection. In: Proceedings of the National Allied Health Conference; 2023 Aug 7–9; Adelaide, Australia.

28 Mokkink L, et al. COSMIN Risk of Bias checklist for systematic reviews of patient-reported outcome measures. Qual Life Res. 2018. doi:10.1007/s11136-017-1765-4.

29 Mokkink L, et al. COSMIN methodology for systematic reviews of Patient-Reported Outcome Measures (PROMs). Amsterdam: COSMIN; 2018.

30 Noor F, et al. Exploration of understanding of integrated care from a public health perspective: A scoping review. J Public Health Res. 2023;12(3):1–21. doi: 10.1177/22799036231181210.

31 Hunter L. Person-centred practice guide to implementing person-centred practice in your health service [Internet]. Unknown; Unknown: 2016. Available from: https://silo.tips/download/person-centred-practice-guide-to-implementing-person-centred-practice-in-your-he.

32 Kirchberger I, et al. Feasibility and psychometric properties of the German 12-item WHO Disability Assessment Schedule (WHODAS 2.0) in a population-based sample of patients with myocardial infarction from the MONICA/KORA myocardial infarction registry. Popul Health Metr. 2014;12:1–23. doi:10.1186/s12963-014-0027-8.

33 van Tubergen A, et al. Assessment of disability with the World Health Organisation Disability Assessment Schedule II in patients with ankylosing spondylitis. Ann Rheum Dis. 2003;62(2):140–45. doi:10.1136/ard.62.2.140.

34 Al Sayah F, et al. Selection of patient-reported outcome measures (PROMs) for use in health systems. J Patient Rep Outcomes. 2021;5(Suppl 2):99. doi:10.1186/s41687-021-00374-2.

35 Foster A, et al. The facilitators and barriers to implementing patient-reported outcome measures in organisations delivering health-related services: A systematic review of reviews. J Patient Rep Outcomes. 2018;2. doi:10.1186/s41687-018-0072-3.

36 Siegelman JN. Reflections of a COVID-19 Long Hauler. JAMA. 2020;324(20):2031–32. doi:10.1001/jama.2020.22130.

Chapter 7

Setting Rehabilitation Goals and Shared Decision-Making in Long COVID Rehabilitation

Emma Tindill, Marlies Wanasili, Karen Dickinson, and Nicole Jackson

---

BOX 7.1   LEARNING OBJECTIVES

By the end of this chapter, readers will be able to:

- Explain the foundational theories that inform goal setting for people with chronic illness (including Long COVID).
- Develop practical strategies for collaborative goal setting tailored to individual needs and contexts.
- Recognise common challenges and supportive factors in the goal setting process.
- Understand how to track rehabilitation progress and respond appropriately if goals are not being met.

7.1 INTRODUCTION

Identifying and setting rehabilitation goals is an essential element of shared decision-making for people with any health condition, including for those experiencing Long COVID. Many people with Long COVID report feeling lost and invalidated by the healthcare system, with little hope for future improvement in their health and wellbeing. Therefore, the shared decision-making process between clinicians and patients must include goal setting to enable patients to feel heard, validated and motivated to progress with their rehabilitation journey. This collaborative process can provide patients with increased hope towards a meaningful "new normal."

DOI: 10.4324/9781003528104-9

7.2 WHAT IS REHABILITATION?

There are many definitions of the term "rehabilitation" with diverse interpretations depending on cultural context and individual experiences. Rehabilitation, as a common concept, is generally understood as treatment aimed to "restore someone to health or normal life through training and therapy…."[1] However, this definition does not reflect the experience of many people with Long COVID who report being unable to truly return to "normal life" while continuing to live with their symptoms.

As described by Karen, her definition of rehabilitation has changed since her initial diagnosis:

> *I have a different definition of rehab now, compared to what I would have when I was first diagnosed. My understanding when I was first doing Long COVID rehab was that it was to get me back to the version of me that I was before having COVID. But now, because I'm understanding the chronic nature of something like this, I understand that the old me doesn't actually exist anymore. So, it's about rehabilitating me or getting me to be the best version, or the most functional version, of myself that I can be now.*
>
> *I don't really like the word "rehabilitation" now. I feel like I'm in "active management of my condition" instead, or something like that. I know I am moving forward but that I'm not getting any better or any worse. It's like you've lost your big toe in an accident. You can learn to walk again but you're never going to get your toe back. I'm missing my toe, but I need to accept that I have to work out ways to live without it, or in this instance, accept ways to live the best I can with Long COVID."*

Karen

Similarly, Nicole states that "it depends where you define rehabilitation is going. My husband has struggled with it because he wants his wife back, but I'm not sure whether we can get there. Life is probably going to look different. I think I can continue to get a lot better than I was but without taking a rehabilitation approach, that's not going to happen."

The World Health Organization defines rehabilitation as "a set of interventions designed to optimise functioning and reduce disability in individuals with health conditions in interaction with their environment."[2] This definition reflects Karen and Nicole's experiences of rehabilitation and further emphasises that health professionals ' -aim, or goal, should not be to "fix" people with Long COVID. Rather, collaborative goal setting and shared decision-making should be prioritised by healthcare professionals to help patients adjust and accept ongoing limitations and adopt strategies to optimise their level of function and participation in daily life.

7.3 WHAT IS A GOAL?

A goal refers to something a patient wants to achieve in the context of their healthcare journey. Goals should be person-centred and address the patient's biological, psychological and social wellbeing. Addressing these core areas encourages the establishment of relevant and meaningful goals and promotes treatment adherence.[3] Reflecting on her rehabilitation journey, Nicole explains that "goal setting is critical to ensure communication between the practitioner and patient, resulting in them being on the same page and working toward the outcome the patient desires and the practitioner believes is realistic. It can also help manage expectations of timeframes and the journey towards the final outcome."

Creating goals enables healthcare professionals and patients to focus their behaviour on meaningful outcomes that positively impact quality of life.[4] Current research also demonstrates that involving patients within the goal setting process increases satisfaction with rehabilitation, as well as confidence and motivation.[4]

Despite goal setting being a core rehabilitation practice, both patients and health professionals experience difficulties in setting meaningful goals.[5] These barriers and challenges are commonly related to health professional skill set, organisational pressures and patient preparedness.[4] Difficulties with goal setting can also be influenced by a patient's lack of knowledge about their condition, and ability to understand the associated symptoms and deficits they are experiencing.[6] Nicole highlights the importance of meeting these needs during goal setting and the health professionals' role in helping people with Long COVID "understand symptoms and their potential for improvement, and the professions who possess the expertise to help them."

Another essential part of the goal setting process involves working with people with Long COVID to increase their sense of self-efficacy, self-management and self-awareness.[7] Support to increase self-efficacy through the provision of education and engaging in open dialogue regarding personal values and beliefs is essential to the development of individually relevant and important goals. In Karen's experience, the process of setting goals took "a good 12 months to shift towards meaningful goals that didn't involve trying to get back to the old me. I had to work with all my therapists to unpack what my actual values were, rather than just defaulting to the things that used to make me happy."

7.4 SHARED DECISION-MAKING

Shared decision-making combines the health professionals' expertise in the management of a condition with the patients' lived experience expertise.[8] Health professionals must engage in a process of actively listening to what the patient values and ensuring the patient feels comfortable with the agreed goals, while also challenging and discussing how realistic goals are to their personal situation. Health professionals must also be willing to try new or different treatment strategies in response to the diversity and unique experience of Long COVID between individuals.

A core component of shared decision-making is validation of the patient's concerns by the health professional. This strengthens the therapeutic relationship and ensures people feel (and are) heard, understood and most importantly, believed. Many people with Long COVID have had the experience of being told they are overly anxious or that their symptoms are not real. To build a trusting and authentic relationship, a safe space must be created to share their experiences with health professionals who truly understand that their experience is unique.

Therefore, shared decision-making must include discussions of what is important to the person with Long COVID, to enable the development of meaningful, achievable and flexible goals. This facilitates a sense of ownership and individual control over their rehabilitation.[9] The foundation of these goals is a thorough assessment to build understanding of the person as an individual. Table 7.1 summarises the skills and knowledge required by people with Long COVID and healthcare professionals to enable goal setting and shared decision-making resulting in tailored interventions. These skills are also needed to unpack the long-term goals typically identified by people with Long COVID into realistic short-term goals and to facilitate personal action plans for goal achievement.[10]

BOX 7.2   PRACTICE POINT

The person with Long COVID is the expert in their own experience of this condition. Integration of lived experience expertise with health professional expertise in assessment and intervention strategies is the hallmark of shared decision-making.

Table 7.1 Roles and Responsibilities Required for Goal Setting and Shared Decision-making

Patient	Healthcare Professionals
Understanding of health condition	Active listening skills
Understanding the expectations of rehabilitation and goal setting process	Motivational interviewing skills
Self-efficacy (including self-awareness and self-management)	Clinical skills and knowledge to provide education and appropriate referral to other professions

7.5 GOAL SETTING FRAMEWORKS

Using frameworks to guide goal setting discussions is beneficial for both people with Long COVID and health professionals, particularly when it comes to tracking and evaluating progress as discussed in this and the previous chapter. The following two frameworks provide a helpful starting point and structure for goal setting with people with Long COVID.

7.5.1 Patient Specific Functional Scale

The Patient Specific Functional Scale (PSFS) was developed by Stratford et al.[11] as a self-reporting outcome measure of function and can be freely downloaded.[12] The PSFS aims to provide health professionals with an efficient framework to guide goal setting for patients experiencing chronic conditions. Although initially designed to be used with people experiencing physical conditions, the scale is applicable to a wide range of clinical presentations, including "invisible" illnesses like Long COVID, which also impact cognitive function.

Patients are initially asked to identify up to five activities they are unable to perform or find difficult due to Long COVID. They then rate the level of functional limitation for each activity on a scale of 0–10. During follow-up assessments, patients reassess these activities using the same scale to monitor their progress over time. The PSFS can be repeated multiple times, allowing for ongoing tracking of improvements. Patients may "graduate" from goals they have completed or achieved. However, goals may also be abandoned if their priorities or functional status change, and new goals added that align with their updated needs.

Ratings are totalled and divided by number of activities to calculate the total score and measure change. However, in the authors' experience, this tool can also be used and explained to patients more simply by directly comparing activity ratings. For example, if the initial score is 3 and the review score is 6, this demonstrates improvement in their ability to complete that activity.

A limitation of many outcome measures is their requirement for goals or activities to be attributed to specific domains of daily living, which results in the patient having to fit their experiences into a predetermined framework. In the authors' experience, the PSFS avoids this problem by allowing patients to describe activities or goals in their own words in a simple table. This approach supports greater goal customisation and can encompass diverse occupational and life domains including physical, functional, social and emotional wellbeing. This simplified measure also effectively supports goal adaptation in response to the symptom and functional fluctuations commonly experienced by people with Long COVID.

Other advantages of the PSFS include its quick completion time (5–10 minutes) and applicability without specialised training. This allows the scale to serve as a valuable tool across different healthcare professions thereby supporting integrated approaches to goal-oriented therapy. However, there are some drawbacks. People with Long COVID may find it difficult to rate their goals on a numerical scale, and it is not intended to capture the impact of specific symptoms. The psychometric validity and reliability of the PSFS have not been formally established, and it should be supplemented with other condition or symptom specific outcome measures for a more comprehensive assessment.

7.5.2 Canadian Occupational Performance Measure

The Canadian Occupational Performance Measure (COPM) is a patient rated outcome measure designed to facilitate goal setting and shared decision-making for people with Long COVID and other conditions.[13] Studies of its application to rehabilitation report that COPM enables patients to focus on and build understanding about their deficits[14] and can therefore enhance self-awareness, a key factor in successful goal setting.

The COPM is based on a semi-structured interview that identifies difficulties in the domains of self-care, productivity and leisure.[15] The person with Long COVID rates their self-perceived importance, performance, and current satisfaction with performance for each issue using a scale from 1 to 10.[15] The sum of scores for performance and satisfaction are divided by the number of issues to derive a total score (see Table 7.2). A meaningful and clinically important change is defined by an increase of two points when scoring is repeated during goal reviews.[15]

Multiple studies have found that patient participation in rehabilitation is dependent on a health professional's ability to facilitate patient-centred practice.[14] An advantage of the COPM is its ability to identify and clarify the patients' needs, values and preferences, which in turn, builds therapeutic partnerships that establish meaningful and collaborative goals.[14] The COPM is also an effective tool for communication amongst multidisciplinary team members and supports an interdisciplinary approach to rehabilitation.[16] Therefore, the COPM can provide a structured, feasible, measurable and comfortable process for goal setting.[16]

Limitations of the COPM include that it can only be completed by Occupational Therapists who have formal training in its administration. The measure can be difficult to administer with people experiencing communication, psychological and or cognitive deficits, who may find its scoring process difficult to understand.[15] This is particularly true regarding the distinction between performance and satisfaction, as these concepts are both abstract and closely related.[15] Health professionals,

Table 7.2 Sample Goals and Canadian Occupational Performance Measure (COPM) Scoring

Goal	Performance (baseline)	Satisfaction (baseline)	Performance (review)	Satisfaction (review)
Standing to shower	5	4	8	6
Prepare and cook dinner	3	1	5	3
Play basketball with my child	1	1	2	2
Sum of scores	9	6	15	11
Total score / number of goals	9/3 = 3	6/3 = 2	15/3 = 5	11/3 = 4.33

therefore, need well-developed communication and active listening skills when explaining the measure to patients in practice.[14] The COPM is well suited to inpatient and community rehabilitation healthcare settings, but acute settings may find it difficult to implement due to greater time constraints and workload pressures.[15]

BOX 7.3   PRACTICE POINT

The COPM and PSFS are outcome measures that support patients to identify individual goals and evaluate their progress in rehabilitation. When considering if these measures are appropriate for your health profession and your patient's needs, clinicians should identify how they can be used to review, evaluate and modify the interventions implemented with people with Long COVID.

7.6 GOAL SETTING STRATEGIES

The following recommendations are founded on the experiences of people with Long COVID and of the authors' experiences as rehabilitation health professionals. The strategies described in this section are intended to provide guidance on potential approaches, acknowledging there are many others available in practice.

7.6.1 Mind Mapping

The first phase of goal negotiation is an opportunity for the patient and health professional to evaluate the current situation and identify problems or priorities for rehabilitation.[17] Mind maps can be useful during initial assessments to elicit activities the person with Long COVID wants and needs to do, and which are personally meaningful to them. They provide a visual representation of significant priorities, key roles, and valued tasks or activities, and can be relatively simple or more complex depending on the depth of discussion during the goal setting process. Figure 7.1 provides an example of a simple mind map.

The mind map approach serves several purposes in the goal setting and therapeutic process, including:

1   Understanding the person as an individual and their key interests and preferences
2   Identifying significant activities completed (pre-illness) in their daily routine

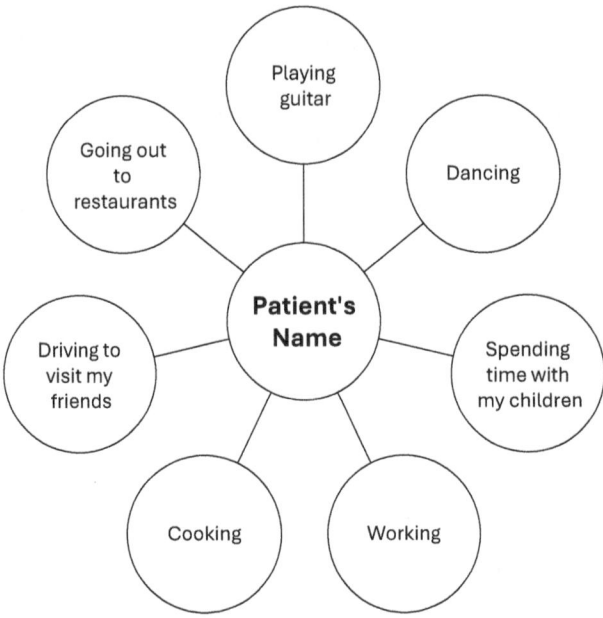

Figure 7.1 Example of a mind map generated during goal negotiation.

3 Prioritising key activities that are rehabilitation priorities
4 Understanding who currently assists the person to participate in activities
5 Breaking down goals into smaller, achievable components
6 Setting realistic timeframes for goal achievement

7.6.2 Identifying Priorities and Setting Initial Goals

A goal setting framework can be applied to support the process of prioritising rehabilitation goals by ranking and comparing roles, tasks and activities. Goals can be set for each priority, which are Specific, Measurable, Achievable, Realistic, and Time-bound (SMART). An example of an initial goal derived from the mind map above could be "I want to be able to cook again." This statement is too broad and needs more detail to become an attainable SMART goal (see Table 7.3).

BOX 7.4 PRACTICE POINT

The mind map (Fig. 7.1) is a useful tool for goal setting and understanding patients as unique individuals. The mind map can also be adapted to focus on a specific goal. For example, if cooking was a priority, consider the key tasks or steps involved that would stem from this circle to enable that goal to be achieved.

Table 7.3 Progressive Development of a Specific, Measurable, Achievable, Realistic and Time-Bound (SMART) Goal

Component	Goal Element
Specific	I want to be able to prepare my own breakfast
Measurable	I want to prepare my breakfast independently every day
Achievable	I will start by preparing breakfast independently 2 days per week
Realistic	I will start preparing breakfast independently using pacing and fatigue management strategies 2 days per week.
Time bound	I will achieve this goal within 4 weeks.

Once SMART goals are developed, expectations can be collaboratively set around when they will be reviewed; for example: "let's spend the next two sessions working on your cooking skills and then review your progress in session three." Always share the completed goal setting tool or framework with the patient to provide something to refer to and support motivation between sessions.

For goal setting to be effective, it is essential for health professionals to acknowledge that rehabilitation is not a linear journey. The uncertainty experienced by people with Long COVID can contribute to goal setting difficulties, because relatively little is known about the condition. From her lived experience, Karen emphasises that "learning to manage the condition or sitting with the discomfort of the condition and with the uncertainty about future recovery" is a skill that patients and health professionals alike must develop to make and support progress.

At times, patients may want to focus exclusively on one role or activity, particularly if their only goal relates to a deeply meaningful or high priority task. A narrow focus, however, may limit a broader rehabilitation journey. Indeed, due to the chronic and unpredictable nature of Long COVID, a variety of goals provides more opportunity to capture tangible evidence of the small improvements needed to achieve larger, long-term goals. Variety can also help people with Long COVID to shift their focus from other goals if progress is halted due to a flare up of symptoms or other barriers to recovery. Variety can be supported by identifying "fundamental goals" (e.g. priorities linked to personal values and relationships) and "specific goals" (e.g. targeted specifically to Long COVID symptoms).[18]

Karen was initially consumed by her long-term goal of returning to work and felt guilty if she used her energy for anything other than pursuing that goal. A useful tool her Occupational Therapist introduced was an activity scheduling worksheet (see Table 7.4). The worksheet emphasises the importance of varied and balanced activities, which can be supported by pacing strategies. Its visual and structured format helps patients plan the even distribution of energy across a variety of activities. The schedule also assists in minimising guilt that people may feel when prioritising activities that may be perceived as unproductive, like social or leisure.

This resource demonstrates the value of a holistic approach to health, wellbeing and goal setting across a range of activity categories to keep people with Long COVID motivated in their rehabilitation journey. Patients are not expected to complete every category every day. It is important for the therapist to advise the patient to spread out participation over the week in response to more holistic goals that can result in improvement across several symptoms or areas of function. For example, a short walk with a friend may address multiple goals at once such as increasing physical activity and socialising once a week. Additionally, this activity could fit into all four categories and clinicians could advise their patients not to schedule another activity on the same day to ensure they are pacing themselves throughout the week. The worksheet clearly illustrates the mutual and interdependent relationship between goals and interventions strategies.

Table 7.4 Activity Scheduling Worksheet Example

Day	Social activity	Leisure activity	Physical activity	Achievement activity
Monday				
Tuesday				
Wednesday				
Thursday				
Friday				
Saturday				
Sunday				

7.6.3 Tracking Progress and Maintaining Motivation

Even with diverse goals, rehabilitation progress for people with Long COVID is often impacted by fluctuations in symptom intensity and duration. These fluctuations can significantly impact both function and the patients' presentation in each session. Rehabilitation sessions can be several weeks apart and therefore the goals identified in the first session may no longer be a priority several weeks later. Changes may also occur due to personal circumstances that shift the priorities of people with Long COVID.

Managing change is where the health professional's skill in tracking progress and supporting patient motivation is crucial, and where the tools and frameworks offered in this chapter offer particular value. Health professionals should regularly check in with patients in follow-up sessions and actively listen to their perceptions of current or future barriers to goal achievement. Reflecting on and referring to initial goals helps both the patient, and the health professional understand current concerns and modify rehabilitation strategies to ensure their ongoing relevance.

Rehabilitation is a long journey that can often feel insurmountable to people with Long COVID. Nicole finds an effective way of staying motivated is to "celebrate the little wins." To do this, she emails her health professionals each time she has made progress, whether that be big or small, which helps her reflect on how far she has come and provides inspiration to keep going. This strategy is a great way for both health professionals and patients to stay motivated and connected in between sessions.

7.6.4 Abandoning a Goal

Despite everyone's best intentions, there will be times when a person's functional capacity or priorities change so much that a goal is no longer feasible. If the goal can't be modified or is simply no longer important to the patient, it is a perfectly valid choice to abandon it and focus efforts and energy elsewhere. Decisions like this are not a "failure" – they simply reflect the uncertainty of Long COVID and life in general.

A replacement goal needs to be created as soon as possible following the same initial framework or process, to support engagement in ongoing rehabilitation by both people with Long COVID and health professionals. These may take more time than the initial goal setting sessions as they also require readjustment of hopes and expectations. Both the patient and the health professional should reflect on any progress made towards the original goal and consider how this might be "translated" or redirected to the achievement of a new goal. The process of setting new goals when patients have achieved initial goals also involves returning to the chosen framework or process. It offers an opportunity to both celebrate progress and acknowledge the hard work the person with Long COVID has done to get to this new level of function. Regardless of the reason for revisiting goals, their holistic nature means several (if not all) will need to be adjusted simultaneously and sufficient time should be allocated for detailed discussion and negotiation.

7.7 CONCLUSION

Goal setting is an essential part of rehabilitation that motivates people with Long COVID to get the most out of their therapy and ensures health professionals provide rehabilitation that optimises function and is relevant to patient needs. Incorporating shared decision-making into every session ensures the provision of effective rehabilitation that more efficiently supports patients to reach their goals. To achieve the best outcomes for their patients, health professionals should actively listen, validate patient's unique experiences, apply goal setting frameworks to their practice and engage in regular reviews through the rehabilitation journey.

REFERENCES

1 Oxford Languages. Oxford English Dictionary. Oxford: Oxford University Press; [cited 2025 Feb 7]. Available from: https://languages.oup.com/google-dictionary-en/.

2 World Health Organization (WHO). Rehabilitation [Internet]. Geneva: WHO; [cited 2025 Feb 7]. Available from: https://www.who.int/news-room/fact-sheets/detail/rehabilitation.

3 Kang E, et al. Person-centered goal setting: A systematic review of intervention components and level of active engagement in rehabilitation goal-setting interventions. Arch Phys Med Rehabil. 2022;103(1):121–30.e3. doi:10.1016/j.apmr.2021.06.025.

4 Crawford L, et al. Facilitators and barriers to patient-centred goal-setting in rehabilitation: A scoping review. Clin Rehabil. 2022;36(12):1694–704. doi:10.1177/02692155221121006.

5 Littooij E, et al. Setting meaningful goals in rehabilitation: A qualitative study on the experiences of clients and clinicians in working with a practical tool. Clin Rehabil. 2022;36(3):415–28. doi:10.1177/02692155211046463.

6 Plant SE, et al. What are the barriers and facilitators to goal-setting during rehabilitation for stroke and other acquired brain injuries? A systematic review and meta-synthesis. Clin Rehabil. 2016;30(9):921–30. doi:10.1177/0269215516655856.

7 Forgea MC, et al. Barriers and facilitators to engagement in rehabilitation among stroke survivors. Rehabil Nurs. 2021;46:340–47. doi:10.1097/RNJ.0000000000000340.

8 Hole B, et al. Shared decision making: A personal view from two kidney doctors and a patient. Clin Kidney J. 2023;16(Suppl 1). doi:10.1093/ckj/sfad064.

9 Rose A, et al. Shared decision making within goal setting in rehabilitation settings: A systematic review. Patient Educ Couns. 2017;100:65–75. doi:10.1016/j.pec.2016.07.030.

10 Baker A, et al. Developing tailored theoretically informed goal-setting interventions for rehabilitation services: A co-design approach. BMC Health Serv Res. 2022;22:811. doi:10.1186/s12913-022-08047-6.

11 Stratford P. Assessing disability and change on individual patients: A report of a patient-specific measure. Physiother Can. 1995;47(4):258–63. doi:10.3138/ptc.47.4.258.

12 PhysioPedia. Patient Specific Functional Scale [Internet]. Unknown: PhysioPedia; [cited 2025 Feb 7]. Available from: https://www.physio-pedia.com/Patient_Specific_Functional_Scale.

13 Vyslysel G, et al. The Canadian Occupational Performance Measure (COPM) as routine practice in community-based rehabilitation: A retrospective chart review. Arch Rehabil Res Clin Transl. 2021;3(3):100134. doi:10.1016/j.arrct.2021.100134.

14 Larsen AE, et al. Enhancing a client-centred practice with the Canadian Occupational Performance Measure (COPM). Occup Ther Int. 2018;2018:5956301. doi:10.1155/2018/5956301.

15 Stevens M, et al. The use of patient-specific measurement instruments in the process of goal-setting: A systematic review of available instruments and their feasibility. Clin Rehabil. 2013;27(11):1005–19. doi:10.1177/0269215513490178.

16 Carswell A, et al. The Canadian Occupational Performance Measure: A research and clinical literature review. Can J Occup Ther. 2004;71(4):210–22.

17 Scobbie L, et al. Goal setting and action planning in the rehabilitation setting: Development of a theoretically informed practice framework. Clin Rehabil. 2011;25(5):468–82. doi:10.1177/0269215513490178.

18 Dekker J, et al. Setting meaningful goals in rehabilitation: Rationale and practical tool. Clin Rehabil. 2020;34(1):3–12. doi:10.1177/0269215519876299.

SECTION THREE
THE INTERDISCIPLINARY LONG COVID TEAM

Chapter 8

The Roles and Responsibilities of Medical Professionals in Long COVID

Melissa Frankcomb, Bruce James Brew, Steven Faux, Alex Holmes, Louis Irving, Tom Marwick, Bernard Shiu, David A. Watters, and Joanne Wrench

---

BOX 8.1   LEARNING OBJECTIVES

By the end of this chapter, readers should be able to:

- Identify key medical specialists involved in Long COVID care.
- Understand how different medical specialists may provide care and treatment for Long COVID symptoms.
- Understand referral indicators for medical professionals for Long COVID symptoms and impacts.

8.1 INTRODUCTION

The myriad of Long COVID symptoms is matched by the wide range of medical professionals who contribute to Long COVID diagnosis, treatment, and management. While no diagnostic test exists for Long COVID, symptoms are well described and can be elucidated with a careful history. This allows for an early diagnosis, facilitates early management, significantly reduces concerns about other causes of the person's symptoms, and improves patient outcomes. Medical professionals are crucial in holistic, person-centred approaches that incorporate and address a patient's biological, psychological, and social needs. Their contribution includes assessing and treating physical symptoms that impair function and quality of life, evaluating mental health needs, and understanding

DOI: 10.4324/9781003528104-11

the patient's broader social environment. Medical professionals also pay close attention to the overlap between these domains.

The General Practitioner (GP) is well positioned to coordinate medical care, including assessment of body system involvement and making the necessary referrals for specialist medical care. Given the common need for input from multiple medical professionals, a collaborative approach to ensure consistency of care is best practice. This requires partnerships with all members of the multidisciplinary rehabilitation team, including nursing and allied health colleagues.

Given the prevalence of Long COVID, all medical professionals will treat patients with this condition, at the very least, for a co-existing health condition. This chapter describes many of the core medical specialists involved in diagnosing and caring for people with Long COVID, including GPs, psychiatrists, perioperative surgical care, cardiologists, neurologists, respiratory physicians, and rehabilitation physicians. We acknowledge this list is not exhaustive, and other specialists with essential roles in treating Long COVID include rheumatologists, immunologists, pain specialists, and gastroenterologists. This chapter should be read with Chapter 9: The Roles and Responsibilities of Allied Health Professionals in Long COVID.

8.2 GENERAL PRACTITIONER

Bernard Shiu

For patients with long term and complicated conditions such as Long COVID, their GP must diagnose and assess symptoms that persist beyond four weeks following COVID-19 infection, including fatigue, breathlessness, or cognitive difficulties. GPs are indispensable in the initial evaluation and ongoing management of Long COVID, coordinating multidisciplinary care, and facilitating specialist referrals (e.g., to cardiologists, respiratory physicians, neurologists, rehabilitation physicians) when necessary. With a comprehensive understanding of a patient's medical history, GPs offer a broader perspective on their long-term care needs.

When symptoms worsen or new concerns emerge, GPs are well-positioned to assess the need for further investigations or adjust the treatment plan accordingly. Their role extends to addressing mental health concerns associated with Long COVID, working collaboratively with psychologists and psychiatrists. Additionally, GPs manage ongoing medication regimens, monitor for side effects, and prevent potential drug interactions by working closely with local pharmacists.

GPs determine when it is appropriate to coordinate chronic disease care, incorporating allied health professionals such as physiotherapists, exercise physiologists, dietitians, and occupational therapists as needed. They also assist patients in accessing disability or insurance support for those with severe, ongoing disabilities due to Long COVID. GPs also help patients manage their Long COVID's social, domestic, and work-related consequences by providing safe and timely guidance around returning to day-to-day activities and work.

In essence, GPs are central to delivering comprehensive and continuous care for long-term COVID patients, ensuring their physical, mental, social, and overall wellbeing is effectively managed.

8.3 RESPIRATORY PHYSICIAN

Louis Irving

Following acute COVID-19 infection, people can have persisting or new respiratory symptoms. Their GP can manage some of these patients, but others can benefit from assessment and management by a respiratory physician.

8.3.1 Post-Acute Lung Injury

Survivors of life-threatening COVID-19 pneumonitis, who have usually required invasive or non-invasive ventilation, are left with diffuse, usually non-progressive pulmonary fibrosis. This typically lessens over many months but may not fully resolve, resulting in reduced lung function and exercise capacity. Management is similar to other forms of chronic lung disease, with an emphasis on cardiopulmonary rehabilitation and prevention of further lung damage. Regular vaccinations to prevent respiratory viruses and early treatment of bacterial lung infections are essential. Some people may require domiciliary supplemental oxygen, particularly in the early recovery period. Organising pneumonia can also follow acute COVID-19 infection. It is usually steroid-responsive but may require prolonged treatment. Respiratory Physicians can assist with weaning steroids or, if necessary, implementing a steroid-sparing agent.

8.3.2 Exacerbation of Pre-existing Lung Disease

As with other respiratory viruses, COVID-19 can exacerbate or worsen underlying asthma, chronic obstructive pulmonary disease, and interstitial lung disease. Diagnosis of exacerbations is usually apparent, and management is the same as for other exacerbations of these conditions. The patient often has a predetermined "action plan" to implement at the first indication of an exacerbation. Ensuring that full recovery occurs after these exacerbations is critical to preserving lung function in people whose respiratory reserve is often already markedly reduced. Tests of lung function such as spirometry, diffusing capacity, and a six-minute walk test are essential for these patients to monitor treatment responses and determine whether they have regained their pre-infection lung function.

8.3.3 Unexplained Dyspnoea and Reduced Exercise Capacity

After relatively mild acute COVID-19, some people develop marked exertional breathlessness and exercise intolerance. This may or may not be associated with fatigue. Physical examination of the respiratory system, static respiratory function tests, and imaging (high-resolution computed tomography and computed tomography pulmonary angiography) are essential because airflow obstruction, diffuse interstitial lung disease, and pulmonary thrombo-emboli are all possible causes of the dyspnoea. Post-COVID cardiac causes of dyspnoea, such as Postural Orthostatic Tachycardia Syndrome (POTS), cardiomyopathy, and arrhythmias, may also need to be considered. An inflammatory myositis affecting peripheral or respiratory muscles causing dyspnoea is possible if creatine kinase, erythrocyte sedimentation rate, C-reactive protein, and autoantibodies are elevated.

If the above causes are not diagnosed, an incremental cardiopulmonary exercise test (CPET) might be considered. This measures maximum exercise capacity (VO^2max) and can detect abnormalities occurring during exercise that are not present at rest. The CPET can also assist in prescribing a safe and effective exercise rehabilitation programme.

8.4 REHABILITATION PHYSICIAN

Steven Faux

Rehabilitation physicians or consultants in rehabilitation medicine have specialist training to assist in the rehabilitation, management, and treatment of people of all ages living with disability. People may be born with these disabilities or activity limitations, or they may acquire them through injury or illnesses such as Long COVID. There are specialist paediatric rehabilitation physicians for people under 16 years, while either paediatric or adult rehabilitation physicians can see those 16–18 years of age as they transition to adult services.

Their role in multidisciplinary rehabilitation teams is to provide medical input, manage or coordinate the management of any medical illness that occurs, and support the team in developing a rehabilitation plan, setting goals, and promoting leadership. In many hospital-based and community teams, rehabilitation physicians act as lead clinicians. They are designated as responsible for providing documentation and certification of rehabilitation episodes of care and their outcomes to insurers, hospitals, and funders.

GPs, allied health professionals, and other specialists often refer complex patients with multiple and various symptoms whose progress does not respond to standard exercise, psychology, or medical treatments. For complex Long COVID patients, rehabilitation physicians work with a team of allied health professionals, nurses, and other medical specialists to design rehabilitation and treatment plans, execute them, and modify them as required. They use medicines, contribute to physical and functional interventions and advise workplaces and insurers of the outcomes of multidisciplinary treatment. In some cases, rehabilitation physicians recommend surgical management or refer patients for further specialist input, such as respiratory medicine or neurology. They will occasionally order complex tests, such as Magnetic Resonance Imaging (MRI), Computed Tomography (CT) scans, or nuclear scans, to clarify diagnoses and monitor treatments provided by the multidisciplinary team. They will also review reports of goal achievement from the interdisciplinary team through a formal and regular case conference protocol. This process ensures that patients progress as expected or needs a medical review for unstable co-morbid illnesses, a failure in medical treatments, or the development of medication side effects. Their qualification and training emphasise the importance of utilising evidence-based treatments and developing goal driven clinical outcomes.

Rehabilitation physicians assess patients with Long COVID to appropriately provide access to established rehabilitation medicine departments in public and private hospitals and outpatient or community-based rehabilitation teams. Patients can be treated immediately, during an acute hospital admission or later from the community as either an inpatient or an outpatient (community patient). Their assessment focuses on criteria for access to multidisciplinary rehabilitation, the likelihood of achieving improved clinical outcomes, and the development of an interdisciplinary rehabilitation plan.

8.5 PSYCHIATRY

Alex Holmes

A psychiatrist is one of a range of mental health professionals available to provide expert assessment and support to patients with Long COVID. A psychiatrist is a doctor who specialises in the assessment and management of mental disorders, including in patients with persistent physical symptoms. A psychiatrist will provide a diagnosis and formulation to understand current symptoms in their psychosocial context. Psychiatric treatment should be integrated with other elements of care.

Seeing a psychiatrist requires a referral from a medical doctor, usually the patient's GP. A referral may be appropriate when the person has a mental disorder, and first-line pharmacotherapy and/or psychotherapy through primary care has not been adequate or effective, or when psychological symptoms are predominant and severe. Referral to a consultation-liaison psychiatrist who specialises in mental health issues concurrent with physical illness may be appropriate when psychological factors are thought to be playing a significant role in the experience or expression of physical symptoms or when questions arise regarding the relevance of pre-morbid psychological vulnerabilities.

A psychiatrist's medical knowledge provides a basis for exploring the complex relationship between physical health and psychological wellbeing. They are also well placed to judge whether physical symptoms can be clearly attributed to physical illness or, conversely, are less in keeping with our current understanding of pathophysiology. This includes assessing patients with medically unexplained symptoms (MUSs), sometimes designated as "functional." Symptoms common in Long COVID, including fatigue, pain, and difficulty thinking, are commonly construed as medically unexplained, and the psychiatrist is asked if these symptoms are "psychological." Many symptoms are multifactorial and are best not thought of as solely physical or mental. A predominant psychological cause for MUS is only considered when there is a component of severe depression or anxiety disorder, in the bodily expression of past trauma, and when the persistence of physical symptoms postpones dealing with pre-existing life challenges (abnormal illness behaviour).

A psychiatrist will make management recommendations based on their diagnosis and formulation. Treatment may include medication individual or group psychotherapy. Suggestions may be made concerning family, occupational, or social stressors. The consultation may be a single assessment, or the psychiatrists may look to develop an ongoing therapeutic relationship. When working with a patient with Long COVID, they will build a shared understanding of the current symptoms and their consequences, provide hope and validation, and promote adaptation and acceptance.

8.6 CARDIOLOGY

Tom Marwick

Many of the most common symptoms associated with Long COVID are nonspecific and potentially cardiovascular in origin.[1] Cardiovascular involvement – including acute events such as myocardial infarction, stroke, myocarditis, and myocardial scarring – may be essential complications of severe acute COVID-19.[2] Acute COVID-19 requiring ventilation is associated with right ventricular dysfunction, an independent predictor of adverse outcome. While known to have lingering effects, these acute changes are not commonly associated with Long COVID symptoms. However, the pre-existing disease and risk that may lead to acute events remain present in patients after acute recovery.

Exercise intolerance, fatigue, shortness of breath, palpitations, racing heart, and chest discomfort are common symptoms of Long COVID. These may be symptoms coinciding with a cardiac diagnosis in addition to Long COVID and need to be evaluated on their own merits. A full cardiovascular history, including the exact nature of chest pain, shortness of breath, and other cardiovascular symptoms, should be gathered to exclude cardiovascular disease and heart failure.

Physical examination should include a cardiovascular examination, paying particular attention to resting and postural changes in blood pressure and heart rate, as POTS is under-recognised in this population (see Chapter 16). A six-minute walk test may be a good adjunct to outpatient evaluation if the practice environment allows, taking into account individual Post-Exertional Malaise. To assess quality of life, an exercise questionnaire such as the Duke Activity Status Index provides an objective picture of functional capacity.[3] See Chapter 11 for further information about assessments of function, participation, and quality of life.

8.6.1 Investigations

A symptom-driven investigation approach, rather than an investigation template, is recommended. A 12-lead Electrocardiogram (ECG) provides information about inappropriate resting tachycardia and the presence of Q-waves if there has been a COVID-related coronary event. If there is suspicion of cardiovascular involvement, an echocardiogram (echo) is the most appropriate test. This can identify impaired ejection fraction, resting wall motion abnormalities, pulmonary vascular disease, and pericardial effusion, to name a few. If the echo shows impaired function and a diagnosis of myocarditis is sought, a cardiac magnetic resonance test may be needed. A Holter monitor may help assess cardiac rhythm irregularities or electrical conduction disease. In patients with exercise intolerance and chest pain, functional testing or CT coronary angiogram may be considered to exclude coronary disease.

8.6.2 Management and Outcomes

Cardiology referral should be guided by underlying disease risk, symptom severity, clinical evaluation findings, and simple tests such as troponin, ECG, and B-type natriuretic peptide. Often, symptoms are found not to be cardiovascular in origin following evaluation. In our experience, approximately 15% of people with Long COVID have abnormal cardiac function. Many of these patients have never been assessed before, and pre-existing pathology, such as unrecognised heart failure, may be the underlying cause of some issues. Often, no pathological cardiac explanation for reduced functional capacity is experienced by Long COVID patients. Therefore, referral to a cardiologist most commonly confirms no underlying cardiac damage, which may be reassuring for some patients. However, if persistent sinus tachycardia is identified, the initial step is the prescription of low-dose beta blockers – titrating to blood pressure and keeping the resting heart rate at an acceptable level for that patient. Treating cardiovascular risk factors is essential in recovering COVID-19 patients because of the association between COVID-19 and cardiometabolic disease and the long "tail" of atherothrombotic events.

8.7 NEUROLOGY

Bruce Brew

Long COVID is very often accompanied by cognitive symptoms, which are frequently referred to as brain fog.[4] This should be distinguished from cognitive symptoms from other causes, especially for people who have severe COVID-19 infection requiring hospital admission (e.g., respiratory failure with hypoxic brain damage, post-Intensive Care Unit syndrome or stroke). Brain fog presents as poor concentration, forgetfulness, and slowed information processing. Significant migraine-like headaches may also accompany it. Despite these impairments being comparatively mild, they often compromise the ability to work and participate in daily life.[5] Most patients slowly improve over months to approximately 2 years. It is unclear how many patients fail to return to their baseline cognitive performance, but anecdotally, it is the considerable minority.

The pathogenesis of Long COVID is only partially understood mainly because studies have considered Long COVID, especially brain fog, to be a stable disease entity. However, clinical observations and emerging data indicate it is a time-dependent, dynamic process with a differing biomarker profile.[5–7] It is unclear whether the same processes drive acute infection and Long COVID.

Nonetheless, the following hypotheses relating to brain fog have been proposed: autoimmunity, residual infection, reactivation of latent herpes virus infection, microthrombi, disturbed gut microbiome, metabolic disturbance, and disturbed resolution biology involving the kynurenine pathway (KP).[8,9] This author favours the latter as it is the only mechanism correlated prospectively with objective cognitive deficits and can underpin the other potential mechanisms. Low level "sanctuary" site infection or viral fragments (not necessarily in the brain) activate the KP both systemically and in the brain, leading to (i) immune tolerance with reactivation of latent herpes infections, autoimmunity, disturbed gut microbiome, a prothrombotic diathesis, as well as (ii) neurotoxicity especially by *N*-methyl-D-aspartate (NMDA)-mediated excitotoxicity and blood–brain barrier impairment.[9] Each of these steps is potentially tractable to intervention.

Patient management should encompass two phases. First, other Long COVID–associated conditions should be comprehensively assessed, including any relationships between brain fog and systemic fatigue, poor sleep, mood disturbance, or recurrent migraine-like headaches. These can be addressed by careful history taking, but often, these are contributing factors in addition to direct brain fog concerns. There is anecdotal evidence for some improvement in fatigue with low dose naltrexone, sleep with orexin antagonists, mood disturbance with selective serotonin reuptake inhibitors, and migraine with Calcitonin Gene-Related Peptide blockers.[10] Second, if brain fog is assessed as not significantly related to any of the above, the approach is primarily cognitive pacing, similar to systemic pacing. Again, anecdotal evidence suggests some may benefit from off-label use of amantadine (as an NMDA antagonist) or selective serotonin reuptake inhibitors independent of mood disturbance (raising serotonin levels).[11]

Currently, management is hampered by the lack of biomarkers, especially concerning the varying pathophysiological changes underpinning the timing from acute infection. Emerging data suggest that the KP should be assessed using the kynurenine/tryptophan ratio[5,9] and MRI brain scans using Diffusion Tensor Imaging and k-trans for blood–brain barrier impairment.[6,12]

BOX 8.2   MELISSA'S LIVED EXPERIENCE OF NEUROLOGICAL SYMPTOMS

I am only 41, but the suffering caused from recurrent, debilitating migraines caused me to question how I could potentially live another 40 years. I wasn't suicidal, I was just looking realistically at the significant negative impact this illness was having on my life and those around me who I love. The suffering was so immense, it was impossible to see a future.

Melissa

8.8 PERIOPERATIVE CARE

David A. Watters

Patients should avoid surgery within at least 7 weeks of an acute COVID-19 infection as there is an increased risk of mortality, pulmonary complications, venous thromboembolism, and unplanned readmissions. People with Long COVID may have an increased risk of perioperative complications depending on the degree of deconditioning and/or impairment of body systems.

8.8.1 Perioperative

As Long COVID is a condition that requires multidisciplinary care, usually coordinated through and delivered by GP providers, it is ideal if people with Long COVID requiring planned surgery are identified on the referral so they can undergo multisystem assessment.[13] Patients contemplating or undergoing surgical procedures do so in the expectation of improved health and function. Long COVID has the potential to impact a variety of postoperative outcomes. However, the risk and nature of any harm will ultimately relate to the body system(s) affected.

All surgical patients should be screened for Long COVID, which requires careful history taking without a diagnostic test. Recognising that, when present, Long COVID can affect the cardiovascular, respiratory, renal, neurological, metabolic, and digestive systems, consideration should be given towards offering targeted prehabilitation (exercise, nutrition, and psychological support) and optimisation of any comorbidities. Given the impact of Long COVID on participation in daily life, these patients are more likely to experience deconditioning, impaired cardiopulmonary reserve, compromised kidney function, or be at risk of postoperative cognitive dysfunction. Preoperative assessment should aim to identify any co-existing system impairments to inform shared decision-making regarding the benefits and potential harm of undergoing surgery. As many Long COVID patients improve over time, there may be an opportunity to delay or defer planned (elective), non-urgent surgical procedures until there is improvement. Valid, proven, and non-surgical options should also be offered before the decision to undergo surgery.[14]

8.8.2 During Surgery

On the day of the procedure, surgery and anaesthesia are likely to continue as normal, with the exception that the co-existence of Long COVID may increase the need for close postoperative monitoring, including high dependency or critical care. The choice of the actual procedure to be performed and whether to perform or protect a gastrointestinal anastomosis may also warrant consideration.

8.8.3 After Surgery

Post COVID-19 pathology also may cause ongoing inflammation and endothelial dysfunction and, therefore, has the potential to increase the risk of venous thromboembolism. There is currently no evidence to support raising the dose of thromboprophylaxis in perioperative patients with Long COVID. Still, consideration should be given to offering extended prophylaxis post discharge, particularly in cancer patients undergoing major resections. Extended prophylaxis is already the standard of care for lower limb arthroplasties. However, given the potential multisystem impacts of the condition, it is also prudent, whenever appropriate, to promote day of surgery chest physiotherapy, resumption of oral nutrition, early mobility, and minimisation of mobility restrictions due to drains, catheters, and other lines.

Around 10–15% of Long COVID patients experience chronic pain. In perioperative care, it is vital to reduce the stress response to relieve acute pain while also avoid the long-term use of addictive analgesics, particularly opiates. The risk of chronic postoperative pain syndromes should be considered, particularly where the patient is already a regular opiate user for pre-existing pain associated with Long COVID or any other condition.

BOX 8.3 PRACTICE POINT: INCLUSIVE AND EFFECTIVE MEDICAL CARE FOR PEOPLE WITH LONG COVID

Based on her lived experience of Long COVID medical care, consider the following tips from Melissa. How might you address these in your clinical practice?

- **Allow adequate time/book double appointments:** "Due to my complex health needs, appointments took a lot of time. I understood how stretched GPs are, and often felt I needed to apologise for taking their time."

- **Patient-centred interventions:** "We are desperate for help and relief from our symptoms, a helpful question could be 'what is impacting you the most? What is causing you the most pain/suffering/anxiety?' and address what paths could be taken to alleviate that issue."

- **Acknowledgement and validation:** "Some patients are hearing from their practitioners' 'I don't believe in Long COVID' or given psychosomatic diagnoses. This can lead to a loss of trust in their health professionals and disillusionment with health care. The first time someone said to me 'I hear you. What you are experiencing is real. You are doing it tough. You can get better. This is how I can help' I cried. No-one had really heard me prior to that, and I questioned whether I was lazy, or making it up."

- **Provide hope:** "When dealing with a life-altering illness that had so many medical unknowns, hope became the lifeline that I clung to. Without it, there was no viable future to look forward to. Hope of a better future, no matter how altered it may be from my past life, was essential to keeping a positive mindset to keep progressing towards a better quality of life."

- **Recognise grief and loss:** "I experienced grief and loss of identity, self-esteem, self-worth and confidence. When I was stripped back from the things I do (my work, hobbies), I had to re-imagine myself away from my illness. Being treated kindly and respectfully as a whole person, keeping in mind who I was prior to my illness, helped me to not be defined by my health, and allowed me to create a new narrative and future – however that looked."

- **Promote inclusion:** "I live rurally and access to medical specialists was a challenge. Telehealth access to medical specialists and allied health shifted me towards rehabilitation and recovery. It is important to consider potential barriers for each individual patient; including people who live remotely, have financial or language barriers, past and current disability, and accessibility issues."

8.9 CONCLUSION

This chapter has provided an overview of various medical specialists' roles in caring for a person with Long COVID. It includes information on possible interventions and when to seek further specialist medical involvement. Primary care services (particularly GPs) are often seen as the "coordinator" of medical care for Long COVID and play the key role of enabling specialist referral where needed. The complex and life altering nature of Long COVID, combined with the diversity of symptoms and emerging evidence base for treatments, means that medical care should be provided in partnership with the multidisciplinary team, the person living with Long COVID and their close others.

REFERENCES

1 World Health Organisation. A clinical case definition of post COVID-19 condition by Delphi consensus, 2021 Oct 6.

2 Chung MK, et al. COVID-19 and cardiovascular disease: From Bench to Bedside. Circ Res. 2021;128(8):1214–36. doi:10.1161/CIRCRESAHA.121.317997.

3 Hlatky MA et al. A brief self-administered questionnaire to determine functional capacity (the Duke Activity Status Index). Am J Cardiol. 1989;64(10):651–54. doi:10.1016/0002-9149 (89)90496-7.

4 Lewthwaite H et al. Treatable traits for long COVID. Respirology. 2023;28(11):1005–22. doi:10.1111/resp.14596.

5 Cysique LA et al. The kynurenine pathway relates to post-acute COVID-19 objective cognitive impairment and PASC. Ann Clin Transl Neurol. 2023;10(8):1338–52. doi:10.1002/acn3.51825.

6 Chaganti et al. Blood brain barrier disruption and glutamatergic excitotoxicity in post-acute sequelae of SARS COV-2 infection cognitive impairment: potential biomarkers and a window into pathogenesis. Front Neurol. 2024;15:1350848. doi:10.3389/fneur.2024.1350848.

7 Phetsouphanh C, et al. Improvement of immune dysregulation in individuals with long COVID at 24-months following SARS-CoV-2 infection. Nat Commun. 2024;15(1):3315. doi:10.1038/s41467-024-47720-8.

8 Monje M et al. The neurobiology of long COVID. Neuron. 2022;110(21):3484–96. doi:10.1016/j.neuron.2022.10.006.

9 Dehhaghi M et al. The roles of the kynurenine pathway in COVID-19 neuropathogenesis. Infection. 2024;52(5):2043–59. doi:10.1007/s15010-024-02293-y.

10 Ozkan E et al. Is persistent post-COVID headache associated with protein-protein interactions between antibodies against viral spike protein and CGRP receptor?: A case report. Front Pain Res. 2022;3:858709. doi:10.3389/fpain.2022.858709.

11 Wong AC et al. Serotonin reduction in post-acute sequelae of viral infection. Cell. 2023;186(22):4851–67.e20. doi:10.1016/j.cell.2023.09.013.

12 Greene C et al. Blood-brain barrier disruption and sustained systemic inflammation in individuals with long COVID-associated cognitive impairment. Nat Neurosci. 2024;27(3):421–32. doi:10.1038/s41593-024-01576-9.

13 Watters DA et al. Long COVID in Victoria. Med J Aust. 2024;221(Suppl 9):s3–s4. doi:10.5694/mja2.52467.

14 Watters DA et al. If the perioperative patient pathway was right, what would it look like? ANZ J Surg. 2024;94(9):1462–70. doi:10.1111/ans.19179.

Chapter 9

The Roles and Responsibilities of Allied Health Professionals in Long COVID

Emily Alexander, Joanne Wrench, Raeya Bognar, Sarah Booth, Kerrie Clarke, Fy Dunford, Danielle Hitch, Victoria Lai, Jennifer Mepham, Chantal C. Mitvalsky, Leigh Seidel-Marks, and Charissa J. Zaga

---

BOX 9.1   LEARNING OUTCOMES

By the end of this chapter, readers should be able to:

- Identify the role of various allied health professionals involved in the care of Long COVID patients.
- Understand how each allied health discipline can address the diverse symptoms that people with Long COVID experience.
- Understand referral indicators for each health profession to maximise access to expert guidance and support for people with Long COVID.

9.1 INTRODUCTION

There is no universal definition for which health professions come under the umbrella term of "allied health," with variability across countries and jurisdictions. For the purposes of this book, we define allied health as a collective term for university educated health professionals that are not medical, dental, or nursing.[1] Each allied health profession has individual specialised knowledge, scope of practice, philosophical basis, and practice culture.[2] Central to all allied health is the ability to practice autonomously and a strong commitment to evidence-based practice.

Allied health professionals have expertise in the prevention, diagnosis, and treatment of a range of health conditions, working across the continuum of care

DOI: 10.4324/9781003528104-12

with care centred around collaboratively generated patient goals. These clinicians have a long-standing central role in rehabilitation where they support recovery, adaptation, and return to participation in daily life, including for people living with invisible conditions like Long COVID.

The following professions covered in this chapter are included under the allied health umbrella: physiotherapy, exercise physiology, occupational therapy, social work, clinical psychology and clinical neuropsychology, dietetics, and speech pathology. The disciplines described in this chapter provide evidence-based therapy individualised to address the most common symptoms and needs of people living with Long COVID. We acknowledge that there are a range of other allied health professionals who may benefit people with Long COVID, including creative and leisure therapists, pharmacy, allied health assistants, and cultural workers. This chapter should be read in conjunction with *Chapter 8: The Roles and Responsibilities of Medical Professionals in Long COVID*.

9.1.1 Interdisciplinary Care

The medical system can be difficult to navigate with some people referred from specialist to specialist with little cohesion or collaboration of care. While this chapter focuses on each allied health discipline separately, health professionals often collaborate closely with each other and medical specialists. Collaborative interdisciplinary care is critical to reduce duplication and streamline assessments and treatment. There is also scope of practice overlap between some allied health disciplines. For example, occupational therapists, speech pathologists, and clinical neuropsychologists can provide cognitive rehabilitation strategies. Likewise, several disciplines may collaborate to enable a particular patient goal. For example, if the goal is to return to work, an exercise physiologist or physiotherapist may provide support around pacing and fatigue management, an occupational therapist could work with employers around job and workplace modifications, social workers may enable access to financial support during the graded return to work, and both clinical neuropsychology and occupational therapy may support cognitive assessment and strategies. Collaboration and agreement on who is providing what element of the rehabilitation plan (and in what order of priority) is essential to ensure patients receive targeted, meaningful, and streamlined care. Minimising therapy overlap and ensuring patients are not overburdened by numerous appointments is crucial and can be supported by allied health therapists working to their full scope of practice.

BOX 9.2 EMILY'S STORY

It was weeks to months after my acute illness and quarantine stay. I had time off work to recover. I felt lost during this time. I made a conscious effort to recover but was plagued by fatigue. I felt so frustrated. Pre-illness I had never experienced lack of energy or mental health issues. I just felt different despite how much I rested. The brain fog crept up on me. For someone who had traditionally been cognitively crisp I was forgetful. I thought getting back into some routine might help, so I decided to do some hours back at work. It was clear that this was not just the normal recovery from a cold or illness.

At work everything felt like a blur. The stimulation was overwhelming. Even reading an email was an effort. I'd read the same sentences repeatedly. My mind was a foggy mess that I couldn't find clarity in. Let alone the anxiety that hung over me. I expected to feel a bit uneasy starting back at work, but this was consuming. I tried to self soothe but it was difficult.

Even after a short shift I would return home fatigued. This was not the normal fatigue you might feel after a workout or a late night. This was different. The fatigue was bone aching and all consuming. It felt like I was attached to a weight that I couldn't free myself from. My mind was not feeling sleepy but exhausted. I would get home from work and need to lie down, at times for hours. You're physically exhausted lying there but not drowsy to sleep, which leaves your mind circling with anxiety as you lie there giving in to your body.

I had been told of the Long COVID clinic at the hospital that I'd worked at, but since leaving hotel quarantine the communication had ceased. I knew I needed to get answers and that meant getting referred to the clinic.

I had several investigations over the following months including appointments with neuropsychology, psychiatry, and respiratory. I completed walk tests and exertional exercise testing and a sleep lab stay.

The neuropsychology testing came back with no focal brain damage and "this will just take time." The sleep lab test also suggested the same. The exertional testing confirmed I had no abnormalities but acknowledged my elevated heart rate. I had ongoing reviews with psychiatry and respiratory consultants to monitor. What I really wanted were answers but unfortunately, there were none. An exercise physiologist was initially helpful in structuring an exercise programme and monitoring my heart rate and fatigue. Balancing fatigue and exercise is still a battle I face three years later.

It got to the point where I felt I couldn't catch a break. I was consumed by my symptoms and felt a shell of what I used to be. I struggled with insomnia and the more I focused on the lack of sleep, the more anxious I became. Dreams were different since COVID they became so vivid and lifelike. Energy conservation and fatigue management have been the major focus of my recovery. If I prioritised work, I'd forfeit a social activity or exercise.

I started seeing a psychologist who specialised in fatigue syndromes. She made me feel supported, understood, and normalised the feelings/ symptoms. Long COVID, like so many other fatigue syndromes are invisible. What you experience internally does not match with what others see. For my work colleagues I appeared my normal self but this was not the case. The long journey of this disease and return to full time work was difficult as my symptoms continued to impact my work. This was difficult as someone who pre-illness was a high achiever. It's also hard to explain the fatigue to others when the response was often "yes well I'm tired too."

On reflection, and being a frontline allied health worker myself, I appreciate that early referrals to specific clinicians provide knowledge, advice and comfort to those going through this journey. I personally would not be where I am today without the support of my psychologist and believe more awareness of Long COVID, the array of symptoms and targeted management plans formulated by allied health professionals is imperative for best patient care.

Emily

BOX 9.2   PRACTICE POINT

What allied health professionals did Emily receive care from and could she have been referred to others for more comprehensive care? Consider your assessments of people with Long COVID – how do you identify which allied health professionals need to be involved?

9.2 CLINICAL NEUROPSYCHOLOGY

Joanne Wrench

Clinical neuropsychology is a sub-specialty of psychology that assesses, diagnoses, and treats people with the cognitive, behavioural, and psychological impacts of brain disorders. This includes detailed assessment of a range of cognitive (thinking) processes such as memory, attention and concentration, language, perception, and problem solving. Clinical neuropsychologists take a wholistic perspective of cognitive and behavioural functioning, including neurological, personal, situational, and affective contributors. Cognitive functioning can be negatively impacted and exacerbated by a range of other medical and psychological processes that are common in Long COVID, for example, psychological distress and trauma, sleep disorders, and fatigue. Clinical neuropsychologists may assist in understanding the complex (and often bi-directional) interplay between these factors.

Cognitive difficulties, including brain fog, are some of the most commonly reported symptoms of Long COVID and clinical neuropsychologists are key members of multidisciplinary Long COVID clinics.[3] The term brain fog does not describe a discrete cognitive process or complaint and may refer to many different cognitive difficulties, including, but not limited to executive dysfunction, slowed processing, attentional difficulties, or memory lapses. Clinical neuropsychologists can assist with "unpacking" diverse cognitive difficulties, informing neurocognitive diagnosis where relevant, as well as supporting targeted treatment recommendations.[4]

While brief cognitive screening measures may be useful in many settings, they tend to under report less severe cognitive changes, and none have been designed for specific use in Long COVID. Neuropsychological assessment can provide a more in depth understanding of subtle cognitive changes as they relate to premorbid estimates for an individual. This, in turn, is more likely to accurately reflect the significant impact these difficulties can have on function and quality of life.

Clinical neuropsychologists are not only "assessors" of cognition; they are well placed to provide a range of cognitive, psychological, and behavioural interventions for people experiencing Long COVID to reduce the impact of cognitive changes and improve outcomes. This includes cognitive retraining, compensatory approaches using behavioural and environmental modifications, and holistic approaches addressing emotional and other noncognitive aspects of functioning. They also work closely with other allied health professionals (in particular, occupational therapy and speech pathology) to deliver cognitive rehabilitation strategies and may support rehabilitation teams with recommendations and strategies to enhance rehabilitation participation and utility.

9.2.1 When to Refer to Clinical Neuropsychology

Consider referral to a clinical neuropsychologist for assessment and management when a person with Long COVID complains of cognitive changes that are impacting daily life, even if brief cognitive screening does not identify impairment. Clinical neuropsychologists can also support with diagnostic clarification, for example, if Long COVID is a differential diagnosis or ruling out other causes of cognitive change.

9.3 CLINICAL PSYCHOLOGY

Kerrie Clarke

Clinical psychologists assess, diagnose, and treat mental health conditions such as anxiety, depression, and post-traumatic stress disorder (PTSD). A clinical psychologist can assess the causes of psychological distress within the context of the person's history and current circumstances. Based on this understanding, they provide treatment to help manage mental health conditions and psychological distress. It is well known that the challenges of living with Long COVID can lead to or exacerbate mental health symptoms including depression, anxiety, and PTSD.[5] Clinical psychologists can play a key role in helping people with Long COVID build on the range of psychological strategies they are already using to cope with the impact of their symptoms.

Clinical psychologists generally provide psychological intervention via individual therapy. At this stage, specific psychological therapies for Long COVID are not yet established.[6] However, clinical psychologists are well placed to offer a variety of psychological interventions to support people with Long COVID manage the mental health impacts of the illness (see Chapter 14). Well-known therapies such as Cognitive Behavioural Therapy (CBT) can help people to manage anxiety, depression, and emotional struggles related to the uncertainty of Long COVID. Other types of psychological therapies include Mindfulness-Based Therapies to manage physical symptoms and to build acceptance and tolerance of these symptoms; Acceptance and Commitment Therapy to build psychological flexibility and help people take meaningful action; and Compassion-Based Therapies to support people to understand and accept feelings of personal suffering through developing kindness towards oneself. It should be noted that CBT and other therapies are not a treatment for Long COVID itself but may offer strategies to help cope with the emotional difficulties that often accompany Long COVID.

Clinical psychologists work closely with other allied health and medical professionals and may offer psychological interventions that support the person with Long COVID to cope with any mental health barriers that may impact their participation in rehabilitation. Clinical psychologists can also facilitate group therapy programmes, including educational sessions about living with Long COVID, enhancing coping strategies, and understanding psychological responses to Long COVID. Therapy can be offered via telehealth or in person.

9.3.1 When to Refer to Clinical Psychology

Consider referral to a clinical psychologist for assessment and management when a person with Long COVID reports distressing psychological symptoms such as trauma, anxiety and/or depression, or exacerbation of previous mental health conditions. Useful mental health screening measures include the Patient Health Questionnaire-9[7] and the Generalised Anxiety Disorder-7.[8] Referral is also appropriate for psychological support to explore or make sense of the experience of Long COVID.

9.4 DIETETICS

Leigh Seidel-Marks

Dietitians are experts in the science of food and nutrition and the impact our diet has on health and wellbeing. Dietitians provide nutrition, biochemical, clinical, and dietary assessment and advice to optimise food intake for symptom management of Long COVID (see Chapter 15), including balancing advice for pre-existing conditions with personal situations such as budget and time constraints. The goal of nutrition intervention for Long COVID is to support symptom management, identification, and correction of nutrient deficiencies and promote an individualised nutritionally adequate intake suitable for the person to meet their nutritional requirements. Advice for those living with Long COVID varies in response to their clinical presentation, individual lifestyle, and personal identity circumstances.

Dietitians commonly collaborate with speech pathologists, occupational therapists, and clinical neuropsychologists to support people living with olfactory impairment, fatigue, and brain fog. Dietitians also work with Exercise Physiologists to support those with a Postural Orthostatic Tachycardia Syndrome (POTS) diagnosis incorporate diet modification, such as a sodium and fluid prescription,[9] or commonly associated gastrointestinal symptoms or food sensitivities.[10] Assessment and correction of malnutrition is another key focus for dietitians when working with people living with persistent symptoms following illness with COVID-19.[11]

9.4.1 When to Refer to Dietetics

Consider referral to a dietitian for assessment and management when a person with Long COVID reports irregular or missed meals (possibly due to ongoing fatigue), changes in their weight, or reduced enjoyment of food. Those newly diagnosed with POTS, reporting gastrointestinal problems or avoiding multiple foods without medical investigation or professional support can also benefit from dietetic input.

9.5 EXERCISE PHYSIOLOGY

Raeya Bognar

Exercise physiology is a specialised healthcare profession that focuses on using exercise and movement to support physical health, manage chronic conditions, and improve overall quality of life. Exercise physiologists are highly trained experts who assess individual needs and develop safe, tailored programmes to address specific health concerns. Their work is particularly relevant for individuals living with Long COVID, including for persistent symptoms such as fatigue, shortness of breath, brain fog, and Post-Exertional Malaise (PEM). There may be some cross over in interventions offered between exercise physiology and physiotherapy in Long COVID care, depending on the interest and expertise of individual clinicians.

Exercise physiologists can design personalised strategies that address pacing and energy management to prevent symptom exacerbation. They carefully monitor progress to ensure that physical activity remains safe and sustainable. This is generally done with regular reviews of baseline and capacity, such as a symptom or activity diary and PEM profile. By addressing the unique challenges of Long COVID, such as fluctuating energy levels and heightened sensitivity to exertion, they help individuals gradually rebuild strength, endurance, and functional capacity.

Beyond exercise prescription, exercise physiologists provide education on self-monitoring and symptom management, empowering individuals to take control of their recovery. Their holistic approach integrates physical, mental, and emotional health, recognising the broad impact that Long COVID can have on daily life. Whether helping someone return to work, resume sport and physical recreation, or simply feel more confident in managing their health, exercise physiologists play a vital role in supporting meaningful recovery.

9.5.1 When to Refer to Exercise Physiology

Consider referral to an exercise physiologist for assessment and management when a person with Long COVID is experiencing persistent fatigue, muscle weakness, breathlessness, reduced physical endurance, physical deconditioning, and/or difficulty managing PEM. Referrals may also be appropriate when patients require a structured plan for improving strength and endurance or need guidance on adapting physical activities to suit their current capacity. By offering evidence-based, patient-centred care, exercise physiologists empower people with Long COVID to navigate their recovery journey and achieve sustainable improvements in health and quality of life.

9.6 OCCUPATIONAL THERAPY

Danielle Hitch

While many associate the word "occupation" with employment, occupational therapists use it to describe activities with personal or sociocultural meaning that support participation in daily life and community.[12] Occupational therapy is a complex, highly skilled, and evidence-based profession that uses occupational engagement to improve health and wellbeing. It enables people to do what they want, need, and must do.

Occupational therapists can adapt or modify occupations using strategies like simplifying and grading tasks, adjusting life roles, and providing cognitive support (see Chapter 12). For example, an occupational therapist will partner with a person with Long COVID to develop a pacing programme that maintains and increases their daily activities.

Occupational therapists are also skilled in modifying social and built environments, such as introducing assistive technology and reorganising spaces. They can facilitate social support by helping people overcome barriers to social participation or by connecting them with community groups and peer networks. They often educate family members and other supporters about Long COVID and how best to support their loved one. Occupational therapists also advocate for accessibility and inclusion in public spaces such as schools, healthcare services, and recreational facilities.

In addition, occupational therapists work with people with Long COVID to improve their physical and mental capacity to engage in meaningful occupations. These interventions include therapeutic activities that incorporate pain management, compensatory techniques, sensory modulation, and re-establishing vital life roles. For example, an occupational therapist can support a person with Long COVID to implement compensatory strategies for attention and memory issues due to brain fog.[13]

9.6.1 When to Refer to Occupational Therapy

Occupational therapy can benefit every person with Long COVID, yet it is often underutilised. Referral to an occupational therapist should be considered whenever symptoms negatively impact on the person's self-care, domestic activities, community participation, or return to work or school. While the focus is on participation rather than symptoms, referral should be considered for people with Long COVID experiencing fatigue, PEM, brain fog, sensory sensitivities, respiratory symptoms, pain, POTS, or mental health issues stemming from the challenges of living with this condition. Early referral supports more effective rehabilitation and better outcomes and should occur at, or soon after, intake into rehabilitation services. While healthcare adds days to lives, occupational therapy adds life to days.

9.7 PHYSIOTHERAPY

Jennifer Mepham, Fy Dunford and Victoria Lai

Physiotherapists use evidence-based techniques to restore movement and function across their lifespan and health journey from inpatient settings to the community, including workplace, school, and sporting environments. With expertise spanning cardio-respiratory, musculoskeletal, and neurological care, physiotherapists play a crucial role in assessing, treating, and managing conditions, including Long COVID.

Physiotherapists collaborate closely with their wider interdisciplinary colleagues to deliver individualised and group-based treatments across various settings, including telehealth, web-based platforms, and in-person services, as soon as it is safe to do so. Using assessment tools such as symptom maps,[14] diaries,[15] and outcome measures, physiotherapists identify symptom cluster presentations and guide the development of targeted treatment strategies. Management plans are tailored following assessment to meet an individual's goals using techniques such as breathing retraining, PEM management, autonomic conditioning for POTS, and safe exercise prescription.

Cardio-respiratory physiotherapists have a key role in the assessment and management of breathing pattern disorders. A thorough respiratory assessment, along with the use of outcome measures, is vital due to the complexity of this dysfunction. Strategies to improve heart or lung function, such as inspiratory muscle training, can be used for those with long-lasting respiratory dysfunction following their acute illness (i.e., those with an Intensive Care Unit [ICU] admission) and for those with co-existing conditions.

Physiotherapists prioritise symptom management to support energy conservation using pacing strategies and screening tools to identify PEM, ensuring management plans prevent symptom exacerbation. Long COVID is a multi-system condition that may present with musculoskeletal symptoms such as muscle/joint pain or balance impairments.

Key considerations for physiotherapists include customising their approach to each patient based on their symptoms, severity, and ability to participate. Careful monitoring and reassessment are frequently undertaken to make sure this is safe. Education is included to ensure people with lived experience are aware of the purpose, empowered to participate in the management, and aware of anticipated outcome of treatments chosen.

9.7.1 When to Refer to Physiotherapy

Consider referral to a physiotherapist for individualised assessment and management of cardio-respiratory symptoms (e.g., breathlessness, cough, breathing pattern disorders), pelvic floor dysfunction, fatigue management (including pacing and return to activities, work, school, or sport), exercise assessment, joint and muscle pain, and screening for safe rehabilitation including management of POTs and PEM. Red flags are carefully considered in all physiotherapy assessments to provide safe exercise progression, particularly with cardiac conditions, PEM, or autonomic dysfunction. Strategies are implemented alongside meaningful education with the common goal that management is sustainable and will endure to improve quality of life.

9.8 SOCIAL WORK

Sarah Booth

Social workers are committed to working side-by-side with people and communities affected by Long COVID, driven by the profession's commitment to social justice and human rights.[16] Long COVID impacts people throughout the community, although disadvantaged groups are overrepresented.[17] The experience of living with Long COVID symptoms commonly leads to increased functional and psychosocial issues including mental health issues, sleep problems, social isolation, productivity loss, greater disability, and increased dependence.[18,19] Despite these challenges, many people affected by Long COVID report difficulty navigating health, income, and disability systems.[20]

When working with people and communities with Long COVID, social workers first develop a comprehensive understanding of their psychosocial situation and consider how different aspects of a patient's life, such as their ethnicity, gender, sexuality, language, and socioeconomic position, may intersect and overlap to increase marginalisation.[21,22]

BOX 9.3 MARGINALISATION AND DISADVANTAGE FROM LONG COVID

Marginalised groups, without the resources to buffer against the functional and psychosocial disruptions of Long COVID, face compounded disadvantages and an increased risk of poverty.[17]

With this understanding, social workers provide a holistic and tailored response, drawing on individual and community strengths and resources while promoting equitable access to health and social services. Interventions may include risk assessments, counselling, advocacy, case management, system navigation, psychosocial education, social connection, and policy development.[22]

9.8.1 When to Refer to Social Work

Consider referral to a social worker for assessment and management when a person with Long COVID, or their family and caregivers, is at risk (e.g., family violence, elder abuse, child at risk, vulnerable adult), experiencing grief and bereavement or difficulties adjusting to health changes, financial, education, or employment issues related to their condition or difficulties with navigating complex systems (including housing, legal matters, aged care, or other welfare institutions). Family and caregiver stress and education, along with emotional and mental health support can also be offered.

9.9 SPEECH PATHOLOGY

Chantal Mitvalsky and Charissa Zaga

Speech pathologists provide assessment and management for patients with Long COVID who may experience changes to voice, swallowing, communication, or upper airway symptoms, which are essential functions for human interaction, health, and nutritional support. Speech pathologists assist in managing patients across the continuum of care, including critically unwell COVID-19 patients in the ICU setting, which may contribute to a high incidence of voice impairments (dysphonia) and swallowing impairments (dysphagia). These are typically attributed to damage to the voice box (larynx) from prolonged intubation, respiratory compromise, deconditioning, or neurological complications.[23] The Royal College of Speech and Language Therapists (RCSLT) report incidence rates of dysphagia (34.7%) and dysphonia (33.3%), followed by laryngeal hypersensitivity (12.0%), upper airway difficulties (8.0%), and cognitive-communication disorder (8.0%) in people with Long COVID.[24]

The speech pathology role in Long COVID ranges from screening and assessment to patient education and the development of tailored therapy programmes for swallowing, voice, and cognitive rehabilitation.[25] Developing suitable evidence-based voice and upper airways treatments for this niche cohort draws on established practices for voice therapy to reduce muscle tension, respiratory training to balance and support the vocal system, and education to reduce throat sensitivity and irritation, as well as the introduction of chronic cough suppression techniques. Treatment practices must be adapted to the unique circumstances of COVID-19 illness, such as permanent lung fibrosis, persistent shortness of breath, upper airway inflammation or irritation, and laryngeal injury in cases of intubation trauma. In some cases, patients may also be referred to ENT for a laryngoscopy to provide visualisation of the voice box and upper airway and receive medical or surgical management for laryngeal injury or upper airway symptoms, such as chronic cough, Gastroesophageal Reflux Disease, or laryngeal hypersensitivity.

Common self-reported Long COVID symptoms include brain fog and word-finding difficulties. Speech pathologists may use pacing exercises, word-finding strategies and cognitive retraining therapies to improve or help manage these cognitive communication difficulties. Additionally, it is within speech pathology scope of practice to provide targeted education and resource development around changes to taste and smell (olfaction), which can impact a person's safety and ability to identify smoke and gas, interest in food, intimacy, and leisure activities.[26]

9.9.1 When to Refer to Speech Pathology

Consider referral to a speech pathologist for assessment and management when a person with Long COVID is experiencing changes to their voice, upper airway, or communication status that are impacting their social wellbeing and work opportunities. Referral should also be considered if they are experiencing swallowing issues that are contributing to poor nutritional intake, chest infections, or discomfort when eating and drinking.

9.10 OTHER ALLIED HEALTH PROFESSIONALS

Many other allied health disciplines can also benefit people with Long COVID depending on their symptoms and functional profile. This includes pharmacy support for medication management, and cultural workers to provide culturally sensitive assessments and interventions. Various Long COVID services also include creative therapies as part of their care. For example, music therapy may support people with breathlessness and mental health issues via voice and breathing exercises, as well as music and relaxation for stress management.[27] Allied health assistants also play a key role in delivery of interventions under the supervision of allied health professionals. For further discussion of interdisciplinary care and care coordination approaches, see Chapters 10 and 18.

9.11 CONCLUSION

This chapter highlights the contributions of a range of allied health disciplines in providing evidence-based and individualised care for Long COVID. There is some overlap between professional boundaries across allied health disciplines, and professionals who work in advanced or extended scope roles may additionally work across these boundaries. Interprofessional collaboration ensures Long COVID rehabilitation is efficient, safe, and effective by referring to appropriate service providers. Timely access to care through coordinated referrals can support symptom management, improve patient outcomes, and enhance recovery. Not all patients know the breadth of allied health disciplines or what they do, and as such, need support to access the right care with relevant referrals and information. This chapter provides a reference guide to when these referrals might be relevant and what supports are on offer.

REFERENCES

1 Department of Health. Review of Australian government health workforce programs. Canberra: Australian Government; 2013.

2 Hitch D, et al. Development of the Translating Allied Health Knowledge (TAHK) framework. Int J Health Policy Manag. 2019;8(7):412–23. doi:10.15171/ijhpm.2019.23.

3 Wrench JM, et al. An allied health model of care for Long COVID rehabilitation. Med J Aust. 2024;221 Suppl 9:S5–S9. doi:10.5694/mja2.52457.

4 Koterba CH, et al. Neuropsychology practice guidance for the neuropsychiatric aspects of Long COVID. Clin Neuropsychol. 2024:1–29. doi:10.1080/13854046.2024.2392943.

5 Thye AY, et al. Psychological symptoms in COVID-19 patients: Insights into pathophysiology and risk factors of Long COVID-19. Biology. 2022;11(1). doi:10.3390/biology11010061.

6 Martinez-Borba V, et al. Guiding future research on psychological interventions in people with COVID-19 and post COVID syndrome and comorbid emotional disorders based on a systematic review. Front Public Health. 2023;11:1305463. doi:10.3389/fpubh.2023.1305463.

7 Kroenke K, et al. The PHQ-9: Validity of a brief depression severity measure. J Gen Intern Med. 2001;16(9):606–13. doi:10.1046/j.1525-1497.2001.016009606.x.

8 Spitzer RL, et al. A brief measure for assessing generalized anxiety disorder: The GAD-7. Arch Intern Med. 2006;166(10):1092–97. doi:10.1001/archinte.166.10.1092

9 Raj SR, et al. Diagnosis and management of postural orthostatic tachycardia syndrome. CMAJ. 2022;194(10):E378–85. doi:10.1503/cmaj.211373

10 DiBaise J, et al. The POTS (Postural Tachycardia Syndrome) epidemic: Hydration and nutrition series. Practical Gastro. 2019;43:14–26.

11 Barrea L, et al. Dietary recommendations for post-COVID-19 syndrome. Nutrients. 2022;14(6). doi:10.3390/nu14061305.

12 Creek J. The core concepts of occupational therapy : A dynamic framework for practice. 1st ed. London: Jessica Kingsley; 2010.

13 Skiffington H, et al. More than "Brain Fog": Cognitive dysfunction and the role of occupational therapy in Long COVID. CardiopulPhys Ther J 2025;36(1):39–49. doi:10.1097/CPT.0000000000000274.

14 Ministry of Health. Clinical rehabilitation guideline for people with Long COVID (Coronavirus Disease) in Aotearoa New Zealand: Revised December 2022 [Internet]. Wellington: Ministry of Health; [cited 2025 Feb 7]. Available from: https://www.health.govt.nz/publications/clinical-rehabilitation-guideline-for-people-with-long-covid-coronavirus-disease-in-aotearoa-new.

15 World Physiotherapy. World PT Day 2021: Activity diary, 2021 [Internet]. London: World Physiotherapy; 2021 [cited 2025 Feb 7]. Available from: https://world.physio/toolkit/world-pt-day-2021-activity-diary.

16 International Federation of Social Workers. Australia: Social Workers respond to COVID-19 pandemic, 2020. Rheinfelden, Switzerland: IFSW; [cited 2025 Feb 7]. Available from: https://www.ifsw.org/australian-social-workers-respond-to-covid-19-pandemi/.

17 Abrams EM, et al. COVID-19 and the impact of social determinants of health. Lancet Respir Med. 2020;8(7):659–61. doi:10.1016/S2213-2600(20)30234-4.

18 Leon-Herrera S, et al. Loss of socioemotional and occupational roles in individuals with Long COVID according to sociodemographic and clinical factors: Secondary data from a randomized clinical trial. PLoS One. 2024;19(2):e0296041. doi:10.1371/journal.pone.0296041.

19 Vartanian K, et al. Integrating patient-reported physical, mental, and social impacts to classify Long COVID experiences. Sci Rep. 2023;13(1):16288. doi:10.1038/s41598-023-43615-8.

20 Croft S, et al. A scoping review of barriers and facilitators affecting the lives of people With disabilities during COVID-19. Front Rehabil Sci. 2021;2:784450. doi:10.3389/fresc.2021.784450.

21 Cohen J, et al. An intersectional analysis of Long COVID prevalence. Int J Equity Health. 2023;22(1):261. doi:10.1186/s12939-023-02072-5

22 Tadic V, et al. The role of social workers in interprofessional primary healthcare teams. Healthc Policy. 2020;16(1):27–42. doi:10.12927/hcpol.2020.26292.

23 Printza A, et al. Dysphagia severity and management in patients with COVID-19. Curr Health Sci J. 2021;47(2):147–56. doi:10.12865/CHSJ.47.02.01.

24 Chalmers S, et al. A retrospective study of patients presenting with speech and language therapy needs within multidisciplinary Long COVID services: A service evaluation describing and comparing two cohorts across two NHS Trusts. Int J Lang Commun Disord. 2023;58(5):1424–39. doi:10.1111/1460-6984.12868.

25 Mohapatra B, et al. Speech-language pathologists' role in the multi-disciplinary management and rehabilitation of patients with COVID-19. J Rehabil Med Clin Commun. 2020;3:1000037. doi:10.2340/20030711-1000037.

26 Elkholi SMA, et al. Impact of the smell loss on the quality of life and adopted coping strategies in COVID-19 patients. Eur Arch Otorhinolaryngol. 2021;278(9):3307–14. doi:10.1007/s00405-020-06575-7.

27 D'Souza AN, et al. Recovering from COVID-19 (ReCOV): Feasibility of an Allied-Health-Led Multidisciplinary Outpatient Rehabilitation Service for People with Long COVID. Int J Environ Res Public Health. 2024;21(7):958. doi: 10.3390/ijerph21070958.

Chapter 10

Bringing It All Together

Integrated and Coordinated Care for Long COVID

Melanie Broadley, Sara Holton, and Danielle Hitch

BOX 10.1 LEARNING OBJECTIVES

By the end of this chapter, readers should be able to:

- Identify the fundamental components of integrated care and describe their application to Long COVID rehabilitation.
- Explore systemic barriers that hinder integrated care for people with Long COVID.
- Evaluate innovative care models to identify strategies for improving care coordination, access, and multidisciplinary care.
- Develop strategies to apply integrated care principles in rehabilitation settings, considering the needs of people with Long COVID and overcoming organisational and systemic challenges.

10.1 INTRODUCTION

People with Long COVID, like those with other chronic conditions, frequently face service gaps. Gaps in care often arise from conflicting priorities, accountability issues, power imbalances, and rigid funding structures.[1] Integrated care enhances continuity in fragmented healthcare systems involving diverse professions and settings that often lack communication or referral pathways.[2]

Integrated care can be understood as a complex adaptive system,[3] where the dynamic interactions between multiple elements create emergent opportunities and challenges that are difficult, if not impossible, to predict. This complexity makes

DOI: 10.4324/9781003528104-13

systematic implementation difficult for individuals and organisations. Various frameworks have been developed to identify the fundamental components of integrated care to ensure the implementation of high quality, patient-centred care. In a scoping review of predominantly European literature, Noor et al.[4] identified four key elements in most models: service delivery, person-centeredness, Information Technology systems, and decision support. These elements include many components, all collectively contributing to integrated care (Figure 10.1).

Integrated care is crucial for individuals with Long COVID due to its complex, multisystem nature.[5] Patients with Long COVID usually need responsive care across primary, secondary, and specialist services to manage their often persistent and fluctuating symptoms.[6] Multidisciplinary approaches to Long COVID rehabilitation were recognised early in the pandemic[7] and have been at least partially implemented[8] in some health services. This chapter examines the current status of integrated care for people with Long COVID, makes recommendations to improve integrated care for this patient group, and presents case studies that showcase innovative approaches adaptable to other settings.

BOX 10.2   PRACTICE POINT

Imagine you have been referred a new patient who lives with Long COVID. Reflect on your assumptions about the services and support they already access or know about. Do you think they experience difficulties managing, accessing, and coordinating, for example, all the health services they access to get Long COVID treatment/support? Do you ask about other healthcare they receive and how they coordinate it during your initial assessments? Are there any things you could do to assist them in managing/coordinating their care?

10.2 CURRENT ISSUES IN ENABLING INTEGRATED CARE FOR PEOPLE WITH LONG COVID

10.2.1 Getting Access to Care and Support

Access to healthcare often marks the end of a long, challenging journey rather than the beginning. Terms like "pathway" or "continuum" suggest a linear process, but people with Long COVID, like those with other chronic illnesses, often face recurring and cyclical interactions with healthcare.[9] These patients may, therefore,

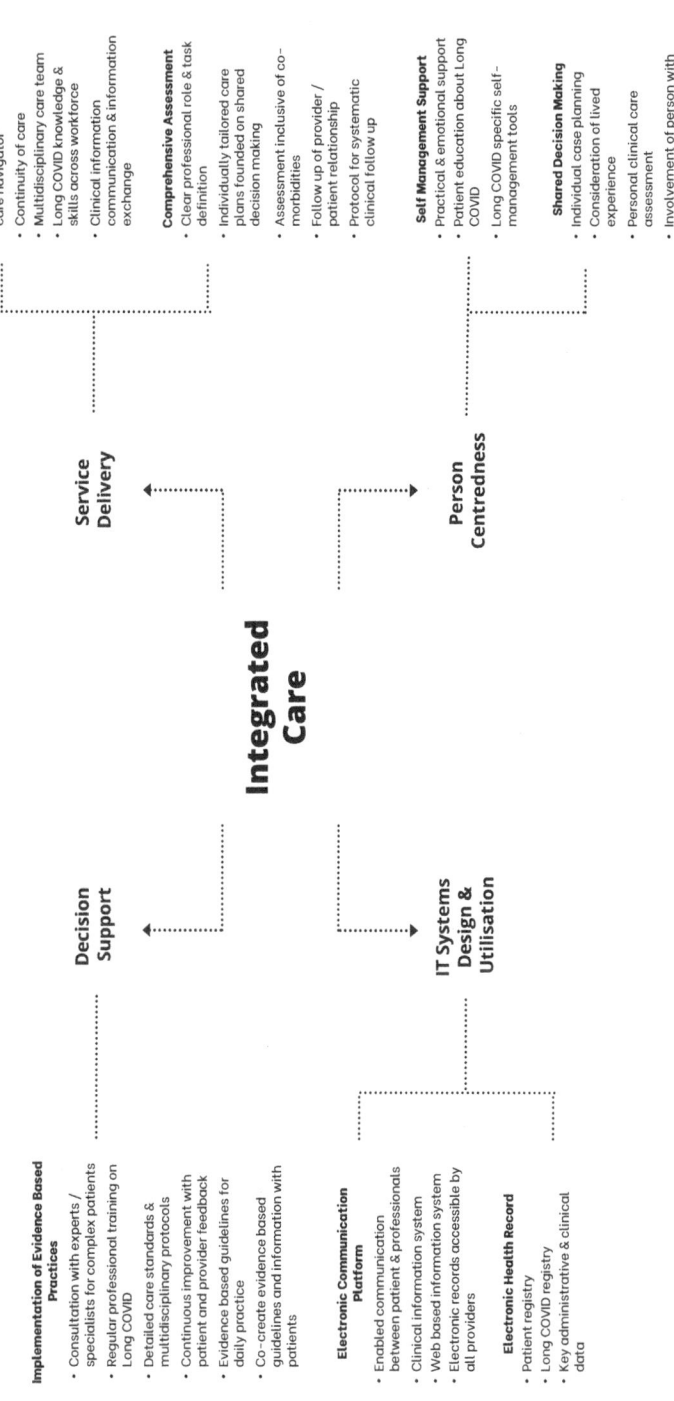

Figure 10.1 Concept map of key integrated care elements. Adapted from Noor F, et al. Exploration of understanding of integrated care from a public health perspective: A scoping review. J Public Health Res 12(3):1–21. Copyright c 2023 by the Authors. Reprinted by permission of Sage Publications, Ltd.[1]

have multiple interactions with the health system and healthcare providers to get the care they need.

Access to secondary and specialist care often relies on relationships with primary care physicians. However, only half of Australians consistently see the same general practitioner (GP), limiting long-term therapeutic relationships essential for referrals.[10] People in rural or remote areas, migrants, and disadvantaged communities also often face significant barriers to accessing primary care.[11–13] As a result, many patients with Long COVID may not be able to access or receive appropriate care, and their symptoms may worsen over time.

One of the most significant barriers to accessing care for people with Long COVID is that their condition does not "fit in" easily into commonly used health condition classification systems. While COVID-19 is classified as a respiratory syndrome,[14] it can affect virtually every body system and health professionals across various specialities often treat Long COVID symptoms. As a result, no single service can meet all the needs of people with Long COVID, and they may not meet the eligibility criteria for existing rehabilitation services.

Emerging evidence suggests three to four Long COVID phenotypes,[15–17] although their constituent features are not consistently described. However, symptom clusters can be identified using clinician and patient rated assessments to inform decisions about appropriate referrals and service access.

People with Long COVID often face new and multiple access barriers throughout their patient journey each time they are referred to another service. A key contributor to these access and care barriers is healthcare "silos," which are organisational obstacles to collaboration, information, and continuity of care between healthcare sites, services, and sectors.[18] Differing eligibility criteria and internal obstacles can further limit patients' access to services, as illustrated by the following experience.

> When I approached my GP about public options, she said there was a physical rehabilitation program at the local hospitals, but people with chronic conditions almost never got appointments because more acute issues (e.g. post-surgery) always took precedence.

Even when people with Long COVID gain access to a rehabilitation service, the health professionals may not have experience or expertise with the condition. This can result in inappropriate or limited care approaches that do not meet the person's needs.

BOX 10.3   PRACTICE POINT

Reflect on how people with Long COVID access your rehabilitation service. What other services or systems have they typically used before being referred? How do you currently assist patients to access services they are referred to after completing rehabilitation?

10.2.2 Barriers to Integrated Care during Rehabilitation

If rehabilitation services accept referrals for people with Long COVID, patients still often face lengthy delays between referral acceptance and initial appointments, especially in publicly funded healthcare.[19,20] These delays can hinder integrated care by preventing early intervention, worsening fragmentation, increasing disability, reducing engagement, and causing cascading delays across the system. While delays often occur in primary care, they are commonly experienced by patients with Long COVID for specialist care.

> When I got accepted into the Long COVID centre, the wait time was any time from four to nine months—and that was three months ago. I don't anticipate hearing from them for quite a while.[20 [p5]]
>
> [The GP] did it as quickly as possible and got me in and then you wait and wait and wait and wait and waiting and waiting. [After 6 months] I followed up with an email saying I haven't received any confirmation... I just don't want it to have gone nowhere. So just tell me that you've got it. And I'm in the queue? ... And then they came back and said, that the first appointments are [a further 6 months away].[21]

Early intervention is vital for rehabilitating people with Post-Acute Infection Syndromes, including Long COVID. Hospitalised patients are advised to have bedside rehabilitation during admission and a comprehensive assessment six to eight weeks post-discharge.[22] However, no guidance exists for non-hospitalised patients, who constitute the majority of people with Long COVID. Extended waiting periods can also worsen health status and outcomes by increasing disability and impairment.[20] Long waiting times for healthcare appointments also deter attendance due to exhaustion and disengagement from the amount of self-advocacy it took to gain access in the first place.[23]

Care coordination is essential to integrated care, but patients often bear the burden of navigating the fragmented healthcare system, organising appointments, and facilitating communication. Care coordination is a specialised, complex task requiring collaboration, communication skills, engagement, and clinical knowledge.[24] Healthcare workers with Long COVID often experience additional challenges as a result of their dual patient-professional identities, which can create dissonance when their lived experience is dismissed.[25]

Managing bureaucracy in healthcare systems can be even more burdensome for those with energy-limiting health conditions. While some people with Long COVID may have the necessary skills to navigate the health system, having to use these skills when they are unwell can exacerbate symptoms such as fatigue and brain fog. Even simple tasks such as transferring medical records from one clinic to another can involve multiple phone calls, emails, payment, and form filling. All of which can significantly impact the "energy budget" of a person with Long COVID.

Primary healthcare professionals act as both advocates and gatekeepers for referrals, and their knowledge and attitudes towards Long COVID can significantly impact integrated care. Patients often report being denied further testing or specialist referrals if initial assessments conducted by primary healthcare professionals appear normal. However, standard tests are not validated for use among people with Long COVID, prompting calls to redefine "normal" biomarkers.[27,28] The limitations of standard rehabilitation tests and assessments and best practices approach to evaluating Long COVID patients are discussed in more detail in Chapter 6.

The complexity of managing unknown aspects of Long COVID can discourage rehabilitation clinicians from working with these patients and can also lead to healthcare professional burnout and demoralisation. Combined with the general impact of the COVID-19 pandemic on clinician health and wellbeing[26], such responses from health professionals can also be a significant barrier to integrated care, as described here,

> *The most difficult thing I've found over and over are clinicians that give up on you because you are too difficult, too allergic, too complex. If a clinician feels they are unable to assist there should be a systematic onward referral rather than just a disappearance or no response. You need to support people to find something else – provided there is something else! Clinicians don't need to be perfect all the time, but they should be open to 'I don't know, but I'll find out.'*

BOX 10.4   PRACTICE POINT

Work through the following questions to reflect on the systemic barriers within your service that could delay rehabilitation for people with Long COVID.

- Are there opportunities to streamline or improve integrated care for your patients?
- How do you enable access to and active engagement in rehabilitation for people with energy-limiting conditions?
- Are there ways to reduce the energy burden of patients who navigate your system?
- How can you alleviate the burden on patients who coordinate their care?
- What steps can be taken to ensure that health professionals in your service are well-informed and empathetic towards the complexities of Long COVID?
- Could you co-design or co-create organisational processes to resolve barriers to integrated care in your rehabilitation service?
- Given the uncertainties of Long COVID, how comfortable are you and your colleagues with providing care?

10.3 IMPROVING INTEGRATED CARE FOR LONG COVID

Existing care models for people with Long COVID typically combine primary care, specialised clinics, and rehabilitation services.[7] Long COVID care models emerged early in the pandemic, often adapting existing services. Specialist clinics led by respiratory, neurology, cardiology, or rehabilitation specialists were common. People with Long COVID contributed to assistive technology,[28] research,[29,30] and self-management platforms like Visible.[31] However, apart from ad hoc input by Long COVID–affected health professionals, clinical models followed traditional templates that are ill-suited to complex and chronic conditions.

Several core features of Long COVID integrated models of care have been identified – hybrid service delivery (i.e., face-to-face and telehealth), scalability to handle the high demand for Long COVID care, and a core team of health professionals with expertise in managing this condition.[32] The pandemic accelerated telehealth adoption[33,] and combining traditional and telerehabilitation is effective for people with Long COVID.[34,35] A key benefit of telehealth is its ability to reduce reinfection risks, an essential concern for many people with Long COVID.[36] These platforms also reduce the cognitive and physical burden of attending face-to-face appointments and, therefore, reduce fatigue. However, access to technology, digital literacy, infrastructure, training, and funding are all potential barriers to telehealth implementation, especially in disadvantaged communities.[37] At the time of writing, further research and economic analysis are needed to enable telerehabilitation's sustainable scalability.

While there is consensus around the value of multidisciplinary contributions to Long COVID care,[7] the integration of different professions into care plans varies significantly. Along with the medical specialists discussed in Chapter 5, physiotherapists, occupational therapists, and psychologists are common multidisciplinary team members.[7,38] However, as outlined in Chapter 6, many other health professionals have the skills and expertise to support people with Long COVID. Following the principles of integrated care, each person with Long COVID should have access to a multidisciplinary team that is personalised to their unique symptom and functional profile. Along with health professionals, this team could include spiritual or pastoral care, cultural practitioners, and other support relevant to individual needs and preferences.

BOX 10.5   PRACTICE POINT

Do you currently practice telerehabilitation? If not, what are the barriers to your service from adopting this mode of delivery? If so, what would you consider the advantages and disadvantages of telehealth from your perspective? Who are the members of your multidisciplinary team? Are there any gaps in the services your team provides (i.e., is there a healthcare profession that you frequently need to make external referrals to?)

10.4 INNOVATIVE APPROACHES TO INTEGRATED LONG COVID CARE

10.4.1 The COVID reCOVeRY (DisCOVeRY) Model of Care[1]

The DisCOVeRY Model of Care is an innovative, co-designed framework addressing people with Long COVID's diverse and complex needs. It has integrated lived, clinical, and academic experience through co-design to ensure relevance, feasibility, and adaptability. Collaboration between multiple stakeholders supports better patient outcomes and promotes meaningful learning for participants.[39]

The DisCOVeRY model was developed in late 2021 by a co-design team of six people with Long COVID and three clinician researchers based in Melbourne, Australia. The process followed Evidence-Based Co-Design (EBCD) principles,[40] using quantitative and qualitative data from patients, healthcare professionals, and international research. An abbreviated EBCD approach incorporated pre-existing data to ensure feasibility during a significant COVID-19 wave and partial redeployment of researchers to frontline duties. Lived experience team members were primary stakeholders, with clinician researchers and healthcare professionals as secondary stakeholders.

Data collection in the first design phase included: (1) functional and quality-of-life outcomes from 127 patients; (2) mixed-methods survey of 85 health professionals about their experiences of treating patients with Long COVID; and (3) narrative interviews with 67 patients to explore lived experiences of Long COVID. The co-design team conducted three two-hour online workshops. Participation was offered either in-person or asynchronously via an online workbook, accommodating fluctuating health status and enabling rural participation. A draft data analysis and international evidence review were presented in the first workshop as a foundation for design. Each workshop focused on a core question, with outputs determined by group consensus (Figure 10.2).

All discussions were recorded and transcribed, with key themes integrated into subsequent workshops. The co-design process, alongside the DisCOVeRY model,

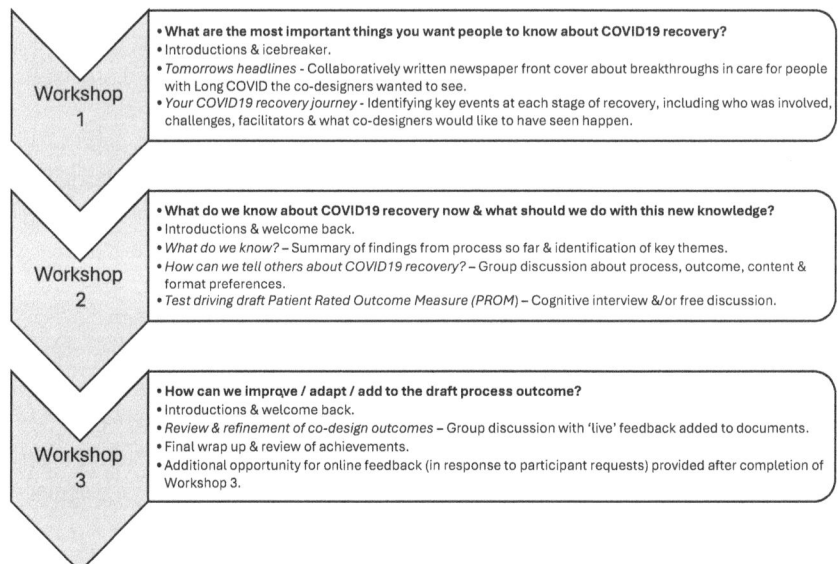

Figure 10.2 Co-Design workshops for the DisCOVeRY model of care.

produced supporting resources, including information videos, infographics, best practice guidelines (outlined in Chapter 1), a patient journey map, a directory of relevant health and other services, and the COVID Check-In patient-rated outcome measure.

The DisCOVeRY model aims to support optimal recovery and prevent or minimise ongoing service or support requirements. Lived experience experts and evidence highlighted the assistance people with Long COVID require accessing services within and beyond healthcare. The model is founded on care coordination, facilitated either independently by accessing a web platform or with the support of a dedicated and independent care coordinator. The pathway taken through this model (see Figure 10.3) represents a single care cycle; entry is via patient or professional referral, and re-entry can occur whenever necessary.

All care will be tailored to individual goals and needs rather than symptom profile or duration, meaning all individual recovery trajectories can be accommodated. The "care and support" concept includes healthcare, psychosocial, vocational, educational, cultural, spiritual, or any other services the person with Long COVID may require. Support and care will be delivered by services already available in the persons' local community, supplemented by any available online or remotely. These services may, therefore, be delivered face-to-face or via telehealth, depending on patient preference and technology availability. Cut-off scores for "clinically significant" disability, based on Australian WHODAS-12 norms,[41] guide decisions about the most suitable care streams. Patients and care coordinators will regularly review care plans so that support evolves in response to patients' changing needs and circumstances. Discharge will be mutually decided by patients and providers, based on personal goals or onward referral to appropriate supports.

The model of care includes evidence-informed and patient-centred components. These include building partnerships with Long COVID peer support groups, communities of practice for healthcare professionals (including journal clubs, case studies, and professional development) and embedded research. Research initiatives arising from the DisCOVeRY model will support rapid evidence translation and continuous service improvement in an "evidence-poor" environment. The governance structure includes a steering committee comprised of equal representation of people with Long COVID and other key stakeholders. These organisation level components of the model will enable the systemic change people with Long COVID seek for sustained and equitable health improvements.

Overall, the DisCOVeRY model of care is designed to be both scalable and inclusive. The flexibility within the model enhances its potential to meet the

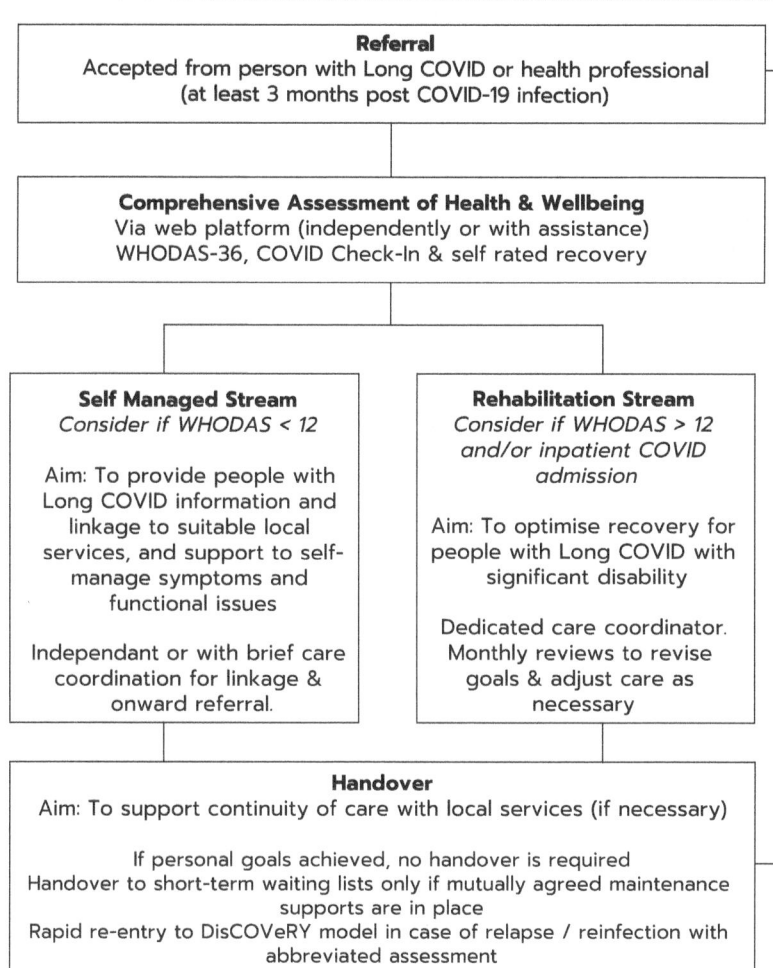

Figure 10.3 The COVid reCOVeRY (DiSCOVeRY) Model of Care.

Note: WHODAS = World Health Organization Disability Assessment Schedule.

needs of disadvantaged populations, and the focus is on access to services and support within the local community. It leverages and makes the most of existing infrastructure, which can enhance efficiency and reduce service duplication. Including lived experience experts within the governance model and peer support initiatives further strengthens its emphasis on patient-centred and culturally responsive care. Its innovative cross-sectoral scope and independence from specific services also offer the potential for its application to other chronic and complex conditions.

10.5 CONCLUSION

Integrated care models have evolved to address the complex needs of people with Long COVID, highlighting the value of multidisciplinary collaboration, care coordination, and patient-centred approaches. Despite advancements, systemic barriers such as healthcare silos, extended wait times, and inequitable access to services persist and amplify the challenges faced by many patients with Long COVID. Innovative approaches, such as the Australian DisCOVeRY model of care, illustrate scalable and inclusive solutions available for use in practice. However, their application to practice may involve overcoming bureaucratic burdens and ensuring equity in resource allocation. Ultimately, advancing integrated care for Long COVID requires continued innovation, co-design with stakeholders, and systemic reform to break down barriers and enhance service delivery. These efforts will benefit people with Long COVID and potentially provide appropriate and feasible care models for supporting others with chronic and complex conditions.

NOTE

1   Content in this section is adapted from "Enabling and Optimising Recovery from COVID-19: A handbook for health professionals and other caregivers of people with Long COVID" by Danielle Hitch, Genevieve Pepin, Kelli Nicola-Richmond & Valerie Watchorn, used under CC BY 4.0.

REFERENCES

1   Spicer N, et al. 'It's far too complicated': Why fragmentation persists in global health. Glob Health. 2020;16:60. doi:10.1186/s12992-020-00592-1.

2   Coughlan CH, et al. How to improve care across boundaries. BMJ. 2020;369:m1045. doi:10.1136/bmj.m1045.

3   Nurjono M, et al. Implementation of integrated care in Singapore: A complex adaptive system perspective. Int J Integr Care. 2018;18:4. doi:10.5334/ijic.4174.

4   Noor F, et al. Exploration of understanding of integrated care from a public health perspective: A scoping review. J Public Health Res. 2023 Jul;12(3):22799036231181210. doi:10.1177/22799036231181210.

5   van der Feltz-Cornelis CM, et al. Integrated care policy recommendations for complex multisystem long-term conditions and Long COVID. Sci Rep. 2024;14:13634. doi:10.1038/s41598-024-64060-1.

6   Fang C, et al. "They seemed to be like cogs working in different directions": A longitudinal qualitative study on Long COVID healthcare services in the United Kingdom from a person-centred lens. BMC Health Serv Res. 2024;24:406. doi:10.1186/s12913-024-10891-7.

7   Decary S, et al. Care models for Long COVID – A living systematic review. First Update – December 2021. SPOR Evidence Alliance, COVID-END Network; 2021.

8 Katz GM, et al. Understanding how post-COVID-19 condition affects adults and health care systems. JAMA Health Forum. 2023;4(7):e231933. doi:10.1001/jamahealthforum.2023.1933.

9 Maas VK, et al. The never-ending patient journey of chronically ill patients: A qualitative case study on touchpoints in relation to patient-centered care. PLoS One. 2023;18:e0285872. doi:10.1371/journal.pone.0285872.

10 Tran B, et al. Overcoming the data drought: Exploring general practice in Australia by network analysis of big data. Med J Aust. 2018;209:68–73. doi:10.5694/mja17.01236.

11 Taylor D, et al. General practice access in regional and remote Australia for ageing populations. Geogr Res. 2020;59:6–15. doi:10.1111/1745-5871.12447.

12 Tillmann J, et al. Determinants of having no general practitioner in Germany and the influence of a migration background: Results of the German health interview and examination survey for adults (DEGS1). BMC Health Serv Res. 2018;18:755. doi:10.1186/s12913-018-3571-2.

13 Smithman MA, et al. Area deprivation and attachment to a general practitioner through centralised waiting lists: A cross-sectional study in Quebec, Canada. Int J Equity Health. 2018;17:176. doi:10.1186/s12939-018-0887-9.

14 World Health Organization (WHO). Naming the coronavirus disease (COVID-19) and the virus that causes it [Internet]. Geneva: WHO; 2020 [cited 2025 Feb 7]. Available at: https://www.who.int/emergencies/diseases/novel-coronavirus-2019/technical-guidance/naming-the-coronavirus-disease-(covid-2019)-and-the-virus-that-causes-it.

15 Kisiel MA, et al. Clustering analysis identified three Long COVID phenotypes and their association with general health status and working ability. J Clin Med. 2023;12:3617. doi:10.3390/jcm12113617.

16 Wong AW, et al. Use of latent class analysis and patient reported outcome measures to identify distinct Long COVID phenotypes: A longitudinal cohort study. PLoS One. 2023;18:e0286588. doi:10.1371/journal.pone.0286588.

17 Blankestijn JM, et al. Long COVID exhibits clinically distinct phenotypes at 3–6 months post-SARS-CoV-2 infection: Results from the P4O2 consortium. BMJ Open Respir Res. 2024;11:e001907. doi:10.1136/bmjresp-2023-001907.

18 Pedersen ER, et al. A multi-dimensional study of organisational boundaries and silos in the healthcare sector. Health Serv Manag Res. 2024;37:200–08. doi:10.1177/9514848231218617.

19 Sunkersing D, et al. What is current care for people with Long COVID in England? A qualitative interview study. BMJ Open. 2024;14:e080967. doi:10.1136/bmjopen-2023-080967.

20 Hawke LD, et al. Swept under the carpet: A qualitative study of patient perspectives on Long COVID, treatments, services, and mental health. BMC Health Serv Res. 2023;23:1088. doi:10.1186/s12913-023-10091-9.

21 Parliament of Australia. Submissions - Submission 493 [Internet]. Canberra: Parliament of Australia; [cited 2025 Feb 7]. Available at: https://www.aph.gov.au/Parliamentary_Business/Committees/House/Health_Aged_Care_and_Sport/LongandrepeatedCOVID/Submissions.

22 Spruit MA, et al. COVID-19: Interim guidance on rehabilitation in the hospital and post-hospital phase from a European Respiratory Society- and American Thoracic Society-coordinated international task force. Eur Respir J. 2020;56:2002197. doi:10.1183/13993003.02197-2020.

23 Karam M, et al. Nursing care coordination in primary healthcare for patients with complex needs: A comparative case study. Int J Integr Care. 2023;23:5. doi:10.5334/ijic.6729.

24 Cruickshank M, et al. What is the impact of long-term COVID-19 on workers in healthcare settings? A rapid systematic review of current evidence. PLoS One. 2024;19:e0299743. doi:10.1371/journal.pone.0299743.

25 Ramers CB, et al. Burnout, compassion fatigue, and the long haul of caring for Long COVID. Open Forum Infect Dis. 2024;11:ofae080. doi:10.1093/ofid/ofae080.

26 Owen R, et al. Time to redefine 'normal' in the context of Post-Acute COVID-19 biomarkers in the assessment of patient outcomes? Physiology 2024;39:S1. doi:10.1152/physiol.2024.39. S1.515.

27 Komaroff AL, et al. Will COVID-19 lead to myalgic encephalomyelitis/chronic fatigue syndrome? Front Med. 2021;7:606824. doi:10.3389/fmed.2020.606824.

28 Dalko K, et al. Cocreation of assistive technologies for patients with Long COVID: Qualitative analysis of a literature review on the challenges of patient involvement in health and nursing sciences. J Med Internet Res. 2023; 25:e46297. doi:10.2196/46297.

29 Turner GM, et al. Co-production of a feasibility trial of pacing interventions for Long COVID. Res Involv Engagem. 2023; 30;9(1):18. doi:10.1186/s40900-023-00429-2.

30 Heaton-Shrestha C, et al. Co-designing personalised self-management support for people living with Long COVID: The LISTEN protocol. PLoS One. 2022; 17(10):e0274469. doi:10.1371/journal.pone.0274469.

31 MakeVisible. MakeVisible: Advancing awareness of invisible disabilities [Internet]. Unknown: MakeVisible; [cited 2025 Feb 7]. Available at: https://www.makevisible.com.

32 Chou R, et al. Long COVID definitions and models of care: A scoping review. Ann Intern Med. 2024 Jul;177(7):929–40. doi:10.7326/M24-0677. Erratum in: Ann Intern Med. 2024 Sep;177(9):1295.

33 Terrell EA, et al. The evolution of telehealth from pre-COVID-19 pandemic through a hybrid virtual care delivery model: A pediatric hospital's journey. Int J Telerehabil. 2021; 13(2):e6432. doi:10.5195/ijt.2021.6432.

34 Cavalcante TF, et al. Models of support for caregivers and patients with the post-COVID-19 condition: A scoping review. Int J Environ Res Public Health. 2023; 20(3):2563. doi:10.3390/ijerph20032563.

35 Satar S, et al. Tele-pulmonary rehabilitation with face-to-face in COVID-19 pandemic: A hybrid modeling. Tuberk Toraks. 2023; 71(1):58–66. doi:10.5578/tt.20239908.

36 Brigo E, et al. Using telehealth to guarantee the continuity of rehabilitation during the COVID-19 pandemic: A systematic review. Int J Environ Res Public Health. 2022; 19(16):10325. doi:10.3390/ijerph191610325.

37 Haque SN, et al. Factors influencing telehealth implementation and use in frontier critical access hospitals: Qualitative study. JMIR Form Res. 2021; 5(5):e24118. doi:10.2196/24118.

38 Ward S, et al. Mapping UK rehabilitation provision for adults after hospital admission with COVID-19. Eur Resp J. 2022;60:1224. doi:10.1183.13993003.congress-2022.1224.

39 Nordin A, et al. Measurement and outcomes of co-production in health and social care: A systematic review of empirical studies. BMJ Open. 2023; 13(9):e073808. doi:10.1136/bmjopen-2023-073808.

40 Goodrich J. Why experience-based co-design improves the patient experience. JHD. 2018;3(1): 84–85. doi:10.21853/JHD.2018.45.

41 Andrews G, et al. Normative data for the 12-item WHO Disability Assessment Schedule 2.0. PLOS One. 2009; 4(12):e8343. doi:10.1371/journal.pone.0008343.

SECTION FOUR

LONG COVID INTERVENTIONS AND MANAGEMENT

Chapter 11

Physical Rehabilitation Techniques for Long COVID

Jennifer Mepham, Angela Maxwell-McRae, and Lynette Hodges

BOX 11.1 LEARNING OBJECTIVES

By the end of this chapter, readers should be able to:

- Describe PEM and physical symptoms in Long COVID.
- Identify evidence-based techniques for physical rehabilitation.
- Reflect on physical activity interventions and their impact on people with Long COVID.

11.1 INTRODUCTION

Physical activity supports health by managing and preventing non-communicable diseases such as cardiovascular disease, cancer, diabetes, and obesity. It also reduces anxiety and depression while boosting wellbeing. However, people with Long COVID experience significant challenges to participating in physical activity, due to the impact of their symptoms.

As outlined in Chapter 2, Long COVID is a multisystem disease with complex symptom clusters that cannot be treated in isolation. Health professionals must recognise the mind-body connection and adopt a holistic approach to health and wellbeing, even when focusing on physical activity. This is crucial for people with Long COVID, who often face dismissal or disbelief about their symptoms and lived experiences.

The exact causes of Long COVID and its physical symptoms remain unclear, but health professionals offering physical rehabilitation play a key role in symptom management and improving quality of life. This chapter presents evidence-based

DOI: 10.4324/9781003528104-15

approaches to physical rehabilitation aimed at alleviating symptoms even when their cause remains unknown. It covers assessments and techniques for managing the physical symptoms of Long COVID, including cardiovascular exercise testing, safety precautions, and movement-based interventions. Post-Exertional Malaise (PEM) is discussed as a key focus for intervention, along with best practice guidelines for assessments and management. All the strategies presented in this chapter are intended to be used in partnership with the lived experience expertise of the patient and within a framework of shared decision-making.

BOX 11.2   PRACTICE POINT

Physical activity is vital for cardiovascular, respiratory, and bone health, and reducing chronic disease risk. Do you discuss your patients' physical activity history during assessment? What were they doing before Long COVID? Reflect on how and why it changed.

11.2 ENHANCING PHYSICAL ACTIVITY FOR PEOPLE WITH LONG COVID: A MULTIDISCIPLINARY APPROACH

Not all health professionals are knowledgeable about PEM or Long COVID, and people with these conditions may need support to find clinicians with appropriate training and experience. Physiotherapists and exercise physiologists play a crucial role in physical rehabilitation for people with Long COVID, given their respective areas of expertise and scope of practice (see Chapter 9). Physiotherapists treat musculoskeletal, neurological, cardiovascular, pulmonary, and pain conditions, while exercise physiologists use exercise to manage chronic conditions and improve health. Both interpret individualised assessments and prescribe evidence-based management plans tailored to patient needs and activity goals.[1] They also address functional capacity issues, enhancing participation in daily life and improve health and wellbeing.

Assessment and intervention by other members of the multidisciplinary team (MDT) complement the leading roles of physiotherapists and exercise physiologists in supporting physical activity for people with Long COVID. For example; occupational therapists implement pacing strategies in daily life and modify environments and tasks to conserve energy. Dietitians provide nutritional plans that support physical activity and implement interventions to address the symptoms of Postural Orthostatic Tachycardia Syndrome (POTS). Social workers address the systemic and psychosocial barriers that limit access to physical activity, while psychologists provide psychological strategies to help patients manage distress related to their physical limitations. The expertise of physiotherapists and exercise physiologists must therefore be integrated with related care provided by multidisciplinary colleagues, to ensure the person with Long COVID receives consistent advice and care (see Chapter 10).

11.3 POST-EXERTIONAL MALAISE

PEM is described by many people with Long COVID as extremely debilitating. PEM symptoms are exacerbated by physical, cognitive, or emotional exertion.[2] Symptoms include fatigue, brain fog, myalgia, sleep disturbances, flu-like feelings, arthralgia, headache, sore throat, and/or tender lymph nodes.[3] Addressing PEM during the first patient interaction is crucial to forming a safe and effective foundation for assessments and interventions.

PEM symptoms typically appear between 24 and 72 hours of exertion. They often last two to seven days but can persist for weeks or months in severe cases.[4] Severity ranges from mild fatigue to complete inability to perform tasks or needing prolonged bedrest. The onset of symptoms occurs during activities of daily living, making it difficult to connect activities to PEM, and the exertion threshold that triggers symptoms can be unpredictable.[4]

The variability of PEM symptom duration and experience can make them hard to predict and manage. Unlike delayed onset muscle soreness from heavy workouts or deconditioning, PEM symptoms do not improve with rest, contrasting to the increased energy and reduced fatigue other people gain from physical activity.[5] Health professionals must recognise the debilitating impact of PEM and avoid attributing symptoms solely to deconditioning or psychological causes to foster respectful therapeutic relationships and shared decision-making.

PEM significantly impacts patients, restricting daily participation and meaningful roles. Some experience PEM from simple activities,[6] making self-awareness of triggers and prevention key to management. Angela has lived with POTS and myalgic encephalomyelitis/chronic fatigue syndrome (ME/CFS) since April 2022 after acute COVID-19.

My main Long Covid symptoms are tinnitus, brain fog, tachycardia and breathlessness, but by far the worst is PEM. PEM feels like my body and brain have shut down. For me it usually starts with my upper arms starting to feel really heavy (like when you have the flu) and then the rest of my body follows. Rolling over in bed feels like a gargantuan effort…(when) I overdo it the deeper I fall into the PEM abyss, the worse the symptoms are and the longer it takes to climb back out of the hole. The biggest issue is that often I have no idea that I am overdoing it. What I can easily achieve one day might cause PEM the next. It is so easy to accidentally push outside my energy envelope.

Angela

Health professionals and people with Long COVID not adequately informed about PEM may unknowingly exceed their energy limits and trigger severe or prolonged episodes by trying to "push through." Repeated PEM can lower baseline functionality, preventing recovery to prior activity levels and creating a cycle of declining health and dependency.[7] Understanding that PEM and deconditioning are not one and the same ensures safe rehabilitation for people with lived experience. In deconditioning, rest relieves symptoms and individuals are able to complete daily exercise, whereas individuals with PEM may experience debilitating symptoms, leaving them unable to participate in life.

BOX 11.3 PRACTICE POINT

Reflect on the PEM symptoms your Long COVID patients have described. How often do they occur? How severe are they? What activities trigger PEM, and how do the symptoms affect their participation in daily life?

BOX 11.4 KEY RECOMMENDATION

All people with Long COVID should be screened for PEM prior to initiating any physical rehabilitation interventions.[8,9]

Screening for PEM ensures silent or poorly understood symptoms are acknowledged, and interventions are safely implemented without exacerbation. To understand the lived experience of PEM symptoms, comprehensive patient reported outcome measures should be used, such as the De Paul Symptom Questionnaire Versions 1 or 2[10,11] and the DePaul Symptoms Questionnaire-PEM short form.[12] The short-form version is ideal for screening when time is limited. These tools help health professionals assess the frequency and severity of PEM symptoms over the past six months. Combined with activity, rest, and sleep tracking via diaries or devices,[13] this data assists identifying and pre-emptively addressing triggers. Identifying the causes of PEM and creating management plans is like finding a missing puzzle piece.

BOX 11.5   PRACTICE POINT

How do you assess if your Long COVID patient is overexerting? Do you use validated measures? How do these assessments shape your clinical reasoning and practice?

11.4 PHYSICAL ASSESSMENT FOR PEOPLE WITH LONG COVID

Comprehensive assessment is essential for physical or movement-based rehabilitation, including screening for urgent medical symptoms and cautions before intervention. The complex nature of Long COVID may mean that the root causes of symptoms remain unidentified despite thorough assessment. When tests are normal or impairments unresolved, physiotherapists, exercise physiologists, and other health professionals can support patients by building skills to manage symptoms, conserve energy, and enhance wellbeing.

11.4.1 Subjective Assessment

Conduct a thorough assessment to screen for red flags needing urgent medical review (see Figure 11.1). Overlapping symptoms may complicate assessment, but tools like the Post-COVID symptom map[1] and activity diaries can identify symptom profiles and PEM triggers.[14] Prioritise assessment by clinical urgency and patient preference and adopt a flexible approach that complements the roles of other MDT members.

A variety of assessments address the many symptoms of Long COVID (see Table 11.1). Physiotherapists and exercise physiologists may also support people with autonomic dysfunction in combination with medical specialists, and these assessments and associated interventions are discussed in detail in Chapter 16.

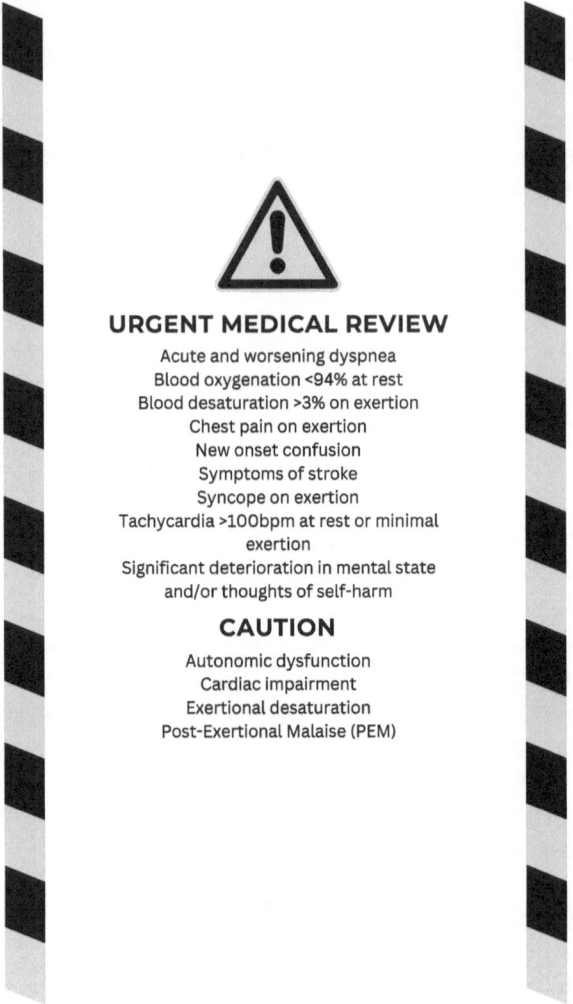

URGENT MEDICAL REVIEW

Acute and worsening dyspnea
Blood oxygenation <94% at rest
Blood desaturation >3% on exertion
Chest pain on exertion
New onset confusion
Symptoms of stroke
Syncope on exertion
Tachycardia >100bpm at rest or minimal exertion
Significant deterioration in mental state and/or thoughts of self-harm

CAUTION

Autonomic dysfunction
Cardiac impairment
Exertional desaturation
Post-Exertional Malaise (PEM)

Figure 11.1 Red flags for urgent medical review and cautions.[15,16]

11.4.2 Assessment Rationale

11.4.2.1 Cardiac Impairment

Physical activity interventions should be implemented with caution in patients with cardiac dysfunction and require ongoing monitoring.[16] Symptoms may include chest pain, tightness, irregular heart rate (HR), tachycardia, excessive breathlessness at rest or with minimal exertion, and fatigue. Cardiac symptoms are common after COVID-19 and may result from microvascular angina, myocardial infarction, pulmonary embolism, pericarditis, or myocarditis.[16,26]

Table 11.1 Physical Assessments for Evaluating Long COVID Symptoms

Impairment/Issue	Assessments
Autonomic	Orthostatic intolerance: Lying and standing BP, NASA 10-minute lean test,[17] Composite Symptom Score 31 (COMPASS 31)[18]
Cardiac	Cardiac risk stratification before resuming exercise Vital sign monitoring (BP, HR)
Fatigue	Activity diary[13] including physical symptoms and functional issues (at least 7 days) DSQ-PEM[10–12,] Fatigue Severity Scale[19]
Musculoskeletal	Pain: Numerical Pain Rating Scale[20]
Respiratory	Screening for • Oxygen saturation • Breathlessness – Nijmegen Questionnaire,[21] Self-Evaluation of Breathing Tool,[22] and the Brompton Breathing Pattern Assessment Tool[23] • Cough – Leicester Cough Questionnaire.[24] Review of medication effects, gastro-oesophageal reflux disease and lung pathology. • Inspiratory stridor or voice changes – Vocal fold Dysfunction Questionnaire[25]

Note: BP = Blood Pressure, HR = Heart Rate.

11.4.2.2 Fatigue Assessment

Fatigue significantly affects daily function and participation and is linked to PEM, POTS, and Mast Cell Activation Syndrome (see Chapter 2). It arises when the cardiorespiratory system cannot meet the muscles' oxygen demands, triggering anaerobic metabolism. However, skeletal anaerobiosis alone does not fully explain the fatigue in Long COVID, and other causes and autonomic dysfunction must be considered. Differentiating fatigue from PEM as distinct, but closely related, symptoms will aid management.

11.4.2.3 Musculoskeletal Impairment

Pain in people with Long COVID may be generalised or focal, changing over time or with exertion. Consider referral to General Practitioner or specialists to exclude rheumatological or autoimmune conditions and for the medical management of pain if required. Consider that assessment and treatment of muscle atrophy and weakness may trigger PEM.

11.4.2.4 Respiratory Impairment

Dyspnoea affects 40% of people with Long COVID, and 20% experience a chronic cough.[27] Other symptoms may include chest tightness or pain, and fatigue.[26] Respiratory dysfunction may result from lung pathology such as fibrosis and small airway disease, perfusion deficits, air trapping, airway inflammation, clotting dysfunction, impaired lung function,[26] breathing pattern disorder,[28] respiratory muscle weakness,[29] and inducible laryngeal obstruction.[30] Consider referral for pulmonary function tests, breathing pattern retraining,[16] or other management by an experienced cardio-respiratory physiotherapist or speech pathologist, if required.[30]

11.5 PHYSICAL ACTIVITY TESTING

Physical rehabilitation in Long COVID focuses on exploring physical activity, fatigue, and factors limiting capability.[31] Cardiopulmonary exercise testing (CPET) protocols are the gold standard for measuring physiological responses. They assess functional capacity and the integration of pulmonary, cardiovascular, and skeletal muscle systems, revealing disturbances in cardiac and respiratory function. Single CPET protocols may not demonstrate impairment and only identify deconditioning. A CPET protocol, when repeated within 24 hours (2dCPET), can differentiate between PEM and deconditioning.[32]

CPET has inherent risks for people with severe PEM, including prolonged symptom exacerbation, reduced baseline function, and potential functional deterioration. People with Long COVID should receive accessible, evidence-based information on CPET risks as part of shared decision-making (see Chapter 21). Moore et al.[33] found people with ME/CFS averaged two weeks to recover from CPET, compared to two days for sedentary controls, with over 10% taking more than three weeks. Hodges et al.[34] report the duration of PEM doubles following a repeated CPET. Understandably, people with Long COVID may decline this assessment to avoid exacerbating PEM.

The risks and benefits of this assessment should be weighed, informed consent obtained, and best practices followed. Health professionals should carefully consider whether the insights gained would meaningfully impact treatment plans, and whether the patient understands PEM well enough to predict and monitor symptoms. However, CPET results may provide validating evidence of the physiological impact of Long COVID, particularly when other test results have been within normal limits. In the absence of CPET, the 6-minute walk test[35] requires minimal equipment and is simple to complete. The following best practices are recommended if CPET is implemented in practice.

BOX 11.6   BEST PRACTICES FOR CPET TESTING IN LONG COVID[26]

- Is exercise testing necessary?[14]
  - Can baseline function be determined from activity diaries?
- Adopt strict inclusion and exclusion criteria for CPET testing.
  - Screen patients rigorously to identify those at risk of severe PEM or complications.
  - Use pre- and post-test outcomes to monitor symptoms for exacerbation.
  - Consider digital tools like symptom-tracking apps to streamline assessments.
- CPET protocols may need to be adapted to minimise the risk of PEM.
  - Conducting CPET sub maximally.
  - Focus on ventilatory and anaerobic thresholds.
  - Use lower starting intensities, smaller workload increments, and clear termination criteria.
  - Always prioritise patient safety.
- Use patient-centred approaches.
  - Explain and discuss the risks of overexertion.
  - Replace motivational phrases (e.g., "keep going as long as you can") with supportive ones like "Stay comfortably within your capacity" and "It's important that you don't overdo it."
  - Clearly outline the purpose, risks, and safety measures of CPET to ensure patients feel heard, understood, and respected.
- Enable accessible testing.
  - Allow patients sufficient time to complete protocols.
  - Provide resting spaces and recovery time after tests.
    Reduce cognitive and physical load by offering pre-assessment completion of outcome measures.
- Provide a COVID safe testing environment
  - Use masks, well-ventilated venues, and infection prevention protocols.

11.6 PHYSICAL INTERVENTIONS FOR PEOPLE WITH LONG COVID

11.6.1 Pacing

Pacing is a key strategy for managing PEM and other symptoms of Long COVID, and for enabling patients to maximise their participation in daily life. It plays an important role in physical rehabilitation. Please see Chapter 12 for an extensive discussion on its implementation.

11.6.2 Respiratory Interventions

Rehabilitation may involve respiratory muscle training (inspiratory and expiratory) without PEM to improve dyspnoea, functional capacity, and quality of life.[29] A systematic review of seven studies showed significant gains in maximum inspiratory and expiratory pressure, quality of life, and reduced dyspnoea.[36] Physiotherapists can manage chronic cough using airway clearance, cough suppression, breathing retraining, and nasopharyngeal hygiene. Studies confirm respiratory telerehabilitation for Long COVID is effective and safe for those unable to attend clinics.[37]

11.6.3 HR Monitoring

Aerobic physical activity is often prescribed using a percentage (50%–70%) of derived age predicted maximum HR (220 minus age).[38] However, people with Long COVID may present with chronotropic intolerance and not have the capacity to reach the predicted maximal HR. Therefore, the maximum HR obtained by cardiopulmonary exercise testing should form the basis of physical rehabilitation rather than a derived percentage HR.

BOX 11.7   PRACTICE POINT

A 37-year-old female with Long COVID completed cardiopulmonary exercise testing, achieving a peak HR of 152 bpm. Using 220-age, what is her age-predicted maximal HR? Would prescribing aerobic activity at 50%–70% differ using her actual HR versus the predicted equation?

It's crucial to base activity recommendations on data from the person with Long COVID, not predicted equations.

HR monitors can help people with Long COVID stay within the anaerobic energy system[14] and improve their physical capabilities. A physiotherapy management model for ME/CFS[39] suggests keeping HR 10% below the anaerobic threshold and using short duration activities (~2 minutes) to reduce strain on the patients' impaired cardiovascular system. In an international ME/CFS study,[40] respondents reported HR monitoring improved their activity management, quality of life, and daily participation. However, potential limitations to HR monitoring include health professional and patient digital literacy, access to wearable devices, and personal preferences.

The Borg rating of Perceived Exertion (RPE) scale[41] offers an alternative for monitoring method for patients on beta blockers or with cardiac/autonomic dysfunction. Maintaining an RPE below levels 13–15 (the anaerobic threshold) is key to managing PEM.[9,39] People living with Long COVID should keep within their energy envelope, the World Health Organization (WHO) Borg CR-10 pacing protocol may provide useful guidance.[42] Establishing a symptom-free baseline within daily activities should be achieved prior to considering return to more demanding physical activity or structured exercise.

BOX 11.8   ANGELA'S STORY

Many people with Long COVID enter rehabilitation with prior knowledge of PEM management practices, but Angela admits her current strategies are sometimes ineffective.

> *Sometimes I choose to do something I know will hit me hard later because I want to live my life. For example, I went to a PINK concert earlier this year. I rested for most of the week leading up to the concert. I wore ear plugs and noise cancelling headphones to the event and went on my mobility scooter. I took snacks, drank electrolytes and did all the things I could to mitigate the sensory overload but I knew I was in for hell afterwards... I loved the concert but there was a massive cost to me and my family.*

Reflecting on this chapter, how would you help Angela find effective strategies to manage her PEM symptoms? What assessment, intervention, and monitoring options might you present as part of shared decision-making?

11.7 CONCLUSION

This chapter emphasises the need for robust symptom assessments to create tailored physical rehabilitation for people with Long COVID. Health professionals must recognise red flags and precautions in physical rehabilitation for Long COVID and conduct thorough screening to ensure safety. Activity tracking underpins rehabilitation by focusing on what is achievable, rather than urging people to "push through." Interventions must be flexible, symptom-titrated, and monitored closely to prevent exacerbations or relapses. If PEM symptoms worsen or fail to improve, the approach should be discontinued immediately. Further research is needed to clarify PEM nuances in Long COVID, as they may differ from ME/CFS.

Treating a condition with limited evidence presents challenges, requiring health professionals to stay updated on research to ensure optimal rehabilitation for people with Long COVID. Listening to patients' lived experiences, acknowledging the uncertainty, and tailoring interventions help ensure compassionate and effective care.

BOX 11.9   ADDITIONAL RESOURCES

For more information on physiotherapy for Long COVID, refer to "Improving the Participation Gap: Physiotherapy for People Experiencing Long COVID" at https://oercollective.caul.edu.au/enabling-optimising-recovery-covid-19/chapter/physiotherapy-and-long-covid/.

REFERENCES

1 Ministry of Health. Clinical rehabilitation guidelines for people with Long COVID (coronovirus disease) in Aotearoa New Zealand. Wellington, New Zealand: Ministry of Health, 2022.

2 Institute of Medicine. Beyond Myalgic Encephalomyelitis/Chronic Fatigue Syndrome: Redefining an illness. Washington, 2015.

3 Chu L, et al. Deconstructing post-exertional malaise in myalgic encephalomyelitis / chronic fatigue: A patient-centred, cross sectional survey. Plos One 2018; 13. doi:10.1371/journal.pone.0197811.

4 Vøllestad NK, et al. Post-exertional malaise in daily life and experimental exercise models in patients with myalgic encephalomyelitis/chronic fatigue syndrome. Front Physiol 2023; 14. doi:10.3389/fphys.2023.1257557.

5 Loy BD, et al. The effect of a single bout of exercise on energy and fatigue states: A systematic review and meta-analysis. Fatigue: Biomed, Health Behav 2013; 1: 223–42. doi:10.3389/fpsyg.2022.907637.

6 Twomey R, et al. Chronic fatigue and postexertional malaise in people living with Long COVID: An observational study. Phys Ther 2022; 102. doi:10.1093/ptj/pzac005.

7 Wormgoor MEA, et al. Focus on post-exertional malaise when approaching ME/CFS in specialist healthcare improves satisfaction and reduces deterioration. Front Neurol 2023; 14. doi:10.3389/fneur.2023.1247698.

8 Kotb N, et al. Post-exertional malaise in pulmonary rehabilitation after COVID-19: Are we not giving enough attention? Can J Respir Crit Care Sleep Med 2023; 7: 93–118. doi:10.1080/24745332.2022.2150722.

9 Gloeckl R, et al. Practical recommendations for exercise training in patients with Long COVID with or without post-exertional malaise: A best practice proposal. Sports Med Open 2024; 10: 47. 20240424. doi:10.1186/s40798-024-00695-8.

10 Jason LA, et al. Test-retest reliability of the DePaul symptom questionnaire. Fatigue 2015; 3: 16–32. 20150108. doi:10.1080/21641846.2014.978110.

11 Bedree H, et al. The DePaul symptom questionnaire-2: A validation study. Fatigue 2019; 7: 166–79. 20190812. doi:10.1080/21641846.2019.1653471.

12 Cotler J, et al. A Brief Questionnaire to assess post-exertional malaise. Diagnostics 2018; 8 20180911. doi:10.3390/diagnostics8030066.

13 World Physiotherapy. Activity diary: Tracking your activity, rest and sleep, 2021 [Internet]. London: World Physiotherapy; 2021 [cited 2025 Feb 7]. Available from: https://world.physio/sites/default/files/2021-06/WPTD2021-ActivityTracker-Final-v1.pdf.

14 Leslie K, et al. A physiotherapist's guide to undestanding and managing ME/CFS. Jessica Kingsley, London, 2023.

15 Greenhalgh T, et al. Long COVID -an update for primary care. Brit Med J 2022; 378: e072117. doi:10.1136/bmj-2022-072117.

16 World Physiotherapy. World physiotherapy response to COVID-19 briefing paper 9- Safe rehabilitation approaches for people living with Long COVID: Physical activity and exercise. London: World Physiotherapy, 2021.

17 Lee J, et al. Hemodynamics during the 10-minute NASA Lean Test: Evidence of circulatory decompensation in a subset of ME/CFS patients. J Transl Med. 2020 Aug 15;18(1):314. doi:10.1186/s12967-020-02481-y.

18 Sletten D, et al. COMPASS 31: A refined and abbreviated composite autonomic symptom score. Mayo Clin Proc 87:12, 1196–120. doi:10.1016/j.mayocp.2012.10.013.

19 Krupp LB, et al. The fatigue severity scale. Application to patients with multiple sclerosis and systemic lupus erythematosus. Arch Neurol 1989; 46: 1121–23. doi:10.1001/archneur.1989.00520460115022.

20 Increasing the reliability and validity of pain intensity measurement in chronic pain patients. Pain 1993; 55: 195-203. DOI: 10.1016/0304-3959(93)90148-I

21 Courtney R, e al. Chapter 6.5 Questionnaires and manual methods for assessing breathing dysfunction. In: Chaitow L, Bradley D and Gilbert C, editors. Recognizing and treating breathing disorders (pp. 137–46). Edinburgh: Elsevier, 2014.

22 Courtney R, et al. Preliminary investigation of a measure of dysfunctional breathing symptoms: The self evaluation of breathing questionnaire (SEBQ). Int J Osteopath Med 2009; 12: 121–27. doi:10.1016/j.ijosm.2009.02.001.

23 Hylton H, et al. Real-world use of the Breathing Pattern Assessment Tool in assessment of breathlessness post-COVID-19. Clin Med 2022; 22: 376–79. doi:10.7861/clinmed. 2021-0759.

24 Birring SS, et al. Development of a symptom specific health status measure for patients with chronic cough: Leicester Cough Questionnaire (LCQ). Thorax 2003; 58: 339. doi:10.1136/thorax.58.4.339.

25 Fowler SJ, et al. The VCDQ--a Questionnaire for symptom monitoring in vocal cord dysfunction. Clin Exp Allergy. 2015 Sep;45(9):1406–11. doi:10.1111/cea.12550.

26 Faghy MA, et al. Using cardiorespiratory fitness assessment to identify pathophysiology in long COVID - Best practice approaches. Prog Cardiovasc Dis 2024; 83: 55–61. doi:10.1016/j.pcad.2024.02.005.

27 Davis HE, et al. Long COVID: Major findings, mechanisms and recommendations. Nat Rev Microbiol 2023; 21: 133–46. doi:10.1038/s41579-022-00846-2.

28 Frizzelli A, et al. An impairment in resting and exertional breathing pattern may occur in Long-COVID patients with normal spirometry and unexplained dyspnoea. J Clin Med 2022;11:20221213. doi:10.3390/jcm11247388.

29 Xavier DM, et al. Effects of respiratory muscular training in post-covid-19 patients: A systematic review and meta-analysis of randomized controlled trials. BMC Sports Sci Med Rehabil 2024;16:181. doi:10.1186/s13102-024-00954-x.

30 Abou-Elsaad T, et al. Persistent shortness of breath in post-COVID-19 patients: Inducible laryngeal obstruction can be a cause. J Voice 2024; 20240222. doi:10.1016/j.jvoice.2024.01.018.

31 Noakes T. Physiological models to understand exercise fatigue and the adaptions that predict or enhance athletic performance. Scan J med Sci 2000;10:123–45. doi:10.1034/j.1600-0838.2000.010003123.x.

32 Hodges LD, et al. Physiological measures in participants with chronic fatigue syndrome, multiple sclerosis and healthy controls following repeated exercise: A pilot study. Clin Physiol Funct Imaging, 2018; 38: 639–44. doi:10.1111/cpf.12460.

33 Moore GE, et al. Recovery from exercise in persons with Myalgic Encephalomyelitis / Chronic Fatigue Syndrome (ME/CFS). Medicina 2023; 59: 571. doi:10.3390/medicina59030571.

34 Hodges L, et al. The physiological time line of post-exertional malaise in Myalgic Encephalomyelitis/Chronic Fatigue Syndrome (ME/CFS). Transl Sports Med 2020; 3: 243–49. doi:10.1002/tsm2.133.

35 The American Thoracic Society. ATS statement: Guidelines for the six-minute walk. Am J Respir Crit Care Med 2002;166:111–17. doi:10.1164/rccm.166/1/111.

36 Calvache-Mateo A, et al. Respiratory training effects in Long COVID-19 patients: A systematic review and meta-analysis. Expert Rev Respir Med 2024:1–11. doi:10.1080/17476348.2024.2358933.

37 Calvache-Mateo A, et al. Efficacy and safety of respiratory telerehabilitation in patients with Long COVID-19: A systematic review and meta-analysis. Healthcare 2023;11:20230912. doi:10.3390/healthcare11182519.

38 Fox SM, et al. Physical activity and the prevention of coronary heart disease. Ann Clin Res 1971;3(6):404–32.

39 Davenport TE, et al. Conceptual model for physical therapist management of chronic fatigue syndrome/myalgic encephalomyelitis. Phys Ther 2010;90:602–14. doi:10.2522/ptj.20090047.

40 Clague-Baker N, et al. An international survey of experiences and attitudes towards pacing using a heart rate monitor for people with myalgic encephalomyelitis/chronic fatigue syndrome. Work 2023;74:1225–34. doi:10.3233/WOR-220512.

41 Williams N. The Borg Rating of Perceived Exertion (RPE) scale. Occup Med 2017;67:404–5. doi:10.1093/occmed/kqx063.

42 Parker M, et al. Effect of using a structured pacing protocol on post-exertional symptom exacerbation and health status in a longitudinal cohort with the post-COVID-19 syndrome. J Med Virol 2022; 95:e28373. doi:10.1002/jmv.28373.

Chapter 12

Optimising Participation in Everyday Life for People with Long COVID

Jenean Whitman, Hayley Scott, Sharon Neale, and Danielle Hitch

---

BOX 12.1 LEARNING OBJECTIVES

By the end of this chapter, readers should be able to:

- Analyse how Long COVID causes activity limitations and participation restrictions.
- Use the International Classification of Function (ICF) framework to assess the complex interplay between personal, environmental, and health-related factors affecting people with Long COVID.
- Develop and adapt evidence-informed strategies such as activity modification, energy conservation, cognitive interventions, and assistive technology to enable participation in meaningful activities.
- Evaluate the importance of lived experiences in shaping interventions and integrate person-centred approaches to improve engagement and self-efficacy in daily life.

12.1 INTRODUCTION

Participation in everyday tasks and activities is vital to human health and wellbeing.[1] Most people take their ability to engage in meaningful roles and activities for granted until illness, life changes, or disasters disrupt it. The COVID-19 pandemic profoundly affected daily life, impacting people's ability to care for themselves, their homes, and their communities.[2] This impact was compounded for people with Long COVID, who experience additional significant disruptions that persist for months or even years.

DOI: 10.4324/9781003528104-16

This chapter outlines evidence-informed interventions that help people with Long COVID regain or adapt their participation in daily life, including task modification, energy conservation, anxiety management, cognitive strategies, and assistive technology. Occupational therapists specialise in the relationship between activity participation and health, though all health professions play a role in supporting people with Long COVID to live their best lives. Through these approaches, this chapter underscores the importance of personalised care for people with Long COVID, which enables improved self-efficacy, confidence, and engagement in daily life. As stated by a participant in our research,[3]

> *The symptoms are what Long COVID is, but the impact it has on my life is what it means.*
>
> Research Participant

BOX 12.2   PRACTICE POINT

Pause and reflect on everything you have done today. What activities did you participate in? Who did you do them with? Where were they done? How often do you do them? Now, recall the last time you were injured or ill. How did it affect your ability to participate in meaningful and enjoyable activities?

12.2 A FRAMEWORK FOR UNDERSTANDING THE IMPACT OF LONG COVID ON DAILY LIFE

The International Classification of Functioning, Disability, and Health (ICF) provides a framework for understanding factors affecting participation in daily life. Developed by the World Health Organization (WHO) in 1980, it offers a standard language and framework for describing influences on health and wellbeing. The ICF measures and describes health and disability at individual and population levels and is endorsed by all WHO Member States as the international standard for describing health and disability.[4] See Chapter 1 for further details on how this textbook aligns with ICF concepts.

The ICF describes the interaction between health conditions and a person's body functions and structures, activities, and participation. It also considers the impact of contextual factors like the environment and personal characteristics. Health conditions refer to diseases or disorders that can be diagnosed, reflecting a Western orientation to health. The health condition of interest here is Long COVID;

however, people may live with multiple conditions, and interventions to increase participation must account for all comorbidities. For example, Postural Orthostatic Tachycardia Syndrome, Mast Cell Activation Syndrome, and other diagnoses may co-occur with Long COVID (as discussed in Chapter 2).

> *I did not have any of the typical comorbidities you hear about with COVID, but since having Long COVID, I have been diagnosed with several other medical conditions including obstructive sleep apnoea, hypermobility spectrum disorder and dysautonomia. Some of these things may have developed later in life, but they seem to have developed much sooner than otherwise expected, probably due to Long COVID.*

> Jenean

Body functions refer to how the body and mind work, including the roles of body structures such as organs and limbs. Problems with these functions or structures, such as fatigue, brain fog, or pain, are known as impairments. Many Western health approaches focus almost exclusively on body structures and functions. However, the ICF innovatively includes contextual factors that may positively or negatively affect activity participation. Environmental factors involve the physical and social surroundings in which people live, including products and technology; the natural and built environment; services and policies, including cultural, economic, and political systems; and social attitudes, supports, and relationships. For people with Long COVID, typical examples include physical barriers (like stairs in a workplace), a lack of specialist services, and negative attitudes from health professionals and the community. Personal factors include gender, age, social background, education, culture, past and current experiences, and personality.

Activity and participation arise from the complex interactions of all ICF components. Activity (also called function) refers to a person's ability to perform daily tasks such as showering, housework, or socialising with family, friends, and others. An activity limitation occurs when someone struggles with or cannot perform these tasks. For instance, a person with Long COVID might struggle to do their laundry due to fatigue or return to work due to brain fog.

While activity focuses on functional ability, participation emphasises meaningful involvement in societal or personal contexts. Participation describes a person's ability to perform essential roles, such as a partner, child, or workmate, and to function in environments like the home, workplace, and community. Participation restrictions occur when people with Long COVID face limitations in performing relevant activities. For example, they may be unable to complete the activities required of their roles as a worker, parent, sporting team member, or volunteer due to the symptoms they experience. These limitations significantly affect their ability to engage in life roles, routines, and health and wellbeing.

The ICF enables health professionals to take a more comprehensive perspective than those offered by biopsychosocial health models and consider broader social and contextual factors influencing recovery. Applying the ICF allows health professionals to provide tailored, contextually relevant interventions that promote meaningful participation and improve the quality of life for people with Long COVID.

BOX 12.3   PRACTICE POINT

Consider someone with Long COVID you know or have worked with. Write some notes about their bodily structures and functions, personal factors, environment, activity, and participation and use these to present the case to your colleagues. You may wish to refer to the ICF browser (https://apps. who.int/classifications/icfbrowser/) for detailed descriptions of all ICF components. From your perspective, what are the potential advantages and disadvantages of applying the ICF to your work with people with Long COVID?

12.3 A MODEL OF FUNCTION AND PARTICIPATION FOR PEOPLE WITH LONG COVID

The activity and participation components of the ICF encompass nine areas of life,[5,6] and those with the highest cognitive, physical, and emotional demands cause the most activity limitation and participation restrictions for people with Long COVID (see Figure 12.1).

Long COVID affects participation in highly individualised ways, fluctuating over time and varying based on life experiences, personal circumstances, and impairments. The order of life areas presented here is a general model and may differ for each person or specific symptoms. For example, a person with POTs may experience the most difficulty with mobility due to the impact of physical exertion and orthostatic intolerance. Health professionals may encounter different functional issues depending on their service setting. For instance, services working with Intensive Care Unit survivors may see more problems in life areas requiring higher physical demands due to critical illness myopathy.[7]

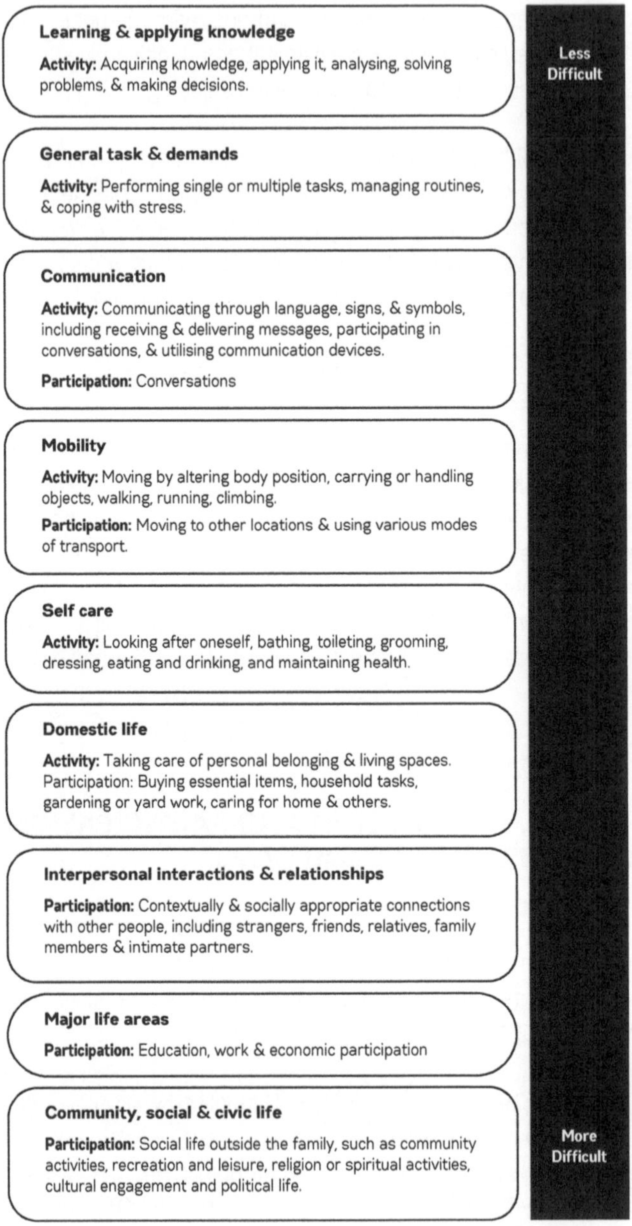

Learning & applying knowledge

Activity: Acquiring knowledge, applying it, analysing, solving problems, & making decisions.

General task & demands

Activity: Performing single or multiple tasks, managing routines, & coping with stress.

Communication

Activity: Communicating through language, signs, & symbols, including receiving & delivering messages, participating in conversations, & utilising communication devices.

Participation: Conversations

Mobility

Activity: Moving by altering body position, carrying or handling objects, walking, running, climbing.

Participation: Moving to other locations & using various modes of transport.

Self care

Activity: Looking after oneself, bathing, toileting, grooming, dressing, eating and drinking, and maintaining health.

Domestic life

Activity: Taking care of personal belonging & living spaces. Participation: Buying essential items, household tasks, gardening or yard work, caring for home & others.

Interpersonal interactions & relationships

Participation: Contextually & socially appropriate connections with other people, including strangers, friends, relatives, family members & intimate partners.

Major life areas

Participation: Education, work & economic participation

Community, social & civic life

Participation: Social life outside the family, such as community activities, recreation and leisure, religion or spiritual activities, cultural engagement and political life.

Less Difficult

More Difficult

Figure 12.1 Model of function and participation for people with Long COVID.

More complex areas of life highlight the subtle and nuanced impact of Long COVID symptoms. As cognitive, physical, and emotional demands increase, minor limitations and restrictions become more apparent. Self-care activities are learnt early in life and rely heavily on routines – structured sequences of activities that reduce effort over time through practice and familiarity. Domestic tasks like housework and gardening require more physical and cognitive effort but are generally not emotionally demanding. These tasks are performed in a familiar environment over which the person has control. Major life areas, as well as community, social, and civic life, exert greater physical, social, and emotional demands and often occur in environments where the person has little or no control. A similar gradient of difficulty exists in interpersonal interactions and relationships, with familiarity with family and friends posing fewer demands than interactions with strangers.

Small deficits may be within the "normal" range on standardised tests but still significantly and meaningfully impact daily life. For example,

> *I've been an engineer all my life, so I've always been pretty 'switched on'. But now I do silly little things all the time, like forget to bring my wallet into the petrol station to pay for my fuel. Might be a little thing to you, but it's so frustrating and humiliating for me.*
>
> Research Participant

Function and participation for people with Long COVID should always include ipsative assessment alongside criterion-referenced or population-normed assessments. For more information about "measuring what matters" for people with Long COVID, see Chapter 6.

BOX 12.4   TYPES OF ASSESSMENT AND OUTCOME MEASUREMENT

Criterion referenced assessment measures and benchmarks a person's current performance against a predetermined set of criteria. They are used to evaluate whether the person has a specific standard of skill or knowledge.

Ipsative assessment compares a person's current performance to their previous performance, focusing on personal progress or change over time. A person's rehabilitation goals provide standards against which progress or change is measured.

Population normed assessment measurement tool that compares a person's current performance against the average performance of other similar people. This average provides a "norm" or population reference and represents what is typical for that group or the general population.

Even a 5% loss of function can have serious consequences for function and participation for individuals, and many people with Long COVID experience more significant deficits. Under-recognition of the impact of mild symptoms can entrench limitations and restrictions, particularly in complex community life areas. Evidence of the longer-term consequences of unaddressed functional and participation issues comes from the 2003 Severe Acute Respiratory Syndrome (SARS) pandemic,[8] also caused by a novel coronavirus. Fifteen years after infection, around 13% of SARS patients remained on long-term sick leave from employment.[9] The lived experience of people with Long COVID highlights how easily its hidden impacts on function and participation can be underestimated, underscoring the importance of proactively treating activity limitations and participation restrictions.

After almost three years with Long COVID, I may appear functional. You might see me lifting weights at the gym twice a week, having coffee with a friend, or attending school events with my kids. What's unseen is the drastic reduction in my activities: from full-time work and frequent exercise (Pilates, swimming, walking, bike riding, and gym six times a week) to two carefully paced gym sessions and gentle at-home Pilates most weeks. Cognitive tasks like medical appointments must be scheduled on separate days to avoid post-exertional malaise or a full crash. What looks functional is only achieved through strict pacing and immense effort, and its only 35%–40% of my pre-Long COVID capacity, even on a good day.

Jenean

BOX 12.5   PRACTICE POINT

The lived experience of people with Long COVID underpins interventions to improve function and participation. Your lived experience informs your clinical reasoning around enabling their participation. Reflect on what you would do if a patient wanted to return to an activity you have never personally experienced.

12.4 STRATEGIES AND INTERVENTIONS TO ENABLE PARTICIPATION IN DAILY LIFE

Many health professions provide strategies and interventions to support participation in daily life for people with Long COVID. However, referral to an occupational therapist should be considered for anyone with Long COVID who is facing difficulties with activity or participation. Occupational therapists are person-centred professionals specialising in the relationship between health, wellbeing, and engagement in meaningful activities and roles[10] (see Chapter 9). Their goal is to enable participation in daily life by enhancing activity performance, modifying activities or environments to promote engagement, or providing support to prevent deterioration.

12.4.1 Activity Modification

Activity modification (or grading) involves adapting activities to help people with Long COVID achieve better function and participation. Tasks can be made more complex to increase therapeutic benefit, such as placing objects further away to improve balance or adding weight to build strength. Tasks can also be made easier, such as using larger handles to compensate for reduced grip strength or simplifying processes to reduce cognitive and/or physical demands.

Activity modification is often mistaken for Graded Exercise Therapy (GET) but differs in focus and application. GET aims to improve physical fitness through structured, incremental increases in exercise intensity, often following a set protocol, regardless of symptom exacerbation. In contrast, activity modification gradually increases engagement in meaningful activities tailored to each person's capacity and symptoms, emphasising energy conservation and avoiding overexertion. This strategy is based on comprehensive task analysis, which breaks down an activity into its component parts to understand its physical, cognitive, sensory, emotional, and environmental demands. This analysis identifies limitations and restrictions and guides tailored strategies to improve participation. Activity modification cannot effectively or safely meet patients' needs or goals without task analysis.

The key to activity modification is finding the right level of challenge for the person's current skill level, enabling optimal improvement. A study of occupational therapy for people with Long COVID[3] reported significant benefits from a safe, graded approach to practising daily activities and building confidence and self-esteem over time. As described by a participant, their path to independently showering began with using a shower seat, "then I practiced standing in the shower." Others in this study requiring daily oxygen were supported to continue performing meaningful activities by raising the bed head height to improve sleep, using a trolley for easier oxygen cylinder access, and carrying objects while cooking.

BOX 12.6 PRACTICE POINT

There are countless ways to implement activity modification, depending on the unique and dynamic interactions between the person with Long COVID, their environment, and the activity they aim to undertake. Consider Jenean's lived experience and identify the various activity modification approaches used to maintain participation,

If you can adapt important activities to be Long COVID-friendly, it can make a big difference. I loved volunteering at my kid's school and previously managed the Treasurer role (3–5 hours weekly) alongside full-time work, but that's no longer possible. Instead, I attend most meetings with careful pacing, take on small admin tasks I can complete over weeks, and help at events in ways that fit my limits, such as short, seated shifts. For one-off events, I plan extra rest before and after, bring a friend to assist, avoid other activities on the day, and use strategies like earplugs, electrolytes, and pacing. While I can't manage music festivals or venues without seating, careful planning allows me to attend seated concerts. I can manage a little more activity on some days for important occasions but need to do less activity the following days to recover back to my baseline.

12.4.2 Managing the Stress of Living with Long COVID

Long COVID is a physiological disorder that is not caused by psychological dysfunction. However, living with this disruptive and unpredictable condition can harm mental health. Dysautonomia can also result in heightened awareness and responsiveness to stimuli.[11]

When your entire life is turned upside down and you must work out new ways to approach everyday life, it has a massive impact on wellbeing.

Jenean

Feelings of fear, anxiety, and being overwhelmed by the thought of completing daily activities are commonly experienced by people with Long COVID. This fear can relate to shortness of breath or the potential for inducing a relapse or "crash" and reduces their ability to complete daily activities and their overall quality of life. Health professionals provide various interventions such as medication, cognitive behavioural therapy, and relaxation strategies to manage these symptoms, as discussed in Chapter 14. Other nonpharmacological strategies can also be used alongside daily activities to maximise function and participation.

For example, an occupational therapist may begin a rehabilitation session with guided visualisation, where the person imagines themselves completing a meaningful activity, such as gardening, without difficulties. Psychoeducation may then be provided about the fear cycle and its impact on gardening to empower the person with Long COVID with information about their condition and challenge distorted perceptions. Once gardening begins, the occupational therapist may guide the person through deep breathing techniques and supported problem solving to prevent symptom escalation. After the activity, they would reflect on the session's success with the person with Long COVID, focusing on which strategies were most effective for future use. This example illustrates strategies before, during, and after an activity to manage fear, anxiety, and being overwhelmed and improve participation in daily life. Collaboration with psychologists and neuropsychologists working with the patient is also recommended to provide additional mental health resources and expertise to optimise participation in daily life for the person with Long COVID.

Many people with Long COVID have already developed their own coping strategies, and these should be incorporated into rehabilitation strategies wherever possible,

> *Work with patients to understand the limits they are likely already very aware of and start off incredibly slowly within those limits. If there is no resulting crash, you can build conservatively from there by including them in all decisions and taking on board their input about what they can and cannot currently manage. Most of us will have a really good idea of what has pushed us over the limit previously and want to avoid those things for self-preservation and to reduce our suffering.*
>
> Jenean

12.4.3 Energy Conservation and Pacing

People with Long COVID often have limited energy and must use it wisely to engage in meaningful activities. Many describe their energy needs using spoon theory, where each unit of energy is a spoon, and activities cost varying spoons.[12] For example, getting dressed may cost one spoon, while housework may cost three spoons. If someone with Long COVID has 12 spoons for the day, they must carefully plan to avoid running out of spoons. In contrast, a healthy person may have 50 or even unlimited spoons.

Self-management strategies like energy conservation and pacing effectively support people with Long COVID to maintain function and participation in daily life. Energy conservation reduces fatigue and enables participation in desired activities, often through pacing. Pacing involves alternating between rest and activity to manage energy levels, prevent overexertion, and minimise the risk of Post-Exertional Malaise. Activities are performed at less than maximum energy capacity by breaking activities into shorter segments and incorporating frequent rest. Prioritising tasks and taking regular breaks help people with Long COVID conserve energy and achieve balanced energy expenditure. As described here,[3]

> It's okay to sit and rest. It's a process. It'll take time and every day, you'll make small steps [which] really helped me build my confidence again.
>
> Taylor[1]

Pacing is a highly individualised intervention tailored to each person's symptoms, triggers, and meaningful activities.[13] Some people focus on maintaining energy levels rather than increasing activity, while others may experience gradual improvements, enabling slow increases in participation. Periods of remission can allow significant activity enhancement. Effective pacing strategies must be customised to meet each person's needs, abilities, and context.

BOX 12.7   THE LIVED EXPERIENCE OF PACING

Pacing is difficult to learn and hard to stick to, but it is arguably the most effective and accessible way to manage symptoms and establish a stable baseline. I have found pre-emptive rest amazingly helpful. I thought breaking up activities by sitting on the couch or doing light tasks while seated was rest, but it wasn't effective at recharging my energy. I've learned that forcing yourself to rest before symptoms increase – even on days you feel comparatively better – can be very effective. Before practising pre-emptive rest, I thought I was doing well with pacing, but when I started tracking my activities, I realised I was doing more than I thought and not resting enough. There's often a gap between the intention to rest and actually doing it. Limited capacity and increased mental load make this even harder.

Tracking daily activities can be eye-opening. I was surprised by how many small tasks I was doing that added up significantly – especially for someone with Long COVID. Recording activity may not appeal to everyone, but even a few weeks or a month can provide valuable insights. The more you understand your energy patterns, the better you can manage activity safely. Clear limits make it easier to stick to helpful boundaries (e.g., only socialising with one friend at a time for an hour in a quiet location). This reduces the mental effort of constantly assessing your capacity, which can be exhausting. Spending ten minutes planning each week's main activities helps me be more productive and avoid big crashes. If symptoms increase, I can review my plan to pinpoint what I overdid. Planning saves energy and makes it easier to manage symptoms effectively.

I do not want anyone to read this and think that pacing is easy. It is incredibly challenging, and we all have some days that are more disciplined than others. Please be extremely kind to yourself through this. Beating yourself up does not achieve anything and is likely to prolong your suffering if you have overdone it. Self-compassion has helped me so much with all of the challenges with Long COVID.

Jenean

The following tips (see Figure 12.2) will support health professionals and people with Long COVID to successfully implement energy conservation and pacing.

BOX 12.8   TYPES OF ASSESSMENT AND OUTCOME MEASUREMENT

For comprehensive information about pacing strategies for people with Long COVID, please read the dedicated chapter in *Enabling and Optimising Recovery from COVID-19: A Handbook for Health Professionals and Other Caregivers of People with Long COVID* (https://oercollective.caul.edu.au/enabling-optimising-recovery-covid-19/).

12.4.4 Assistive Technology and Environmental Modifications

Assistive technology is an umbrella term for products or systems that enable people to maintain or improve independence and daily functioning.[14] A wide

General Tips

- Identify the times of day when fatigue is worse, and the activities that cause excess fatigue.
- Schedule activities based on patterns of energy levels throughout the day.
- Divide or spread activities across the week to avoid over-exertion on a single day.
- Allow full rest days in between activities when necessary.
- Schedule high-priority activities first to ensure there is enough energy to do the things that are most important and meaningful.
- Allow enough time to complete activities and take rest breaks between them.
- Don't wait to feel tired before taking a rest. Rest is most effective when applied before fatigue occurs or worsens.
- Conserve energy during routine tasks to reserve energy for activities that bring joy and purpose.
- Switching between cognitive and physical tasks may increase available energy and productivity.

Example Energy Saving Strategies

- Use pre-cut or prepared vegetables to minimise food preparation.
- Performing activities sitting wherever possible.
- Organising items in one place to avoid multiple trips.
- Use assistive technology (like grabbers or battery-operated scrubbing brushes) to reduce physical effort.
- Delegate tasks to formal or informal carers.
- Use timers and alarm reminders to support pacing strategies.

Key Questions for People with Long COVID

- Am I doing more than I thought?
- Am I actually resting enough between activities, and not just intending to?
- How often do I check in with myself to see how I'm feeling?
- How many major activities can I manage in a day? Do some activities need more spacing (e.g., I can't exercise on consecutive days—does this apply to cognitive tasks too)?
- How much should I reduce my load after stress, strong emotions, or an acute illness like a cold?

Figure 12.2 Tips for pacing and energy conservation.

variety of assistive technology is available, classified as either simple or complex. Simple assistive technology, such as a shower chair, is low cost, low risk, and easily sourced. In contrast, complex assistive technology is high-cost, high-risk, and requires significant time and resources to source due to often being custom-made, such as a power wheelchair. When prescribing assistive technology, Occupational

Therapists consider the environment where the product or system will be used. This may involve recommendations for simple or complex modifications to the home, workplace, or community, such as installing shower rails to support balance and fatigue or ensuring appropriate seating in the community for rest breaks while shopping.

These interventions can effectively support function and participation for people experiencing Long COVID. For example, "Sam"[3] reflected on the benefits of simple assistive technology in supporting them to participate in self-care activities, "Getting down to the toilet was hard, took too long. Now I use a higher seat [also known as an over toilet frame] which makes life easier." Other assistive technology products helpful for people with Long COVID include long-handled aids, like a long-handled sponge to reduce bending in the shower, oxygen holders for community transport, kitchen trolleys to avoid carrying heavy items, and noise-cancelling equipment. Many people also develop strategies to use equipment in new ways in place of access to rehabilitation services.

> I put a little stool on wheels in the kitchen so I can whiz around doing things without standing. I sit on the floor to unstack the dishwasher because my dysautonomia is triggered by bending down. I also hang washing on an indoor rack and sit down to fold washing. It's all about finding ways to reduce your load.
>
> Jenean

An emerging area of practice is using assistive technology and equipment to support people with Long COVID with sensory modulation. Long COVID affects many of the sensory systems, and people with this condition often report feeling more sensory disturbances, such as increased sensitivity to light and sound.[15] Sensory modulation strategies are effective for people experiencing a range of health issues, but further research is needed to confirm their effectiveness for people with Long COVID. However, these strategies are already being adopted to enable activity and participation.

> Some things that I have found helpful are taking advantage of quiet hours at shopping centres, wearing sunglasses inside if the lights are too bright and using ear plugs. I like the Loop earplugs that allow you to still hear things and join in on conversations but block out or at least dull a lot of the background noise.
>
> Jenean

12.4.5 Reducing the Cognitive Load of Activity and Participation

Occupational therapists commonly provide cognitive interventions to remediate or compensate for concentration, memory, and executive functioning issues. These interventions are embedded within activities meaningful to each person with Long COVID and are individually tailored. A common problem is brain fog, describing symptoms such as word-finding difficulties, concentration issues, memory impairment, and disorientation.[16] Cognitive strategies to increase activity and participation must address multiple limitations simultaneously. While Chapter 13 discusses cognitive interventions and supports in detail, the following strategies (Figure 12.3) are particularly relevant to enhancing activity and participation.

Tips for Managing Cognitive Load

- Use imagery mnemonics, such as acronyms (e.g., "TBA") to enhance memory recall
- Break complex information into smaller, manageable chunks to improve retention.
- Write everything down to reduce reliance on memory.
- Set phone reminders for deadlines, appointments, and preparatory tasks.
- Schedule tasks, including work, exercise, planning, and rest periods, in a calendar app.
- Assign specific locations for documents and tools to create an organised workspace.
- View rest as a productive activity that will support better activity participation.
- Use timers to prevent overcommitting to tasks and avoid fatigue.
- Plan cognitive-heavy tasks or meetings in the morning when focus and clarity are strongest.
- Recognise how fatigue impacts on cognition and problem-solving and adjust expectations accordingly.
- Communicate cognitive limitations to others, such as needing time or specific conditions to perform at your best.
- Celebrate small achievements, such as completing rest periods or managing tasks effectively.
- Accept limitations and focus on strategies to maximise functionality.

Figure 12.3 Tips for reducing the cognitive demands of activity and participation.

12.5 CONCLUSION

As the COVID-19 pandemic continues, the impact of Long COVID on participation in daily life has become increasingly evident. It is now clear that this condition can cause significant activity limitations and participation restrictions for all people with Long COVID, regardless of their acute or ongoing symptom severity. This chapter has outlined the complex interplay of factors that shape these challenges and explored strategies to enhance participation. By addressing limitations and restrictions holistically, health professionals – particularly occupational therapists – can support people with Long COVID to regain meaningful engagement in life, fostering self-efficacy, confidence, and improved quality of life. This chapter reaffirms the need for proactive, person-centred approaches to ensure that the invisible burdens of Long COVID are acknowledged and addressed effectively.

NOTE

1   'Taylor' is a pseudonym.

REFERENCES

1 Law MC. Participation in the occupations of everyday life. Am J Occup Ther. 2002;56(6):640–49. doi:10.5014/ajot.56.6.640.
2 Tull MT, et al. Psychological outcomes associated with stay-at-home orders and the perceived impact of COVID-19 on daily life. Psychiatry Res. 2020;289:113098. doi:10.1016/j.psychres.2020.113098.
3 Scott HM, et al. Occupational therapy practice for post-acute COVID-19 inpatients requiring rehabilitation. Aust Occup Ther J. 2024;71(6):940–55. doi:10.1111/1440-1630.12976.
4 Ziauddeen N, et al. Characteristics and impact of Long Covid: Findings from an online survey. PLoS One. 2022;17:e0268052. doi:10.1371/journal.pone.0264331.
5 World Health Organization. International Classification of Functioning, disability and health (ICF). Geneva: World Health Organization; 2001.
6 Australian Institute of Health and Welfare. ICF Australian user guide. Version 1.0. Canberra: AIHW; 2003.
7 Tortuyaux R, et al. Intensive care unit-acquired weakness: Questions the clinician should ask. Rev Neurol. 2022;178(1–2):84–92. doi:10.1016/j.neurol.2021.12.007.
8 Centre for Disease Control and Prevention (CDC). SARS basic fact sheet 2004 [Internet]. Atlanta: CDC; [cited 2025 Feb 7]. Available from: https://stacks.cdc.gov/view/cdc/13498.
9 Zhang P, et al. Long-term bone and lung consequences associated with hospital-acquired severe acute respiratory syndrome: A 15-year follow-up from a prospective cohort study. Bone Res. 2020;8:8. doi:10.1038/s41413-020-0084-5.

10 World Federation of Occupational Therapists (WFOT). Definitions of occupational therapy from member organisations [Internet]. Geneva: WFOT; [cited 2025 Feb 7]. Available from: https://www.wfot.org.

11 Baguley IJ, et al. Dysautonomia after severe traumatic brain injury: Evidence of persisting overresponsiveness to afferent stimuli. Am J Phys Med Rehabil. 2009;88:615–22. doi:10.1097/PHM.0b013e3181aeab96.

12 Miserandino C. The spoon theory [Internet]. But You Don't Look Sick: Unknown; [cited 2025 Feb 7]. Available from: https://butyoudontlooksick.com/articles/written-by-christine/the-spoon-theory/.

13 Long COVID Physio. Pacing [Internet]. Long COVID Physio: Unknown; [cited 2025 Feb 7]. Available from: https://longcovid.physio/pacing.

14 World Health Organisation. Assistive technology. Geneva: WHO; [cited 2025 Feb 7]. Available from: https://www.who.int/news-room/fact-sheets/detail/assistive-technology.

15 Hayes LD, et al. More than 100 persistent symptoms of SARS-CoV-2 (Long COVID): A scoping review. Front Med. 2021;8:750378. doi:10.3389/fmed.2021.750378

16 Jennings G, et al. Comprehensive clinical characterisation of brain fog in adults reporting Long COVID symptoms. J Clin Med. 2022;11(12):3440. doi:10.3390/jcm11123440.

Chapter 13

Cognitive Rehabilitation for Long COVID

James Lewis, Joanne Wrench,
Jodie McGregor, and Karen Felder

BOX 13.1   LEARNING OBJECTIVES

By the end of this chapter, readers should be able to:

- Describe the types of cognitive difficulties experienced by people with Long COVID and their impact on function.
- Understand how to assess for cognitive impairments, including barriers to participation and how to use subjective and objective measures.
- Understand a range of possible cognitive rehabilitation strategies using restoration of function and compensatory strategies.
- Appreciate the complex interplay between mood, fatigue, and cognitive difficulties.

13.1 THE COGNITIVE IMPACTS OF LONG COVID

Neurocognitive sequelae of COVID-19 became apparent early in the pandemic, with acute impacts prominent in Intensive Care Unit and hospitalised COVID-19 patients. Cognitive difficulties were initially linked to secondary neurological complications, such as delirium, stroke, and hypoxic brain injury associated with severe COVID-19 illness. As the pandemic progressed, it became clear that people with no known neurological event were also experiencing cognitive impacts. Termed by patients as brain fog, these cognitive impacts lasted months after COVID-19 infection and were increasingly described by people who had "mild" acute illness.[1]

DOI: 10.4324/9781003528104-17

BOX 13.2 WHAT IS BRAIN FOG?

Brain fog is not a medical term, but it is a well understood and accessible way for people with Long COVID to describe cognitive "clouding" or changes to normal cognitive functioning. Brain fog is often associated with slowed thinking, difficulty concentrating, and memory lapses.

Health professionals should carefully unpack what brain fog means for each person because it encompasses a range of cognitive difficulties. Evaluation may be via clinical interview and/or cognitive assessments.

In addition to acute neurological injury (e.g., stroke or hypoxic brain injury), hypothesised mechanisms for cognitive changes in Long COVID include metabolic disturbances, persistent inflammatory or abnormal immune responses, and latent viral persistence.[2,3] Cognitive function can also be impacted by mood, sleep, and fatigue difficulties common in Long COVID.[4,5]

Research on the prevalence of cognitive difficulties in Long COVID is confounded by considerable variability in study design, including sampling, measurement, and timeframes. Despite this, there is growing consensus that cognitive difficulties are one of the most reported symptoms of Long COVID, with an estimated prevalence of around 20–50%.[6] Severity of acute illness is linked to Long COVID cognitive difficulties; however, many people with initially "mild" COVID-19 still report highly impactful cognitive changes.[7]

13.1.1 Types of Cognitive Difficulties in Long COVID

There is no "diagnostic pattern" of cognitive deficits in Long COVID. Studies report varied impairments across all domains of cognitive functioning, including memory, executive functioning, attention, speed of processing, language, and perception.[8,9] The most commonly identified deficits in formal assessment are executive dysfunction (e.g., problem-solving, shifting between competing demands, working memory), along with reduced attention and processing speed. These reflect self-reported "brain fog" and may negatively impact other cognitive processes, such as memory. At a group level, deficits tend to be in the order of 6–10% reduction when compared to normative data.[7,9]

13.1.2 Course of Cognitive Difficulties

Like most Long COVID symptoms, the course of cognitive deficits over time is variable. Many people have improvement over time, whilst others find delayed onset of difficulties or periods of recovery followed by re-emergence of symptoms. This may occur over the longer term (months) or even day to day (good and bad days). There is some evidence that symptoms present at six months remain at two to three years.[10]

13.2 ASSESSMENT OF COGNITION IN LONG COVID

Cognitive screening tests may not reliably detect cognitive impairment in Long COVID[11] and subjective reports of cognitive concerns alone may not be good predictors of cognitive test performance.[8] An assessment approach that includes subjective and objective measures (see Chapter 6) of cognitive changes as well as measures of fatigue, functional participation, and psychological factors such as depression and anxiety is advised.[12] Comprehensive neuropsychological assessments may be helpful in identifying and characterising cognitive difficulties for some people.

13.2.1 Clinical Interview

The dismissal or minimisation of cognitive concerns is commonly experienced by people with Long COVID, leading to mistrust in the healthcare system. Taking the time to listen and acknowledge self-reported difficulties is fundamental to building trust within the therapeutic setting. It can be challenging for many people with Long COVID to describe the fluctuating and variable impact of their cognitive symptoms,[13] finding ways to support the individual to articulate their experience is important.

Key information to obtain includes the course of the person's symptoms across acute post-infection (< 4 week), subacute (4–12 week), and chronic (>12 week) periods. Importantly, clinical interviews can help determine if symptoms are new or an exacerbation of a pre-infection condition and can help inform the next steps and approach to cognitive assessment and rehabilitation.

13.2.2 Cognitive Assessment

Not all people with Long COVID cognitive difficulties require, or can manage, full neuropsychological assessment. Fatigue is a significant limiting factor to participation. Supporting access to cognitive testing via telehealth can be helpful to reduce the impact of fatigue as well as some of the physical and emotional challenges of in-person appointments. Brief and targeted assessments adding tests from relevant domains as needed, self-report questionnaires (e.g., Cognitive Functioning Self-Assessment Scale)[14] to supplement interviews for the person to complete at their own pace, shorter and multiple sessions, and scheduling of sessions at times during the day when the person tends to feel more alert may also be helpful. Attentional tasks conducted at the beginning and end of testing session can also be useful to monitor for any potential effects of fatigue.[12]

Assessment may initially focus on the cognitive domains typically impacted by Long COVID including processing speed, attention, memory, and executive skills. Including measures with and without a time component may support accurate interpretation by reducing the potential impact of fatigue.

Interpreting test findings in the context of the person's pre-infection baseline is particularly important in Long COVID, given changes may be subtle.[7,15] For example, a person of high pre-infection baseline cognitive functioning may not show cognitive impairments when compared to normative data but may notice reduced abilities when compared to their usual level. Acknowledging the contribution of fatigue and mood on everyday cognitive functioning is also essential.

13.2.3 Feedback

Validation of cognitive complaints and patient experience is a critical part of feedback and psychoeducation, particularly given the frequent reports of medical "gaslighting" experienced by Long COVID patients. Focusing on test performance relative to pre-infection levels and "inefficiency" rather than "impairment" may be helpful to frame subtle changes noted on assessment. Discussions around how tests only offer one measure of function may also be helpful when test performance and subjective experiences of cognition differ.

13.3 FUNCTIONAL IMPACTS OF COGNITIVE CHANGES IN LONG COVID

BOX 13.3 "I HAD A BEAUTIFUL BRAIN, AND I JUST NEVER REALISED"

For the first year I had the experience of not being able to hold a thought in my head. In place of my thoughts, there was just emptiness. It was startling. I couldn't read or watch TV. I spent a lot of my day staring straight ahead.

> I was completely dependent on my husband to fill out forms, make appointments, and have simple phone conversations. It was like I ceased to exist. Even 2.5 years on I can't call the dry cleaner to arrange delivery or call my mum to wish her happy birthday.
>
> I still find it hard to process information, make decisions, follow conversations, multitask, and process emotions. I feel drained after five minutes of typing. I had a beautiful brain, and I just never realised. The frustration is daily and endless. I'm constantly having to say, no sorry I can't call to say hi, or talk briefly to the pharmacist or the accountant. All the minutiae of life that we take for granted. Every day I need to weigh up – do I take a shower or order the shopping. I need to do both to survive.
>
> Karen

Cognitive changes associated with Long COVID often negatively impact a person's daily functioning and quality of life. This includes difficulty returning to pre-infection activities such as work, study, and social activities.[16] Daily activities involve multiple cognitive functions, often placing high demand on an individual's cognitive resources. Table 13.1 outlines some of the common functional impacts of cognitive changes, all of which are compounded and heavily impacted by fatigue and other psychological impacts of Long COVID. Cognitive and physical fatigue are also linked, highlighting the shared "energy bucket" for all forms of activity. For further information about the functional impact of Long COVID, see Chapter 12.

13.3.1 A "Hidden" Impairment

Cognitive difficulties may not be obvious or noticed by others. Their "hidden" nature means they may be underappreciated by health professionals, friends, family, and other close contacts, which can undermine their ability to provide support and understanding. Others might assume the person is functioning normally or is overstating the difficulties they experience, further isolating those affected.

> *My parents and friends would tell me I was looking well, thinking that was a helpful thing to say. I felt anything but well and trying to explain my cognitive fatigue was impossible. I was just too tired … Hearing that I looked well made me feel isolated and panicked … What I really needed to hear was 'Rest. Breathe. I understand. Take your time.' Often if I stopped and rested for 5–10 minutes I could keep going.*
>
> Karen

Table 13.1 Functional Impacts of Long COVID Cognitive Difficulties

Functional Area	Impact
Work	Difficulties keeping up with task demands or the physical requirements of employment. Even subtle cognitive impairments may require workplace modifications or reductions in hours, with some people with Long COVID needing to cease employment or retrain in a new field.
Social	Finding large groups and social gatherings overwhelming, difficulty following multiple conversations and word-finding difficulties impact social participation and can lead to social isolation.
Relationships and caring responsibilities	Being cognitively and emotionally overwhelmed with the demanding tasks of parenting and/or providing care to others. Difficulties with multitasking, organising, and keeping up with the "mental load" of parenting responsibilities.
Daily tasks	Difficulty planning and organising daily household, financial, and other tasks.
Health access	Communication expectations (e.g., complex instructions), face-to-face appointments, and lengthy medical forms are barriers to healthcare access. This may limit medical support for both Long COVID and other health concerns.

BOX 13.4 LIVED EXPERIENCE PERSPECTIVES: RECOMMENDATIONS FOR SUPPORTING ACCESS TO CARE FOR PEOPLE WITH LONG COVID COGNITIVE CHANGES AND FATIGUE

Provide practical solutions that acknowledge individual limitations. For example, quiet areas to await appointments, opportunities to recline/lie down, scheduling rest breaks, considering the timing, and length of appointments.

Build trust through understanding. Validate the patient experience and acknowledge that appointments can be overwhelming. A supportive, non-judgmental approach will help foster trust.

Adopt a collaborative approach. Encourage the patient to bring written notes, including questions, health information, and progress, to help guide the appointment and take time to review these together.

Offer alternative communication channels. Ask if people would prefer to complete part of the appointment via email (e.g., forms) or other medium including telehealth.

Provide a review process before finalising decisions. At the end of the appointment, summarise key points and send these to the patient in writing for review and confirmation.

Challenge ableism in care. Consider how usual practices such as forms and phone calls can be adjusted to be more inclusive and effective for those living with cognitive challenges.

13.4 COGNITIVE REHABILITATION MODELS IN LONG COVID

Cognitive rehabilitation approaches can be broadly distilled into three main categories: (1) cognitive retraining/restoration using mental/sensory stimulation, drills, and exercises, (2) compensatory approaches using behavioural and environmental modifications, and (3) holistic approaches that address emotional, motivational, and other noncognitive aspects of function, in addition to cognitive aspects.[17]

Cognitive rehabilitation is founded historically in the care of acquired brain injuries (such as traumatic brain injury) and has an extensive evidence base.[18] This includes models of recovery that inform the most appropriate rehabilitation approach to use for each patient and injury. As an example, severe brain injuries with little likelihood of neurological recovery may favour use of compensatory approaches, whilst cognitive retraining approaches may be used in milder injuries.

To date, there are no validated theoretical models of Long COVID to inform whether restoration of function or compensation is more effective for each patient and as such guidelines do not favour specific cognitive interventions.[12] However, initial evidence indicates that cognitive rehabilitation programmes may improve outcomes for people with Long COVID.[19]

Cognition is not divorced from emotion, motivation, or other noncognitive functions and must be considered within its psychosocial context. Strategies in other chapters of this book can also potentially benefit cognitive functioning, including pacing and fatigue management, interventions for low mood and anxiety, and approaches to managing pain/headaches or other physiological issues (e.g., Postural Orthostatic Tachycardia Syndrome). Some of the principles to consider when implementing cognitive rehabilitation are listed below.

BOX 13.5   COGNITIVE REHABILITATION TIPS FOR SUCCESS

A strong therapeutic alliance between the clinician and patient is fundamental to cognitive rehabilitation.

Rehabilitation is not something we "do" or "give" to people. It is a two-way, interactive, and collaborative process that should reflect both the health professional's experience and knowledge in healthcare, and the patient's knowledge of themselves, their symptoms, and their experiences.

Develop a shared formulation of the patient's cognitive symptoms. This might include exploring which domains of cognitive functioning are most affected in a patient's everyday life, what coping strategies are currently being used, and whether the problems are exacerbated by psychosocial factors such as low mood or anxiety.

Formal cognitive assessment is only part of the story. Although formal assessment of cognition can help rehabilitation, it is not always able to sufficiently pinpoint or fully explore the everyday problems faced by the person.

Be led by functional needs and goals. The interventions and strategies chosen and applied should be guided by the cognitive symptoms experienced in everyday life as identified and described by the patient.

Start small with measurable goals. Focus initially on basic tasks and progress as appropriate towards more cognitively demanding activities. It's usually best to start with strategies that are simpler to learn and implement.

Flexibly adopt approaches. Goals may change over time, and so too might the rehabilitation approaches. For example, a patient forgets details of conversations at work and sets a goal to improve their memory. The initial rehabilitation approach might use external memory strategies (e.g., taking notes). As rehabilitation progresses, supporting fatigue and sleep may assist.

Work collaboratively with colleagues. Liaise with allied health and medical colleagues involved in the patient's care about opportunities to align your work with theirs.

13.5 COGNITIVE REHABILITATION STRATEGIES FOR LONG COVID

13.5.1 Breaks and Rest

Adding in regular breaks for rest can help sustain functioning throughout the day, especially during cognitively demanding tasks. Evidence suggests that generally, the longer the break, the greater the boost on performance.[20] For many people with busy lives and competing demands, this can be difficult to implement – with some worrying that taking regular breaks will slow them down or be counterproductive.

The following strategies may be helpful:

- Psychoeducation, including that attention and concentration naturally work best in short bursts.
- Set regular break times. For example, instead of waiting until overwhelmed, breaks can be scheduled every half-hour or hour.
- The length of the break might depend on the tasks. Highly depleting tasks typically need longer breaks (i.e., greater than 10 minutes).
- Low-stimulation activities, such as listening to calming music, sitting in silence, deep breathing, or practicing a brief mindfulness exercise, are recommended during periods of rest.
- Some people may also find low intensity physical exercise helpful, such as going for a short walk (if appropriate and being mindful of the risk of Post-Exertional Malaise).

BOX 13.6   PRACTICE POINT

Cognitive rehabilitation is not just *doing*. It is also about pacing, resting, and *not doing*.

> *For me, the meditation, timeouts, and not doing have been far more impactful. Sometimes it's not about what you do—it's about what you don't do. There is a real pitfall in people doing too much to try and rehab their cognition … in doing too much they often actually worsen.*
>
> Karen

13.5.2 Reducing Sensory Overload

Background noise and other sensory stimulus can contribute to cognitive fatigue and be distracting. Sensory stimulation can be reduced by moving to a quiet part of the office or working from home, using noise-cancelling headphones, playing white noise, avoiding strong scents (e.g. perfumes) or adjusting the lighting.

13.5.3 Organisational and Memory Strategies

There are a range of strategies that can help patients *optimise* cognitive functioning by "working smarter, not harder." Below are some examples of common strategies, but there are also many others:

- Split larger tasks into small, manageable steps to help reduce the sense of overwhelm and overload.
- Encourage patients to identify a small number of essential tasks that they want to prioritise and focus on these first.
- Organisational aids such as a diary, calendar, or notebook can support memory function. Additionally, there are a range of AI, web- and phone-based memory aids (e.g., online calendars, reminders and alarms, notetaking and audio recording apps) that may be helpful.
- Explore how interruptions and distractions (e.g., notifications on phones and computers) can be reduced.
- Encourage patients to focus on one task at a time rather than attempting to multitask, with a pause between tasks to provide a "reset."

BOX 13.7   PRACTICE POINT

Cognitive rehabilitation strategies are "person specific," based on prior use and experience, cognitive strengths and weaknesses, individual preferences, and stage of recovery. Reflect on the list of compensatory strategies for supporting organisation and memory. Do you use any of these strategies in your daily life? Which ones would you find helpful? Are there any you don't think would be useful for you?

13.5.4 Metacognitive Skills Training

Metacognitive skills involve "thinking about thinking" and are one of the few evidence-based strategies for executive dysfunction.[18] These skills help promote goal-directed behaviour through conscious control of thoughts and actions. They can be particularly helpful for patients who describe making "careless mistakes" or not taking in information because they had been "zoning out."

Patients are encouraged to periodically "stop and think" whilst they complete a task. A range of strategies can be used including thinking aloud and self-monitoring using prompts, for example, What is my goal at the moment? Am I on task? Is there a strategy I can use here to help me? How I am feeling emotionally and physically? Do I need to take a break?

13.5.5 Somatic Awareness

Being able to tune in to one's body and somatic experiences is an important component to effectively using compensatory strategies. Patients can start this process by closing their eyes, taking some deep breaths, noticing and then describing an unpleasant feeling in their body, for example, noticing tension in their chest or pain when experiencing frustration or anxiety about their memory lapses or brain fog. Learning to notice these experiences (pain, heaviness, fatigue, fogginess, and tension) through regular practice can help work towards a proactive rather than reactive response to symptoms, which may help avoid crashes or cognitive overload.

13.5.6 Sensory Modulation

Attention and concentration are closely linked to arousal states. When under-aroused and feeling sluggish, it can be hard to maintain focus and attention can wander or drift. Equally, when over-aroused, internal thought processes can feel scattered, and attentional focus might move around quickly and be easily distractible. Learning to modulate arousal states by using the senses can help with attention and concentration issues related to fatigue, brain fog, and anxiety.

Patients can explore their sensory preferences to work out what sensory inputs are calming (when they feel over-aroused) and what sensory inputs are alerting for them (when they feel under-aroused). Movement, touch, smell, taste, sound, light, and temperature can all be explored as ways to modulate arousal. For example, many people find listening to instrumental music can help modulate their arousal – higher energy/tempo music is typically alerting, and lower tempo/energy is typically calming. Occupational Therapists complete validated sensory profiles and can also assist in implementing these interventions.

13.5.7 Emotional Regulation

Modalities such as Acceptance and Commitment Therapy (ACT) and Dialectical Behaviour Therapy incorporate a range of distress tolerance and emotional regulation skills such as self-soothing, grounding, mindfulness, deep breathing, progressive muscle relaxation, and self-compassion. These skills can be modelled and practiced in session and used when patients notice distress or dysregulation is impacting on cognitive functioning.

13.5.8 Acceptance of Symptoms

Cognitive abilities are integral parts of identity and sense of self. The way people see themselves and what they value can be related to their cognitive abilities (e.g., "I am a good listener to my friends," or "I am good at solving problems at work"). When cognitive abilities change, these aspects of identity can be challenged. It can be extremely distressing to no longer feel or experience the same competency around cognition.

Accepting these changes is understandably difficult. ACT can help change the relationship with distress and help build acceptance of a new "normal." This process takes time, but the three pillars of ACT (reducing experiential avoidance, increasing awareness of the present moment, engaging in valued actions) can all help reduce distress resulting from cognitive difficulties and help patients stay in the present moment, which can in turn help with memory and concentration.

13.5.9 Thought Analysis

It is not uncommon to have an increased sensitivity to cognitive failures with changed cognitive functioning, which can add to distress. In this context, it is common to experience thoughts such as "I'll never get my brain back" or "I'm always going to forget things." Exercises that help break down thoughts can be helpful to maintain a balanced perspective and regain a sense of control. Typically, this process might involve:

- Validating the patient's experience and acknowledging the fear and frustration that accompanies cognitive difficulties.
- Encouraging identification and further examination of specific thoughts related to distress (e.g., "I'll never get my brain back"), and the emotional and behavioural consequences.
- Encouraging reflection with questions like "What evidence do you have this is true" and "What evidence do you have this is not true?"
- Support noticing any fluctuations in cognitive difficulties and what factors may exacerbate symptoms (e.g., stress, fatigue) as well as considering what cognitive tasks may be unchanged.
- Regular practice of these exercises both in session and for "homework" can help patients integrate a range of thoughts and experiences about their cognition to maintain a balanced perspective.

13.5.10 Cognitive/Brain Training

Cognitive training is based on the idea that cognitive abilities such as problem-solving, reasoning, attention, executive functions, and working memory can be improved by exercising the brain with practice of specific tasks, the same way that physical fitness is improved with exercise. Research is mixed about whether this type of training translates or generalises to improvements in real-world functioning,[21] and research specifically in relation into cognitive training for Long COVID is still in its infancy. However, any potential benefits are likely to be limited by the high levels of cognitive fatigue people experience. For many people, it may be better to conserve energy for more meaningful activities.

13.6 EMERGING MEDICAL INTERVENTIONS FOR LONG COVID COGNITIVE CHANGES

There are a range of medical therapies for Long COVID currently being researched and evaluated[22] with the aim to treat underlying biological causes of the cognitive symptoms. Some therapies that have garnered interest include non-invasive brain stimulation, hyperbaric oxygen therapy, palmitoylethanolamide supplementation, and low-dose naltrexone.

Whilst these therapies might have potential, clinical evidence is still evolving, and more rigorous, large-scale studies are necessary to establish long-term effectiveness and safety in Long COVID. Due to a general lack of therapeutic options for people with Long COVID, many of these novel, untested therapies are being sought out and trialled by people living with cognitive changes either via self-medicating or off label prescriptions.

13.7 CONCLUSION

The cognitive sequalae of Long COVID are common and varied. They have a significant functional impact across social, work, study, and personal aspects of daily life. Whilst the aetiology of these difficulties continues to be researched, current approaches to rehabilitation include a broad range of interventions commonly used in other cognitive health conditions. These include a range of compensatory strategies for cognitive impairment, as well as holistic interventions to support adjustment, coping, and acceptance.

REFERENCES

1 Callard F, et al. How and why patients made Long Covid. Soc Sci Med. 2021;268:113426. doi:10.1016/j.socscimed.2020.113426.

2 Greene C, et al. Blood-brain barrier disruption and sustained systemic inflammation in individuals with Long COVID-associated cognitive impairment. Nat Neurosci. 2024;27(3):421–32. doi:10.1038/s41593-024-01576-9.

3 Moller M, et al. Cognitive dysfunction in post-COVID-19 condition: Mechanisms, management, and rehabilitation. J Intern Med. 2023;294(5):563–81. doi:10.1111/joim.13720.

4 Klinkhammer S, et al. A biopsychosocial approach to persistent Post-COVID-19 fatigue and cognitive complaints: Results of the prospective multicenter NeNeSCo study. Arch Phys Med Rehabil. 2024;105(5):826–34. doi:10.1016/j.apmr.2023.12.014.

5 Cavaco S, et al. Predictors of cognitive dysfunction one-year post COVID-19. Neuropsychology. 2023;37(5):557–67. doi:10.1037/neu0000876.

6 Ceban F, et al. Fatigue and cognitive impairment in Post-COVID-19 Syndrome: A systematic review and meta-analysis. Brain Behav Immun. 2022;101:93–135. doi:10.1016/j.bbi.2021.12.020.

7 Stenberg J, et al. Preliminary findings on cognitive dysfunction in university-educated patients after mild COVID-19 disease. Arch Rehabil Res Clin Transl. 2023;5(4):100294. doi:10.106/j.arrct.2023.100294.

8 Knapp SAB, et al. Neurocognitive and psychiatric outcomes associated with postacute COVID-19 infection without severe medical complication: A meta-analysis. J Neurol Neurosurg Psychiatry. 2024;95(12):1207–16. doi:10.1136/jnnp-2024-333950.

9 Hampshire A, et al. Cognition and memory after COVID-19 in a large community sample. N Engl J Med. 2024;390(9):806–18. doi:10.1056/NEJMoa2311330.

10 Taquet M, et al. Cognitive and psychiatric symptom trajectories 2–3 years after hospital admission for COVID-19: A longitudinal, prospective cohort study in the UK. Lancet Psychiatry. 2024;11(9):696–708. doi:10.1016/S2215-0366(24)00214-1.

11 Schild AK, et al. Multidomain cognitive impairment in non-hospitalized patients with the post-COVID-19 syndrome: Results from a prospective monocentric cohort. J Neurol. 2023;270(3):1215–23. doi:10.1007/s00415-022-11444-w.

12 Widmann CN, et al. Improving neuropsychological rehabilitation for COVID-19 patients: Guideline-based advances. Zeitschrift fur Neuropsychologie. 2023 June 1;34(2): 57–70. doi:10.1024/1016-264X/a000373.

13 Ladds E, et al. Persistent symptoms after Covid-19: Qualitative study of 114 "long Covid" patients and draft quality principles for services. BMC Health Serv Res. 2020;20(1):1144. doi:10.1186/s12913-020-06001-y.

14 Annunziata MA et al. Cognitive Functioning Self-Assessment Scale (CFSS): Further psychometric data. Appl Neuropsychol Adult. 2018;25(1):1–4. doi:10.1080/23279095.2016.1225575

15 Ladds E, et al. Cognitive dysfunction after COVID-19. BMJ. 2024;384:e075387. doi:10.1136/bmj-2023-075387.

16 Wrench JM, et al. An allied health model of care for Long COVID rehabilitation. Med J Aust. 2024;221 Suppl 9:S5–S9. doi:10.5694/mja2.52457.

17 Wilson BA. Cognitive rehabilitation: How it is and how it might be. J Int Neuropsychol Soc. 1997;3(5):487–96.

18 Cicerone KD, et al. Evidence-based cognitive rehabilitation: Systematic review of the literature from 2009 through 2014. Arch Phys Med Rehabil. 2019;100(8):1515–33. doi:10.1016/j.apmr.2019.02.011.

19 Braga LW, et al. Long COVID neuropsychological follow-up: Is cognitive rehabilitation relevant? NeuroRehabilitation. 2023;53(4):517–34. doi:10.3233/NRE-230212.

20 Albulescu P, et al. "Give me a break!" A systematic review and meta-analysis on the efficacy of micro-breaks for increasing well-being and performance. PLoS One. 2022;17(8):e0272460. doi:10.1371/journal.pone.0272460.

21 Simons DJ, et al. Do "Brain-Training" programs work? Psychol Sci Public Interest. 2016;17(3):103–86. doi:10.1177/1529100616661983.

22 Gorenshtein A, et al. Intervention modalities for brain fog caused by Long-COVID: Systematic review of the literature. Neurol Sci. 2024;45(7):2951–68. doi:10.1007/s10072-024-07566-w.

Chapter 14

Psychosocial Support and Interventions for Long COVID

Alex Holmes, Kerrie Clarke, and Jessica Lee

BOX 14.1   LEARNING OBJECTIVES

By the end of reading this chapter, you should be able to:

- Understand the psychological and psychosocial challenges of living with Long COVID.
- Identify psychological principles in providing healthcare to people with Long COVID.
- Consider the role of specialist mental health support as part of multidisciplinary care.

14.1 INTRODUCTION

The experience of Long COVID affects a person on a physical level, which has a psychological impact and affects daily life. Thus, it is helpful to conceptualise the psychological challenge of Long COVID within a framework that recognises the complex interplay between biological, psychological, and social factors in determining health. A patient-centred approach to care includes forming a thorough picture of the individual symptoms, how they affect their life, and the factors that may increase distress related to their symptoms. Psychological distress is common when a person develops a new illness, and this distress can increase as symptoms persist. Family and friends are sufficient support for most people. Primary health professionals who provide supportive and person-centred care, especially in the absence of curative treatments, will also assist people living with the symptoms of Long COVID. In this support, it is crucial not to misattribute the cause of Long COVID as a psychological condition or insinuate that symptoms are

DOI: 10.4324/9781003528104-18

self-generated. Some people, especially those with severe or persistent symptoms, may develop secondary mental health disorders such as anxiety and depression that may require specialist assessment and treatment.

14.2 PSYCHOLOGICAL RESPONSES TO LONG COVID

Everyone will respond differently to Long COVID. Furthermore, a person's response to their illness may change over time, especially when facing typical cycles of improvement and setbacks. A move towards acceptance of the condition as it is experienced in the here and now is adaptive, especially when there is no clear indication as to when recovery might occur. In Jessica's experience, this process occurred in three phases (Figure 14.1):

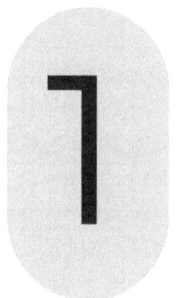

"I'M SICK"
It is not just a case of just a few more weeks to recover, as I had hoped

"THIS IS GOING TO TAKE TIME"
There was no quick fix to get my old life back. I have resigned from my job. I'm not improving fast. I have to adjust my life and mindset to this reality, especially around being patient.

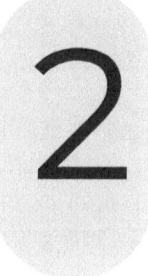

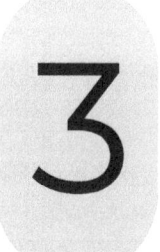

"I NEED TO CHANGE MY APPROACH"
I need to re-navigate and think differently. I need to accept changes and create new goals, new things to bring me joy.

Figure 14.1 A lived experience of adapting to Long COVID.

14.2.1 Anxiety and Depression

Depression and anxiety are common responses to the experience of Long COVID.[1] People may experience depressive symptoms such as low mood, decreased self-worth, and feelings of guilt at not being able to engage in everyday tasks due to the physical impact of the illness. People with Long COVID have described cycles of "doing a bit more" or "pushing a bit harder" during periods of "feeling better," often followed by a period of increased fatigue and decreased function. These cycles can lead to feelings of hopelessness and self-criticism and further exacerbate low mood and depressive symptoms. In some situations, external pressures from family or work lead people to feel unsupported or not believed, which may increase a sense of worthlessness and being a burden on others.

There is an overlap between the somatic symptoms of anxiety, such as tachycardia, and symptoms of Long COVID. Many people with Long COVID experience post-exertional malaise (PEM), which worsens after activity. The "boom and bust" cycles of symptoms, especially fatigue, can lead to anxiety about increased activity leading to PEM. Some people with Long COVID may avoid activity to lessen their fear of triggering PEM. Whilst this strategy has some benefits, it can then lead to secondary anxiety and depressive symptoms if the person avoids engaging in meaningful activities. The identification and treatment of anxiety symptoms that are exacerbating Long COVID symptoms may reduce the avoidance of activity.

14.2.2 Grief and Loss

The experience of Long COVID often entails unexpressed losses. The ability to live within the world is limited not only by physical distress and impaired function but also by a narrowing of focus towards physical symptoms. People report a loss of agency, value, and purpose in their personal and professional lives. They lose connection with family and the workplace. Leisure, exercise, and socialisation are markedly reduced. Communication, trust, and intimacy can be profoundly affected. These losses lead to various emotions, commonly sadness and anger, but may also challenge the individual's sense of identity and self-worth.[2]

> *When you lose your job, you can't see your friends, go to the gym, play with your kids, or support your family, it's hard. It's easy to question your worth, value, and contribution to the world. You often lose the things that gave your life joy, purpose, and by default, good mental health. It can be incredibly isolating.*
>
> *There is a disconnect from the person you are now, and the person you used to be, your identity is challenged.*
>
> Jessica

14.2.3 Cognitive Symptoms

People with Long COVID often report a decline in cognitive ability (see Chapter 13). A sharp decline in a wide range of cognitive abilities can impair function in both work and personal roles. The relationship between cognitive and psychological symptoms is complex. Difficulties with concentration and clarity of thought may result in vigilance and anxiety about cognitive performance and intolerance of normal errors. Clinical experience suggests that those who were previously cognitively active, especially as part of their work, find brain fog challenging to tolerate. Identifying and understanding specific cognitive areas of concern and providing simple exercises to address these may be useful, alongside validating the frustration related to the lost capacity.

14.2.4 Experience of the Healthcare System

An essential determinant of the psychological response to Long COVID is people's experience within the healthcare system. People with Long COVID are vulnerable to being isolated or marginalised. People can feel that their symptoms are not being taken seriously. When patients are informed that there is "no medical cause" for their symptoms, they commonly feel that they are not being believed, are being told it is "in your head'," or even that they are "making it up'." Hence, well-meaning offers of psychological help may be inadvertently construed as implying that the symptoms are psychological.

> It's a challenge not being taken seriously, having symptoms dismissed as depression, anxiety or "all in your mind". When not believed, it's easy to question and gaslight yourself wondering, 'Am I really feeling this way?', 'Am I making it up? 'Do I just need to think positive and all this would go away?', 'Deep down do I actually want to be sick?'. Being focused on symptoms creates a hyper-focus on your limitations and loss, which solidifies your identity as a 'sick person'.
>
> Jessica

14.3 PSYCHOSOCIAL INTERVENTIONS IN GENERAL HEALTHCARE

There are essential psychological elements in all healthcare interactions in Long COVID. The interplay of physical symptoms, psychological distress, and feelings of loss creates a complex landscape. A holistic and multidisciplinary approach will prompt professionals to consider a multi-faceted approach to treatment.

Professionals need to be attuned to anticipatory anxiety and avoidance, the distress and loss arising from persistent symptoms, and the potential for patients to feel invalidated and unheard. Acknowledging losses and supporting narratives involving hope and acceptance can promote agency and help people regain control over their recovery. Interactions that are experienced negatively can increase helplessness, a sense of isolation and decrease hope.[3]

When a healthcare practitioner validates the person's symptoms of Long COVID, the person feels supported and is more able to communicate openly. Measures such as providing a low stimulus environment and allowing pauses in consultations enhance validation. Advocacy and support with applications for allowances and additional services, which can be difficult and time-consuming, are highly valued. An open mind regarding the cause of symptoms, avoiding psychological reasons for symptoms that do not easily fit anatomical or pathological explanations and encouraging exploration of mind-body linkages can further enhance the working relationship. People with Long COVID can be hypervigilant to new or changing symptoms. Professionals must respond to and validate new concerns with reassurance and appropriate exploration and investigations when necessary.

These simple comments made by medical professionals have helped me feel seen, heard and validated: 'That sounds really tough', 'I'm sorry you're going through this', 'That doesn't sound like fun at all', 'I bet you're sick of all these tests', 'You are doing so well dealing with all this'.

Jessica

BOX 14.2   PRACTICE POINT: USEFUL PSYCHOLOGICAL PRINCIPLES IN HEALTHCARE INTERACTIONS

- Maintain a reliable, consistent, and tolerant therapeutic alliance with a key practitioner.
- Focus on "care over cure" and working together as a team.
- Understand what works for that person.
- Accept shared uncertainty, frustration, and disappointment.
- Provide helpful knowledge updates in simple terms and offer new treatments or investigations when appropriate.
- Emphasise the population level trajectory towards recovery.
- Explore and develop concepts of recovery relevant to the individual.
- Promote mind-body connections.
- Acknowledge concerns that symptoms may be misconstrued as psychological.

14.3.1 Challenges for Health Professionals

Irrespective of the speciality, a common aim of health professionals is to provide effective treatment that reduces suffering. The experience of recovery in Long COVID is often cyclical, and effective and reliable evidence-based treatments are not yet on offer. Improvement may lead to a sense of recovery or mastery, whilst relapse may result in feelings of loss of control, uncertainty, and an understandable degree of frustration. It can be challenging for health professionals to navigate this journey with the patient.

Professionals may respond to relapse or lack of improvement in different ways. There may be repeated efforts through additional investigations, referrals, or trials of novel treatments. "Doing something" or "trying something" is often valued by patients, construed as "not giving up" and evidence that they are not being marginalised or abandoned. Alternatively, professionals may distance themselves, feeling like "I do not have anything more to offer." This may unconsciously provide relief from feeling ineffective or help limit empathy fatigue. It may also shield them from more open expressions of disappointment or frustration levelled at them or the healthcare system.

Patients with Long COVID identify the maintenance of a non-judgemental, receptive, and pragmatic relationship as being of great value to their recovery, "It has been invaluable to have medical professionals who have treated me like a whole person — not just a set of symptoms." Current experience suggests a focus on care rather than cure can counter isolation, promote hope, and mitigate against the development of secondary mental health disorders. It is also a foundation to discuss and triage novel therapies and provide valuable updates on current knowledge.

14.3.2 Themes of Recovery in Long COVID

People use different coping strategies to manage everyday life with Long COVID.[3] Identifying these strategies can help health professionals attune their support and interventions. Table 14.1 summarises some common themes in Long COVID recovery.[2,3] These themes may be revisited at different times during the recovery journey at times of relapses, when new symptoms appear, or when new comorbid diagnoses are made.

> *Realising this powerful mind/body connection, it became essential to learn to regulate my nervous system, both through body work (breathing, yoga, time*

in nature, meditation, and gentle movement) and mindset work (challenging thoughts, unpacking worst-case scenarios, using positive visualisation).

Jessica

Table 14.1 Common Themes Within the Cycle of Psychosocial Recovery and Targets for Healthcare Practitioner Intervention

Theme	Suggested Interventions
1. Seeking reassurance and knowledge	• Describe and delineate individual symptoms and how the individual perceives and understands them. • Provide validation of the experience of symptoms, especially when test results are normal or inconclusive. "A normal test does not mean that you are not unwell." • Provide information about the prevalence and duration of common symptoms of Long COVID. • Early referral to allied health intervention if appropriate. • Screen for mental health symptoms and refer when appropriate. • Consider linking to social support groups in the local community (if available). • Discuss managing exposure fatigue and possible distress when interacting with online communities.
2. Developing increased awareness and understanding of symptoms	• "Everyone experiences Long COVID a little bit differently, so it's important to find an approach that works for you." • Offer resources for self-monitoring, for example, (1) smartwatches to monitor activity, sleep, and heart rate, or (2) a diary, wall chart, and mind map linking physical, emotional, and social interactions. • Be mindful of the balance of self-monitoring and hypervigilance to symptoms and triggers. • Explore mind-body linkages.
3. Developing strategies for living with Long COVID	• Acknowledge a person's attempts to find what works for them. • Offer strategies for particular symptoms. • Enhance the use of helpful coping strategies and highlight success. • Indicate that different strategies may work at various times. • Emphasise participation in meaningful and joyful activities.

	• Explore how the person can try to balance expectations and capacity. • Explore the timing of return to work or change of career. • Enhance supportive and validating social connections. • Offer realistic hope for recovery and for overcoming symptoms. • Build acceptance as an active stance that allows the person to take action on what is possibly related to where they are at in their recovery.
4. Dealing with setbacks	• Validate the cyclical nature of recovery. • Focus on previous success. "We've been here before, and you've gotten better." • Re-screen for mental health symptoms if indicated. • Review needs for enhanced allied health support.

14.3.3 Supporting Families and Other Informal Supports of People with Long COVID

Social support networks are essential in recovery from illness and should be considered in recovery planning for people with Long COVID. Families, carers, and supporters benefit from learning about Long COVID. It is helpful for them to understand the cyclical nature of recovery and the role of the various health professionals involved. This knowledge can help family members and other supporters manage recovery expectations, especially concerning the patient's capacity to work or undertake their usual family roles. Family interventions may also be useful in some circumstances.

14.4 MENTAL HEALTH DISORDERS AND LONG COVID

Mental health disorders, especially depression and anxiety, are common in the general population and are more likely to occur in those with persistent physical illness. Previous mental illness, family history of mental illness, adverse developmental experiences, or trauma may predispose a person to develop a mental health disorder. Screening tools can be used in routine care to identify symptoms of depression and anxiety and can be administered by most health professionals. The Patient Health Questionnaire-9[4] and the Generalised Anxiety Disorder-7[5] are useful screening measures for Long COVID. These tools may also assist in determining the need for referral to a mental health specialist.

14.4.1 Diagnosis of Mental Health Disorders in Long COVID

Major depression and anxiety disorders are more common in people with Long COVID, with a prevalence rate of 23%.[1] Diagnosis is based on the severity of the symptoms, the presence of clearly abnormal symptoms and/or the inability to engage in everyday activities due to these symptoms. It can be difficult, however, to determine if a mental health disorder is present due to the overlap of physical symptoms of Long COVID with the diagnostic criteria for the mental health disorder. Table 14.2 outlines considerations when exploring mental health diagnosis in Long COVID.

Table 14.2 Psychological Response to Illness and Indicators of Mental Health Diagnosis in Long COVID

Symptoms	Response to Illness	Mood and Anxiety Disorders
Low mood	Absent or Intermittent	Depressed most of the day, nearly every day
Loss of enjoyment	Secondary to reduced function	Markedly diminished interest or pleasure in all/almost all activities most of the day, nearly every day
Worry	Uncertainty about recovery Able to turn thoughts elsewhere	Excessive anxiety and worry more days than not. • "I am terrified that if I do anything, I will get worse." Finds it challenging to control the worry • "I cannot stop my mind."
Fear	Related to loss of function and life roles and societal concerns about re-infection	This leads to significant avoidance and impacts participation in daily life
Frustration and/or irritability	Frustration about function, participation, and uncertainty	Pervasive and uncharacteristic irritability

Guilt	Secondary to reduced role function	Strong ideas of failing others
Worth	Secondary to reduced role function	Strong beliefs of uselessness or worthlessness
Hopelessness	Proportional to symptom trajectory	Hopelessness. • "I cannot see my way out."
Suicidality	Absent	Thoughts of life not worth living or suicide.
Energy and motivation	Pervasive fatigue Is motivated but has no energy	Feeling unmotivated, lacking energy, described as a lack of interest or motivation. Restless and having trouble relaxing
Sleep	Related to physical symptoms of Long COVID.	Change from regular pattern, excessive or disrupted sleep
Cognition	Brain fog fluctuates with fatigue.	Unable to think or make decisions coloured by pessimism and thoughts of mental incapacity.
Physical symptoms	Occur in the absence of corresponding anxious thoughts and feelings.	Episodic somatic symptoms of anxiety (racing heart, chest discomfort, shortness of breath, sweating, dizziness) associated with feelings of dread or catastrophe.

14.4.2 Diagnostic Considerations for Post-traumatic Stress Disorder

A diagnosis of post-traumatic stress disorder (PTSD) is less common in Long COVID than depression and anxiety. Most post-traumatic symptoms have been observed in people who had a severe infection requiring prolonged hospital admission and ventilator support. Specific signs of PTSD include flashbacks, nightmares, avoidance of triggers (i.e., not attending medical appointments), avoiding thinking or talking about the trauma experience, and poor memory of the event. If these symptoms are evident, health professionals should discuss them with the patient and refer them to specialist mental healthcare.

14.4.3 When to Refer for Specialist Mental Health Care

Health professionals may consider referral to specialist mental healthcare in various circumstances. Referral should be considered if the patient is describing distressing psychological symptoms, exacerbation of previous mental health conditions, or is above the threshold on screening. Some patients may request extra psychological support to explore or make sense of their experience. When raising the topic of a mental health referral, the practitioner needs to be mindful of inadvertently implying the person's symptoms are psychological. Referrals regarding holistic care and optimising wellbeing are best discussed as crucial to aiding recovery.

Where possible, health professionals should refer to mental health professionals who have experience in either working with Long COVID or other chronic health conditions. Clinical and health psychologists can offer a range of psychological strategies based on an individual formulation of the person's psychological symptoms. Referral to a psychiatrist should be considered when first line pharmacotherapy and/or psychotherapy through primary care has not been adequately effective or when psychological symptoms are predominant and severe.

Considering patient preferences is essential. Patients may prefer specific types of professionals, and finding a mental health practitioner who fits their needs can enhance the therapeutic relationship. Many individuals with Long COVID have reported that mental health support is beneficial as part of a multidisciplinary treatment approach. Therefore, referral to specialised mental healthcare should occur within an integrated medical and allied health support network that emphasises various interventions.

14.5 SPECIALIST MENTAL HEALTHCARE IN LONG COVID

14.5.1 Psychological Therapies

Whilst specific psychological therapies tailored for Long COVID are not yet established, general psychological interventions have shown promise in alleviating symptoms of depression, anxiety, and PTSD.[6] In approaching psychological interventions, mental health professionals should start with a collaborative formulation of the individual's biological, psychological, and social experiences and articulate their definition of recovery. This will help professionals avoid applying psychological therapies known to be effective in other disorders without adapting them to the unique characteristics of Long COVID.

Due to the physical limitations experienced by patients with Long COVID, delivery of psychological interventions via telehealth increases access to treatment. Audio-visual content that can be reviewed and repeated can complement interventions, particularly if the person experiences brain fog and cognitive difficulties.[6] Patients should be offered rest breaks and the opportunity to meet their sensory and energy needs (e.g., keeping their camera off, lying down during appointment).

14.5.1.1 Acceptance and Commitment Therapy

Acceptance and commitment therapy focuses on building psychological flexibility skills to help people take meaningful action, even in the context of unwanted or painful experiences.[7] A person's level of psychological flexibility can affect how they relate to their experience of Long COVID.[8] Psychological inflexibility correlates with depression, anxiety, insomnia, and symptom duration.[9] Table 14.3 provides suggested ACT interventions in Long COVID.

14.5.1.2 Mindful Self-Compassion

Mindful self-compassion is an intervention that combines the skills of mindfulness and self-compassion. It aims to help people understand and accept feelings of personal suffering by developing kindness towards themselves.[10] It targets self-judgment and stigma related to Long COVID, promoting healthier behaviours and improving communication about personal needs.[8]

14.5.1.3 Cognitive-Behavioural Therapies

Cognitive-behavioural therapy (CBT) offers patients mechanisms to cope with symptoms of Long COVID rather than treating the symptoms themselves. CBT is widely available in the community for the treatment of psychological symptoms. Early evidence has shown that CBT is effective in reducing anxiety, depression, and stress and improves coping and quality of life. CBT programmes for Long COVID have focused on enhancing sleep–wake cycles, unhelpful beliefs and fears about symptoms, and increasing social support and activity levels.[11] CBT can also assist patients dealing with anxiety about re-infection or over-focusing on physical symptoms using mindfulness, exposure, and cognitive restructuring techniques. There is limited evidence that CBT improves symptoms of Long COVID, such as fatigue and poor concentration.

Table 14.3 Application of ACT for Psychological Symptoms Associated with Long COVID

ACT Process	Interventions
Encouraging openness to experience	• Differentiate the thoughts and feelings about the symptoms from the symptoms themselves. "You notice that when you experience post-exertional fatigue, you think you have caused more damage?" • Identify attempts to suppress unwanted emotions, thoughts, memories, and bodily sensations. "Is there anything you do that gives you some relief in the short term but actually makes it worse in the long term?" • Determine the level of acceptance of symptoms. "How much do you struggle against the symptoms you're currently having? What impact does that have on other areas of your life?" • Explore what is in their control and what is out of their control.
Awareness of the present moment	• Promote awareness of thoughts, feelings, sensations, and being in the present moment. "Can you describe your experience in this moment?" • Explore limiting beliefs resulting from comparisons with pre-COVID self. "How much do you think about what you were like before you had COVID?" • Encourage focus on increasing awareness of times they have felt "better" or when symptoms are stable
Engaging in valued actions	• Identify values. "What is most important to you about how you live?" • Explore the flexible nature of values-based living • Setting goals in line with values. "What small thing might you do today that is in line with X value?"

14.5.2 Pharmacotherapy

Antidepressants are effective in treating anxiety and depression in patients with chronic illness. Studies in Long COVID are yet to be conducted. To date, however, clinical experience suggests that antidepressants are helpful when core depressive symptoms are present (persistent low mood, lack of enjoyment, irritability, feeling stuck, and not coping). Treatment commonly leads to improved mood and coping, with enhanced activity and function, but with little or no change to Long COVID symptoms. For anxiety disorders, antidepressants can reduce rumination and uncontrollable worry. This may be particularly useful if there is anxiety about activities that may exacerbate Long COVID symptoms and secondary avoidance. Professionals must be mindful of patients balancing increased activity with the risk of PEM.

14.2.5.1 Selective Serotonin Reuptake Inhibitors

Selective serotonin reuptake inhibitors (SSRIs) are the most common type of antidepressant prescribed. The choice of SSRI may be based on the patient's past use or practitioner preference. It should be noted that when commencing any new medication, care needs to be taken to normalise early side effects that may be misconstrued as new symptoms of Long COVID to decrease the risk of non-adherence. For example, patients can experience nausea and vomiting, temporarily exacerbating gastrointestinal symptoms of Long COVID. Other side effects include exacerbation of headaches, restlessness, or increased anxiety. When anxiety is pronounced, the short-term use of a benzodiazepine, such as diazepam, may be indicated.

14.5.2.2 Other Antidepressant Medications

Serotonin noradrenaline reuptake inhibitors have been suggested to assist in the management of pain; however, to date, when used in patients with Long COVID and pain, they have shown unclear benefits over SSRIs. Mirtazapine may be indicated for patients with sleep disturbance and decreased appetite; however, it may compound fatigue. Amitriptyline (Endep) can be used in 25 or 50 mg doses for persistent pain, including in Long COVID. When used as an antidepressant, doses above 75 mg are usually required but this can result in side effects such as drowsiness, dry mouth, and dizziness.

14.6 CONCLUSION

Long COVID represents a novel challenge for people living with the illness and for health professionals. The psychological burden of persistent symptoms varies across individuals and their contexts, and most psychological support can be provided through personal and family networks. The evidence for effective, evidence-based interventions, albeit increasing, remains limited. All health professionals working with patients with Long COVID have an essential role in supporting mental health and wellbeing. This is best done through understanding and validating their symptoms and notions of recovery and taking a person-centred and multi-focused approach to treatment. When secondary psychological disorders develop, psychological and pharmacological therapies are effective. Still, they should be delivered in a multidisciplinary context and avoid the implication that Long COVID is a psychological disorder that only requires mental health intervention.

REFERENCES

1 Seighali N, et al. The global prevalence of depression, anxiety, and sleep disorder among patients coping with Post COVID-19 syndrome (Long COVID): A systematic review and meta-analysis. BMC Psychiatry. 2024;24:105. doi:10.1186/s12888-023-05481-6.

2 Leggat FJ, et al. An exploration of the experiences and self-generated strategies used when navigating everyday life with Long COVID. BMC Public Health. 2024;24(1):789. doi:10.1186/s12889-024-18267-6.

3 Thurner C, Stengel A. Long-COVID syndrome: Physical-mental interplay in the spotlight. Inflammopharmacology. 2023;31(2):559–64. doi:10.1007/s10787-023-01174-4.

4 Kroenke K, et al. The PHQ-9: Validity of a brief depression severity measure. J Gen Intern Med. 2001;16(9):606–13. doi:10.1046/j.1525-1497.2001.016009606.x.

5 Spitzer RL, et al. A brief measure for generalised anxiety disorder: The GAD-7. Arch Intern Med. 2006;166(10):1092–97. doi: 10.1001/archinte.166.10.1092.

6 Martinez-Borba V, et al. Guiding future research on psychological interventions in people with COVID-19 and post COVID syndrome and comorbid emotional disorders based on a systematic review. Front Public Health. 2023;11:1305463. doi:10.3389/fpubh.2023.1305463.

7 Hayes SC, et al. Acceptance and commitment therapy: An experiential approach to behavior change. New York: Guilford Press; 1999.

8 Tudor L, et al. Post-covid-19 syndrome: Self-compassion and psychological flexibility moderate the relationship between physical symptom load and psychosocial impact. Acta Psychol. 2023;241:104093. doi:10.1016/j.actpsy.2023.104093.

9 McCracken LM, et al. Health, wellbeing and persisting symptoms in the pandemic: What is the role of psychological flexibility? J Contextual Behav Sci. 2022;26:187–92. doi:10.1016/j.jcbs.2022.10.003.

10 Neff K. Self-compassion: The proven power of being kind to yourself. New York: William Morrow; 2015.

11 De Luca R, et al. Psychological and cognitive effects of Long COVID: A narrative review focusing on the assessment and rehabilitative approach. J Clin Med. 2022;11(21):6554. doi:10.3390/jcm11216554.

Chapter 15

Nourishing the Path to Recovery

Nutrition and Long COVID

Jane Willcox, Mary Mangos,
Paige van der Pligt, and Leigh Seidel-Marks

BOX 15.1 LEARNING OBJECTIVES

By the end of this chapter, readers should be able to:

- Summarise evidence-based nutrition management for Long COVID symptoms that support recovery.
- Understand the importance of treating and preventing malnutrition in people living with Long COVID.
- Guide dietetic referral for nutrition assessment and management and provide practical nutrition tips for people living with Long COVID.

15.1 INTRODUCTION

Nutrition plays a critical role in the risk of acquiring COVID-19, and in Long COVID management and recovery. People with Long COIVD may experience different forms of malnutrition arising from pre-existing conditions, their acute COVID-19 infection or their Long COVID symptoms. Optimal nutrition is therefore crucial for recovery.

Even without signs of malnutrition or Long COVID symptoms that impact nutrition intake, people with Long COVID may benefit from optimising nutrition intake to support their recovery. Optimal nutrition status plays a crucial role in immune system support, tissue and muscle recovery and maintenance, inflammatory

DOI: 10.4324/9781003528104-19

responses, energy provision, mental and cognitive health, gastrointestinal health, and prevention of secondary complications.

Working with people living with Long COVID follows the standard nutrition assessment (dietary, biochemical, anthropometric, clinical) and management approach. Due to individual variations in symptom presentation, it's crucial to recognise personal goals and set realistic expectations for recovery management. Many people struggle with getting their condition recognised and accessing support, and the uncertainty of living with Long COVID affects mood, appetite, and nutrition. Validating lived experiences and the impact of persistent symptoms, while providing information about recovery, is central for building trust and fostering positive change.

This chapter outlines the evidence supporting the role of nutrition in Long COVID and provides direction for health professionals working with people experiencing moderate to severe Long COVID in the ambulatory setting. For people who required intensive medical support for acute COVID, including intensive care, medical nutrition therapy may be best provided by acute care dietitians.

15.2 MALNUTRITION AND LONG COVID

Malnutrition is defined as deficiencies or excesses in nutrient intake, imbalance of essential nutrients or impaired nutrient utilisation. The triple burden of malnutrition includes undernutrition, overweight and obesity, and micronutrient deficiencies,[1] each with underlying causes that promote inadequate dietary intake of essential foods and nutrients. Evidence across studies has reported the prevalence of malnutrition ranging from 22% at four to five months post-acute COVID-19[2] to 36% at six months.[3] Malnutrition may represent both a cause and a consequence of Long COVID.[2] Poor dietary intake and malnutrition is associated with oxidative stress, which negatively impacts the immune system,[4] significantly increasing susceptibility to bacterial and viral infection.[5] On the other hand, common symptoms of Long COVID (such as fatigue, loss of appetite, and alterations to taste and smell) are associated with reduced food intake, weight loss or gain and a resulting higher risk of malnutrition.[2] Persistence of weakness, myalgia and arthralgia even six months post hospital discharge has also been observed in outpatient groups coupled with both undernutrition and obesity.[6,7]

Malnutrition has significant, adverse effects on people with Long COVID. It increases risk of reinfection in the post-acute period,[7] worsens clinical outcomes,[8] increases chance of readmission to hospital and length of hospital stay[5] and has been associated with increased risk of mortality.[7] As such, monitoring nutrition status and malnutrition risk is critical in assessing recovery from acute disease[2,3,9] and in aiding prevention of negative long-term health outcomes. Ongoing nutritional assessment and management in people with Long COVID should be prioritised to aid best health outcomes for these people.

> *My COVID-19 story started in September 2022 with fever, body pain, asthma, and persistent coughing for 10 days. Unfortunately, other symptoms then progressively developed including fatigue, brain fog, headaches, low mood, muscle pain, heavy legs, low blood pressure and dizziness, speech difficulties, heart palpitations, sore throat, and hair loss resulting in my Long COVID diagnosis. Unable to work my husband became my carer while working fulltime. Recovery has been slow, and I am still not fully recovered.*
>
> Mary

15.3 NUTRITION SCREENING AND REFERRAL TO A DIETITIAN

Dietitians are tertiary qualified clinical nutrition experts who specialise in medical nutrition therapy (see Chapter 9) and work with individuals to optimise health through food and nutrition management. A dietitian is trained to implement personalised advice and management to address specific disease states, symptoms, nutrient deficiencies, and complex dietary needs. Dietetic accreditation programmes exist in many countries, ensuring commitment to best practice through assurance of qualifications and ongoing professional development.

Referral to a dietitian is recommended (and not limited to) for:

- Severe and protracted malnutrition (e.g., significant weight loss or gain)
- Nutrition deficiencies
- Complex nutrition needs (e.g., chronic conditions, functional impairment)
- Issues and/or symptoms impacting the ability to eat (e.g., reduced appetite, treatment side effects, fatigue)
- Specialised life stages (e.g., pregnancy, sports training).

When referring to a dietitian, a letter outlining the reason for referral, medical history, medications and recent biochemical tests will support prioritisation and assessment. Dietitians can also see people without a medical referral.

Assessing people living with Long COVID follows the standard nutrition assessment approach, however close attention should be directed to understanding the lived experience of symptoms for people with Long COVID to support the development of client goals (see Chapter 7). The following guidelines outline how dietitians and other health professionals contribute to nutritional screening and assessment for people with Long COVID, which makes the most of their respective skills and expertise (see Box 15.2).

BOX 15.2   LIVED EXPERIENCE RECOMMENDATIONS FOR HEALTH PROFESSIONALS

- Advise on nutrition's role in the management and recovery of Long COVID and refer to a Dietitian.
- Work with people with Long COVID to understand how easy or challenging it might be to implement changes.
- Provide one suggestion at a time with realistic optimism for suggestions made. This includes sharing both risks and benefits.
- Show empathy and compassion along a person's Long COVID journey. For example, "It makes sense that you feel disappointed with implementing that change."

Mary

15.4 NUTRITION FOR RECOVERY

Recovery time from COVID-19 is variable and depends on disease severity, preexisting comorbidities and age.[11] Chronic, low-grade inflammatory and immunologic states can persist for weeks, months or even years in people living with Long COVID. It is, therefore, crucial that nutrition interventions target inflammation in the recovery process because a healthy diet is essential for the production of antibodies, reduced oxidative stress, and reduced inflammation.[5] Recent attention has been given to the usefulness of various dietary patterns such as the Mediterranean Diet,[12] which have been found to exhibit anti-inflammatory properties and aid in the recovery of COVID-19.[13] The Mediterranean Diet is largely comprised of healthy, unsaturated fats, fruits, vegetables, wholegrains, and fish.[13] While observational studies report positive associations between consumption of a Mediterranean Dietary pattern and better health outcomes,[14] there is insufficient evidence to suggest a single dietary approach to aid Long COVID recovery. Rather, a personalised approach to symptom management and optimising nutritional status is the overall priority in management and care. Correcting nutritional deficiencies and providing individualised care to reduce the risk of malnutrition, while also potentially helping to reduce inflammation and strengthen the immune system, are the cornerstone of nutrition management for people with Long COVID (Figure 15.1).

1. Person's nutrition-related medical history

• Pre-existing conditions (e.g. diabetes, cardiovascular disease, coeliac disease, autonomic dysfunction etc).
• Medication and vitamin and mineral supplement use (note medication with impact on nutritional status).
• Current Long COVID symptoms (see Chapter 1) and concerns that may impact nutrition status
   (e.g. fatigue, loss of taste/smell, appetite changes, gut changes, anxiety, autonomic dysfunction).

2. Clinical examination and history

Anthropometry
• Height, weight, BMI (if appropriate)
• Weight history: Trends before and after COVID diagnosis (e.g. weight loss)
• Body composition analysis if available (muscle mass, fat mass)

Physical examination
• Signs of nutrient deficiencies (e.g., pallor, hair loss, skin changes).
• Functional assessment (e.g., muscle strength, fatigue levels).

Biochemical data
• Relevant nutrients (e.g. vitamin D, B12, iron).
• Inflammatory markers (e.g. CRP, ESR).
• Relevant metabolic markers (e.g. blood glucose, lipid profile)

Malnutrition screening
• Risk for malnutrition and undernutrition (e.g. Malnutrition Screening Tool[10])

3. Consider referral to a Dietitian

Using the information outlined above consider discussing onward referral for detailed nutrition assessment and education to support recovery.

4. Nutrition assessment

• Changes to appetite or eating with Long COVID onset and recovery
• Special individual eating pattern (e.g. vegetarian, vegan, gluten-free etc)
• Typical daily intake (including meals, snack, drinks and supplements)
• Meal timing and frequency
• Relationship with food (e.g. disordered eating patterns pre or post COVID, impact of taste changes)
• Access to food, socioeconomic status and impact on food intake and capacity to prepare meals

5. Personalised nutrition plan

• Discuss the person's nutrition goals and desire, capability and capacity to make nutrition changes.
• Discuss the importance of nutrition in recovery
• Co-set goals based on nutrition assessment and person goals. Encourage realistic goals and a positive relationship with food and their body.
• Encourage balanced and varied food pattern and adequate hydration – consider individual access to food and living circumstances
• Manage nutrition related Long COVID symptoms as indicated
• Supplement based on the deficiencies identified

6. Monitoring and follow up

• Agree on follow up period and monitoring
• Assess any new or ongoing symptoms
• Assess progress and adjust nutrition plan as required
• Coordinate with multi-disciplinary team (e.g. medical practitioner, dietitian, occupational therapist, psychologist, social worker)

Health Professionals

Nutrition Professionals

Figure 15.1 Nutrition screening and assessment for Long COVID.

Ensuring people are supported to achieve adequate intake of energy, macronutrients, and micronutrients from a variety of healthy food groups, including fruit and vegetables, grains, cereals and legumes, lean meat, chicken, fish, and reduced-fat milk and dairy foods, is essential. Inclusion of important nutrients including protein, carbohydrate, dietary fibre, unsaturated fats (e.g., omega-3 fatty acids), zinc, selenium, B vitamins, vitamins C and D, and antioxidants such as polyphenols and flavonoids[12,14,15] can assist in reducing inflammation, malnutrition risk, sarcopenia, and poor recovery outcomes (Figure 15.2).

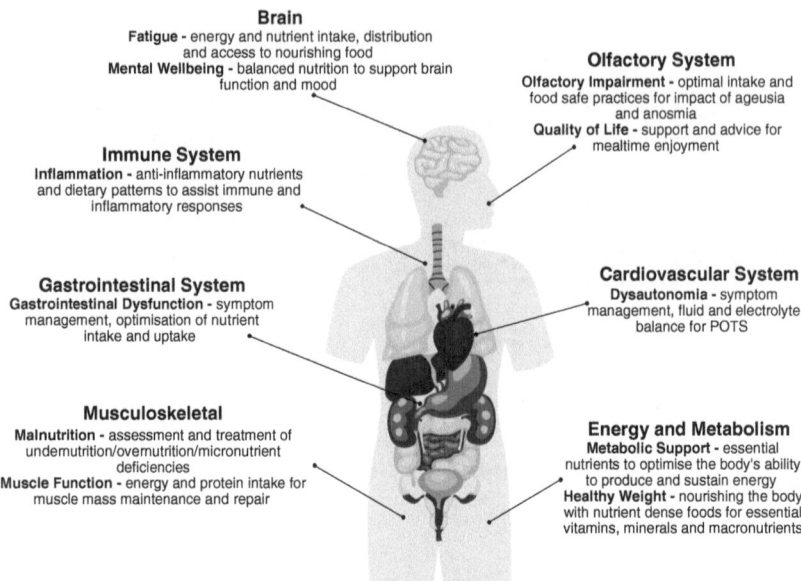

Brain
Fatigue - energy and nutrient intake, distribution
and access to nourishing food
Mental Wellbeing - balanced nutrition to support brain
function and mood

Olfactory System
Olfactory Impairment - optimal intake and
food safe practices for impact of ageusia
and anosmia
Quality of Life - support and advice for
mealtime enjoyment

Immune System
Inflammation - anti-inflammatory nutrients
and dietary patterns to assist immune and
inflammatory responses

Cardiovascular System
Dysautonomia - symptom
management, fluid and electrolyte
balance for POTS

Gastrointestinal System
Gastrointestinal Dysfunction - symptom
management, optimisation of nutrient
intake and uptake

Musculoskeletal
Malnutrition - assessment and treatment of
undernutrition/overnutrition/micronutrient
deficiencies
Muscle Function - energy and protein intake for
muscle mass maintenance and repair

Energy and Metabolism
Metabolic Support - essential
nutrients to optimise the body's ability
to produce and sustain energy
Healthy Weight - nourishing the body
with nutrient dense foods for essential
vitamins, minerals and macronutrients

Figure 15.2 The role of nutrition in supporting bodily functions for recovery.

A personalised approach to nutrition management, which considers a person's co-morbidities, culture and way of living, sociodemographic factors, current nutrition status, and their personal Long COVID journey, is critical. This can be provided via dietitian-led care as part of a comprehensive multi-disciplinary management plan.

> *Having had experience working with dietitians in the past, I had some understanding about the importance of nutrition in promoting my recovery and managing symptoms. I did seek Long COVID recovery support with medical professionals and what I experienced was often 'hit and miss', and very discouraging as my symptoms worsened.*
>
> *Along with scant information for Long COVID management, the different medical professionals either did not mention nutrition or provided a list of different 'diet options' with no direction. Restrictive diets, including intermittent fasting and low histamine, were challenging, made no difference or worsened my symptoms.*
>
> *What helped me was more trial and error and doing my own research online. What is currently working well for me? Eat regularly, adding salt to water and food, limiting coffee to one in the morning, always having healthy snacks accessible, continuing my Mediterranean diet and avoiding alcohol.*
>
> Mary

15.4.1 Balanced Food and Nutrition

In the Long COVID clinic we would recommend general healthy, balanced eating for people which would surprise them. They were even more surprised when eating this way improved their health and wellbeing.

Leigh

A wide variety of food is required to deliver the energy, protein, carbohydrates, fibre, fluids, vitamins, and minerals required for recovery. Regular dietary recommendations are appropriate for people with Long COVID, and country-specific healthy eating guidelines should be consulted for the best approach to achieving a balanced diet (see Box 15.3).

BOX 15.3   ESSENTIAL NUTRITION COMPONENTS TO SUPPORT RECOVERY FROM LONG COVID

- Protein at each meal for muscle repair and recover may include lean meats, fish (at least twice per week), eggs, beans, lentils, tofu, nuts, and low-fat dairy foods.
- Fruit (2 serves) and vegetables (5 serves) each day for vitamins, minerals, and fibre. Frozen, fresh, or tinned options are all good.
- High fibre and low glycaemic index carbohydrates at each meal for slow-release energy and gut health includes oats, barley, whole grain breads and cereals, basmati rice, some fruits, and vegetables.
- Healthy fats daily such as extra virgin olive oil, fish, and nuts.
- Nutrient dense foods provide a high amount of nutrients for their energy (e.g., fruits, vegetables, low fat dairy, lean proteins, whole grains, and nuts). Limit "empty foods" without key nutrients (e.g., soft drinks, confectionary).
- Encourage plenty of water to prevent dehydration.
- Limit caffeine containing drinks, alcohol, and sugar sweetened beverages.

While low-histamine and gluten-free diets are seen as helpful by some, there is currently no evidence to support their use in routine practice. However, the following evidence-based recommendation can support people with Long COVID to eat when they are feeling unwell (see Box 15.4).

BOX 15.4   NUTRITION TIPS TO SUPPORT ENERGY CONSERVATION AND FATIGUE MANAGEMENT

- **Small frequent meals**, including breakfast, for consistent energy and to prevent fatigue with eating large meals.
- **Healthy snacks** such as berries, cut up fruit and vegetables, yoghurt, and nuts for when tired.
- **Healthy convenience foods** and pre-prepared meals, for example, frozen vegetables, canned beans, and rotisserie chickens are convenient and save effort.
- **Encourage asking for help with accessing food**, meal preparation, or planning and preparing meals in advance.

15.4.2 Vitamin and Mineral Supplements

An evidence-based approach is important for nutrition supplementation including vitamin and mineral supplements and nutraceutical (bioactive) compounds. If nutrition deficiencies are identified during clinical, dietary, and biochemical assessment, additional supplementation may be required to support for diet and lifestyle alterations. Currently, there is insufficient evidence supporting the use of routine vitamin or mineral supplements, probiotics or nutraceuticals for Long COVID recovery. For people eating only small amounts, who are at risk of micronutrient malnutrition, a general multivitamin may be recommended to no more than 100% of daily recommendations for single nutrients.

There is also caution against the excessive use of supplements. When advising people, emphasise that taking supplements without a clear medical indication can pose significant risks. These include potential interactions with prescribed medications, the possibility of reaching toxic levels of certain nutrients, and adverse effects on organ function. A dietitian, following a thorough assessment, is best suited to determine any necessary supplementation safe and is tailored to their individual health needs.

15.5 NUTRITION FOR SYMPTOM MANAGEMENT

15.5.1 Nutrition and Olfactory Dysfunction

Olfactory change is a common symptom of Long COVID. Part or whole loss of taste (ageusia) and smell (anosmia) can be a short-term (transitory) or ongoing. These changes can make food taste bland, significantly impacting the enjoyment of food, the desire to eat, food choice, appetite, and food intake.

One person with olfactory dysfunction spoke about the complete loss of food enjoyment and the great sadness that her "culture had been taken" from her.

Leigh

Nutrition management of olfactory dysfunction is crucial due to the risk of reduced enjoyment of food compromising food intake leading to nutrition imbalances. There are risks associated with the consumption of unsafe or spoiled foods leading to food borne illness. Further, depressed mood, anxiety and reduced quality of life from a changed psychosocial relationship with food may occur.[16] The following evidence-based tips (Box 15.5) will support people with Long COVID to manage olfactory dysfunction.

BOX 15.5   NUTRITION TIPS TO SUPPORT OLFACTORY CHANGES

FOR THE HEALTH PROFESSIONAL

- Explore the loss of taste or smell and its impact on eating behaviour including food choice, appetite, and food intake and potential malnutrition. Discuss why it is important to optimise safe nutritional intake.

FOR THE PERSON WITH OLFACTORY CHANGES

- Experiment with different flavours. Use herbs, spices, and other flavour enhancers (e.g., condiments – mustard, pickles, chutneys, tomato sauce)
- Try different food textures, such as crunchy, creamy or crispy foods, and different colours.
- Eat in a relaxed environment and concentrate on the colour, texture, smell, and your taste memory of the food.
- Monitor weight and talk to a dietitian to prevent nutrition deficiencies if food intake is a concern.
- Be food safe by checking expiry dates and have others check if food has spoiled. Label food when opening to keep track of its age.
- Work with a Dietitian to identify strategies to cope with loss of taste or smell and to ensure a balanced food intake.

15.4.2 Nutrition and Fatigue

Inadequate nutritional intake may be one of the mechanisms behind underlying fatigue, with inadequacies in nutrients including energy, protein, carbohydrate, iron, vitamin B12, vitamin D, and fluid. In turn, fatigue can make it difficult to maintain

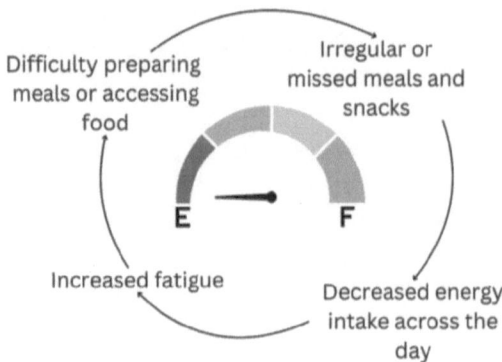

Figure 15.3 Fatigue nutrition cycle.

an adequate food and nutrient intake due to reduced energy to access, prepare and eat food, impaired cognitive function, appetite changes, or gastrointestinal associations (e.g., irritable bowel syndrome, Postural Orthostatic Tachycardia Syndrome [POTS]) (Figure 15.3).

> *I would wake up in the morning and have to decide if I had enough energy to eat or have a shower.*
>
> Mary

The cycle starts with difficulty preparing or accessing food, leading to decreased food intake, resulting in decreased energy intake and energy continuing the cycle.

This may lead to people with Long COVID opting for quick, convenient foods of poor nutritional value. In addition to enquiring about sleep quality and duration, the following evidence-based recommendations (Box 15.6) provide health professionals and people with Long COVID with nutritional strategies to manage fatigue.

BOX 15.6 NUTRITION TIPS TO SUPPORT LIVING WITH FATIGUE

FOR THE HEALTH PROFESSIONAL

- Discuss the link between nutrition and fatigue to elicit potential nutrition-related contributions to fatigue.
- Measure and correct any nutrition deficiencies.
- Examine food intake to understand adequacy of macronutrients (energy, carbohydrate, protein, fat) and micronutrients (vitamins and minerals) and fluid.

- Refer to a Dietitian for detailed assessment.
- Discuss tips to optimise nutrition intake when experiencing fatigue.

FOR THE PERSON WITH FATIGUE

- Drink plenty of water to prevent dehydration, which can worsen fatigue.
- Eat small frequent meals, including breakfast, to provide consistent energy and prevent fatigue with eating large meals.
- Choose nutrient dense foods that provide a high amount of nutrients for their energy (e.g., fruits, vegetables, low fat dairy, lean proteins, whole grains, and nuts). Limit "empty foods" without key nutrients (e.g., soft drinks, confectionary).
- Keep healthy snacks handy such as cut up fruit and vegetables, yoghurt, and nuts.
- Take advantage of healthy convenience foods and pre-prepared meals, for example, frozen vegetables, canned beans, and rotisserie chickens are convenient and save effort.
- Ask for help with meal preparation and plan and prepare meals in advance so there are nutritious meals ready to go.
- Focus on the nutrients you are lacking that have been identified by a health professional. Eat foods that help boost that nutrient or take supplements if this is recommended.
- Limit caffeine particularly in the later part of the day, which can make it difficult to sleep.

15.6 NUTRITION AND POSTURAL ORTHOSTATIC TACHYCARDIA SYNDROME

POTS is a type of cardiovascular autonomic dysfunction seen in Long COVID (see Chapter 16). It can significantly impact nutrition intake and status, with nutrition also playing a role in management and recovery of POTS. Dysautonomia may result in gastrointestinal symptoms including nausea, abdominal pain, gastroparesis and early satiety, or feeling full, leading to reduced food intake or nutrient malabsorption. The fatigue, low energy and low blood pressure POTS causes can contribute to lack of appetite and energy for accessing and preparing food. Medications for POTS treatment may also change appetite and interact with other nutrients, while additional sodium and fluid may alter electrolyte balance or blood pressure.

It took me a while to fully understand that increasing my electrolyte and fluid intake would make a difference to my blood pressure. I had to work hard at it.

Grace

A multidisciplinary structured approach (see Chapter 10) to POTS including dietetic interventions is required to aid increase in blood volume and blood pressure, prevent sarcopenia, reduce gastrointestinal symptom impact, and promote overall Long COVID recovery. Dietitians can provide nutrition-related strategies to help optimise POTS management. The following evidence-based tips (Box 15.7) will support people with Long COVID to employ nutritional strategies when managing POTS.

BOX 15.7   NUTRITION TIPS TO SUPPORT LIVING WITH POTS

FOR THE HEALTH PROFESSIONAL

- Discuss the impact of POTs on nutrition and elicit potential nutrition-related reasons contributing to symptoms.
- Discuss the nutrition-related strategies to optimise POTS management.

FOR THE PERSON WITH POTS

- Drink plenty of water to increase blood volume with recommendations of 3 litres of water daily[17] and increased sodium recommendations. Drinking 500 ml of water before getting out of bed may help some.
- Increase salt (sodium chloride) intake to help increase blood volume. Varying for individuals, salt can be increased gradually to three to ten grams daily (two teaspoons of table salt is approximately ten grams) using ordinary table salt, electrolyte or salt tablets, or electrolyte solutions.[17] To make an electrolyte drink add 6 level teaspoons (30 g) of sugar and ½ level teaspoon of salt (2.5 g) into 1 litre of water, flavouring with cordial can help with palatability.
- Choose salt containing foods that are higher in nutrients or can be added to other nutrient dense foods. For example, soya sauce, ketchup or tomato sauce, pickles, olives, salted nuts, salted popcorn, commercial soups, and wholegrain bread.
- Eat small frequent meals, including breakfast, containing protein, and low glycaemic index carbohydrates (e.g., beans and legumes, most fruit and vegetables, wholegrain bread, pasta) to slow blood diversion to the gastrointestinal system.
- Check food intolerances or triggers with some people with POTS reporting different food triggering symptoms. Keep a food diary with the associated triggers.

- Limit or avoid alcohol with the potential for worsening with possible blood vessel dilation and diuretic effect.
- Be cautious of caffeine in coffee, tea, and caffeine energy drinks. Some people may experience a worsening of symptoms such as tachycardia.
- Consult with an accredited dietitian experienced with POTS to create a nutrition management plan that suits individual needs, circumstances, and symptoms.

15.7 NUTRITION AND GASTROINTESTINAL SYMPTOMS

Common gastrointestinal symptoms of Long COVID include loss of appetite, nausea, dyspepsia, diarrhoea, constipation, irritable bowel syndrome, and abdominal pain. These symptoms may be episodic or chronic and can significantly impact nutrition status and quality of life. Nutrition plays an important role in both the pathophysiology and management of these symptoms.

> *I experienced digestive bloating, pain and constipation and a worsening of symptoms in response to dairy, soy, alcohol and eating carbohydrates such as gluten free bread, pasta and rice. I was bedbound most of the day relying on others for my nutrition and other needs."*
>
> Mary

> *I kept saying that I was not digesting food properly with my gut moving slowly. This was put down to anxiety at the start and I am relieved to find out that this was related to Long COVID.*
>
> Jenny

Tailored nutrition assessment and advice is fundamental to supporting recovery and must balance the multifactorial nature of symptom management with maintaining nutritional adequacy. Referral to an experienced dietitian should be considered to ensure people with Long COVID living with these symptoms receive high quality and effective care. However, the following evidence-based recommendations (Box 15.8) provide health professionals and people with Long COVID with guidelines for managing Long COVID–related gastrointestinal symptoms

BOX 15.8 NUTRITION RECOMMENDATIONS FOR MANAGING LONG COVID–RELATED GASTROINTESTINAL SYMPTOMS.

FOR THE HEALTH PROFESSIONAL

- Detailed symptom history: Discuss the onset of symptoms including duration, frequency and severity of symptoms and any potential triggers. Differentiate between pre-morbid, COVID, and post-COVID symptoms. Enquire about previous nutrition education or advice.
- Evaluate nutrition intake and status: Assess for malnutrition, weight change, and dehydration. Enquire about changes in food intake, changes in appetite and elimination of food groups. Consider the need for referral to a dietitian for a full assessment.
- Exclude other potential causes or gastrointestinal conditions including inflammatory bowel disease, and coeliac disease or POTS (Chapter 17) via usual diagnostic pathways.

FOR THE PERSON WITH GASTROINTESTINAL SYMPTOMS

- Keep a record of symptoms, food eaten, and any other potential triggers.
- Discuss referral to a dietitian for tailored advice.
- Stayed hydrated by sipping water and electrolyte drinks as required thought the day. Avoid caffeine.
- Focus on small, frequent meals to reduce the digestive load, bloating and nausea.
- Anti-nausea strategies can include sipping water, ginger tea, or ginger supplements.
- Reduce stress at meals by making them as relaxing as possible and allow enough time to eat without rushing.
- Choose easy-to-digest foods for a short time, such as low-fibre foods such as white rice, toast, and popped rice cereal. Limit overly spicy, fried, or fatty foods, as well as alcohol, as they can exacerbate gastrointestinal discomfort.

15.8 CONCLUSION

Health professionals should discuss the role of nutrition in Long COVID management and recovery and refer to a Dietitian when appropriate. Working together will help both the health professional and the person with Long COVID to better understand the implementation and outcome of nutritional changes. Providing one suggestion at a time, realistic optimism about implementing recommendations and sharing both potential risks and benefits will support individual recovery. Importantly, health professionals should demonstrate empathy and compassion for the journey of people with Long COVID, especially when hoped for recovery may be slow. With the right advice and support, it is possible to continue to enjoy meals and eating while still promoting healing and recovery.

A meal is more than the sum of its parts or nutrients; it provides joy, fosters human connection, and creates opportunities to share love, culture, and memorable moments around the table.

REFERENCES

1 Prentice AM. The triple burden of malnutrition in the era of globalization. Nestle Nutr Inst Workshop Ser. 2023;97:51–61. doi:10.1159/000529005.

2 Tosato M, et al. Malnutrition in COVID-19 survivors: Prevalence and risk factors. Aging Clin Exp Res. 2023;35(10):2257–65. doi:10.1007/s40520-023-02526-4.

3 Gérard M, et al. Long-term evolution of malnutrition and loss of muscle strength after COVID-19: A major and neglected component of Long COVID-19. Nutrients 2021;13(11):3964. doi:10.3390/nu13113964.

4 Younes S. The role of nutrition on the treatment of COVID 19. Hum Nutr Metab 2024;36:200255. doi:10.1016/j.hnm.2024.200255

5 Kurtz A, et al. Long-term effects of malnutrition on severity of COVID-19.Sci Rep. 2021;11(1):14974. doi:10.1038/s41598-021-94138-z.

6 Souza JA, et al. Patients with post-COVID-19 syndrome are at risk of malnutrition and obesity: Findings of outpatient follow-up. Rev Nutr. 2022;35:e220015. doi:10.1590/1678-986520 2235e220015.

7 Ponce J, et al. Association between malnutrition and post–acute COVID-19 sequelae: A retrospective cohort study. JPEN 2024, doi:10.1002/jpen.2478.

8 Lee C-Y, et al. Malnutrition and the post-acute sequelae of severe acute respiratory syndrome Coronavirus-2 infection: A multi-institutional population-based propensity score-matched analysis. Life 2024;14(6):746. doi:10.3390/life14060746.

9 Levy D, et al. Long-term follow-up of sarcopenia and malnutrition after hospitalization for COVID-19 in conventional or intensive-care units. Nutrients. 2022;14(4):912, doi:10.3390/nu14040912.

10 Serón-Arbeloa C, et al. Malnutrition screening and assessment. Nutrients. 2022;14(12):2392. doi:10.3390/nu14122392.

11 Rizvi AA, et al. Post-COVID syndrome, inflammation, and diabetes. J Diabetes Complicat. 2022;36(11):108336. doi:10.1016/j.jdiacomp.2022.108336.

12 Angelidi AM, et al. Mediterranean diet as a nutritional approach for COVID-19. Metab Clin Exp. 2021;114. doi:10.1016/j.metabol.2020.154407.

13 Milton-Laskibar I, et al. Potential usefulness of Mediterranean diet polyphenols against COVID-19-induced inflammation: A review of the current knowledge. J Physiol Biochem. 2023;79(2):371–82. doi:10.1007/s13105-023-00914-1.

14 Barrea L, et al. Dietary recommendations for Post-COVID-19 Syndrome. Nutrients. 2022;14(6):1305. doi:10.3390/nu14061305.

15 Schloss JV. Nutritional deficiencies that may predispose to Long COVID. Inflammopharmacology. 2023;31(2):573–83. doi:10.1007/s10787-022-01088-0.

16 Speth MM, et al. Mood, anxiety and olfactory dysfunction in COVID-19: Evidence of central nervous system involvement? Laryngoscope. 2020;130(11), 2520–25. doi:10.1002/lary.28964.

17 Raj SR, et al. Diagnosis and management of postural orthostatic tachycardia syndrome. CMAJ. 2022;194(10):E378–85. doi:10.1503/cmaj.211231.

Chapter 16

Management of Postural Orthostatic Tachycardia Syndrome

Naomi Whyler, Raeya Bognar, Nathan Butler, Jennifer Smallridge, and Emma Tippett

---

BOX 16.1 LEARNING OBJECTIVES

By the end of this chapter, readers should be able to:

- Understand the key characteristics and symptoms of Postural Orthostatic Tachycardia Syndrome (POTS).
- Identify effective lifestyle modifications that aid in the management of symptoms.
- Describe and understand the pharmacological interventions available to improve symptoms.
- Appreciate the significance of patient education and self-management techniques in enhancing treatment outcomes.
- Apply a multidisciplinary approach to support individuals with POTS to improve their overall quality of life.

16.1 INTRODUCTION

Dysautonomia is characterised by dysfunction of the Autonomic Nervous System (ANS), which governs many vital processes that operate involuntarily, that is, automatically without conscious thought. These include heart rate (HR), blood pressure (BP), digestion, pupil response, kidney function, and temperature regulation. This intricate system is essential for maintaining the body's internal environment, and disruption can profoundly impact daily life. People with dysautonomia often struggle to regulate this critical system, leading to symptoms of light-headedness, fainting, nausea due to BP fluctuations, irregular HR, and

DOI: 10.4324/9781003528104-20

gastrointestinal disturbance. In severe cases, this can lead to malnutrition and other life-threatening complications. The most common dysautonomia diagnosis is Postural Orthostatic Tachycardia Syndrome (POTS).

Dysautonomia is not rare. Before the COVID-19 pandemic, the prevalence of POTS was estimated between 0.2% and 1% of the United States population, or 1 in 500 people.[1] Data from other countries is lacking, and the prevalence of all types of dysautonomia worldwide is difficult to estimate. It predominantly affects people born female (80%) and most often impacts daily life between 15 and 50 years of age.[1] Approximately 80% of people with Long COVID present with dysautonomia-like symptoms[2]; therefore, being able to identify and manage it is essential for interdisciplinary care and validation for the individual.

BOX 16.2   PRACTICE POINT

Reflect on your current knowledge about dysautonomia. Have you come across this in your clinical practice in the past? What else would you like to know about these conditions?

16.2 PATHOPHYSIOLOGY OF DYSAUTONOMIA AND POTS

The pathophysiology of dysautonomia in Long COVID involves complex interactions between the ANS and various physiological processes disrupted by COVID-19 infection. Theories about the underlying mechanisms are multifaceted (see Chapter 2), involving neurotropism, autoimmunity, persistent inflammation, and neuro-immune-endocrine dysregulation (Figure 16.1).

While the dysautonomia pathophysiology in Long COVID is complex and not currently well-understood, its causes may overlap with other conditions like Myalgic Encephalomyelitis/Chronic Fatigue Syndrome (ME/CFS) and mast cell activation syndrome (MCAS)[1] potentially due to shared vascular pathological processes and vasoactive mediators.[6] POTS is also associated with joint hypermobility,[1] chronic migraines and irritable bowel syndrome.[7] It can be triggered by other conditions, including infectious agents and hormonal changes such as the onset of puberty and pregnancy.[1] It can also overlap with autoimmune conditions such as Autoimmune Autonomic Ganglionopathy.[1] Understanding the mechanisms connecting these disorders will be essential to developing diagnostic and therapeutic strategies for Long COVID patients.[8]

Neurotropism	Autoimmunity	Inflammatory Responses	Cardiovascular Autonomic Imbalance	Neuro Immune Endocrine Dysregulation
• COVID19 invades the central autonomic centres e.g. hypothalamus and medulla either directly (neuronal, haematogenous routes) or indirectly[3]	• Autoantibodies to receptor and glycoproteins on cellular membranes lead to autonomic dysfunction[3]	• Persistent inflammation and cytokine storms cause sympathetic overactivity and parasympathetic underactivity[3,4]	• Lower heart rate variability suggests impaired vagal activity and sympatho-vagal imbalance[5]	• Reduced hypothalamic-pituitary-axis (HPA) axis activity and altered neurotransmitter levels (dopamine, serotonin) affect autonomic function with pro-inflammatory sympathetic activity and anti-inflammatory parasympathetic activity leading to 'inflammaging' or chronic inflammation[4]

Figure 16.1 Current theories about underlying mechanisms for dysautonomia caused by COVID-19 infection[3-5].

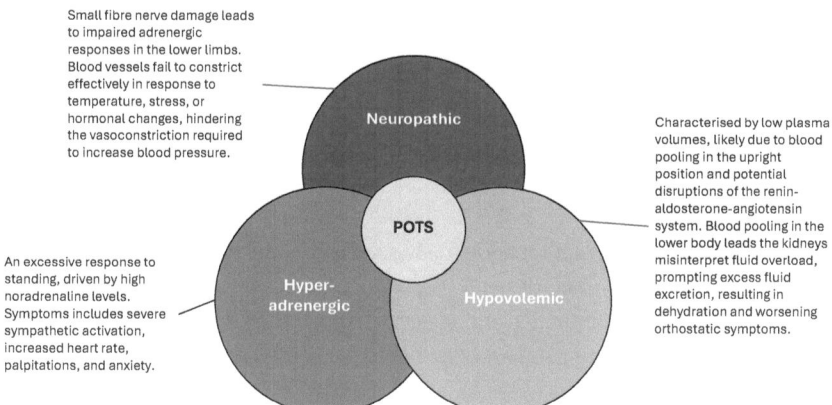

Figure 16.2 Postural Orthostatic Tachycardia (POTS) classifications.[9,10]

POTS can be classified into three interrelated subtypes, and patients will sometimes experience more than one[9,10] (Figure 16.2).

16.3 CLINICAL PRESENTATION OF POTS

The clinical presentation of POTS is wide-ranging due to the impact of dysautonomia on multiple body systems.[1] It should be suspected in those with cardiovascular symptoms and signs, which include palpitations, dizziness, orthostatic tachycardia (significantly increased HR upon standing), presyncope (the sensation they are about to faint), chest pain, dyspnoea, and acrocyanosis (persistent blue or purple skin discolouration). These symptoms are often accompanied by others, such as heat intolerance, headaches, cognitive dysfunction, anxiety, sleep disorders, gastrointestinal disturbances, sensory overwhelm, and fatigue.[1]

16.4 DIAGNOSIS OF POTS

Both people with Long COVID and POTS frequently experience frustrating delays and barriers to diagnosis, which can cause significant physical, emotional, and social distress. Once suspected, however, POTS can be diagnosed using objective diagnostic criteria, which can validate their lived experience and inform treatment pathways.

POTS is diagnosed when the HR increases by 30 beats per minute (bpm) upon postural changes from lying to sitting or sitting to standing.[1] A change of 40 bpm is required for those aged 12–19 years.[1] A postural BP drop of 20 millimetres of mercury (mmHg) is diagnostic of orthostatic hypotension rather than POTS.[1] However, even when diagnostic criteria are not met, many people with Long COVID experience symptoms and signs of dysautonomia and benefit from similar management strategies.

Every person with persistent fatigue following COVID infection should be assessed for POTS, preferably by their General Practitioner. Objective measures like the 10-minute National Aeronautics and Space Administration (NASA) Lean Test and Tilt Table Testing (TTT) are used for diagnosis.[1] The NASA Lean Test is the most straightforward and most accessible test to perform, requiring only a BP measuring device (sphygmomanometer) and a wall.

TTT is considered the gold standard for POTS diagnosis and is commonly used in research trials and sometimes in clinical assessments. However, it is not required for diagnosis and can be challenging for many to access, causing delays in diagnosis and management. Access barriers include financial cost, geographical barriers, especially in rural and remote areas, and, notably, the additional patient burden and energy expenditure required to travel and undergo an intensive test. The physiological stress of TTT may exacerbate symptoms in the short to medium term, limiting the patient's abilities to perform activities in daily life. These considerations inform decisions about which assessment is best for the person with Long COVID and their health professional.

Subjective measures can also be used alongside objective measures or where objective measures are unavailable due to resourcing or access barriers. The Malmö POTS Score[11] (MAPS) is a free, readily accessible and usable test containing twelve questions that evaluate the impact of POTS symptoms from a 0–10 scale (0 = no symptoms, 10 = pronounced symptoms). These symptoms include dizziness, palpitations, breathing, chest pain, headache, concentration challenges, muscle pain, nausea, gastrointestinal challenges, abnormal tiredness, and insomnia.

Alternatively, the Composite Autonomic Symptom Score[12] (COMPASS-31) is a validated screening tool for POTS, which measures 31 items across six domains of autonomic function: orthostatic intolerance, vasomotor, secretomotor, gastrointestinal, bladder, and pupillomotor. A high score indicates worse autonomic dysfunction, with a total score of 0–100. The measure has excellent internal consistency and is also freely available online.

BOX 16.3   PRACTICE POINT

Reflect on the barriers and facilitators to diagnosing suspected dysautonomia. How could you incorporate accessible testing into your practice? What challenges do you anticipate facing when doing this? How might improving access to diagnosis help your patients with Long COVID?

16.4.1 Common Comorbidities and Interactions

Following diagnosis, other potential conditions commonly associated with dysautonomia should be considered. Fatigue is a cardinal symptom of a phenomenon widely experienced in Long COVID – Post-Exertional Malaise (PEM). PEM refers to symptoms that worsen with physical, cognitive, or emotional exertion, including brain fog, myalgia, sleep disturbances, flu-like feelings, arthralgia, headache, sore throat, and/or tender lymph nodes.[13,14] POTS is a condition while PEM is a symptom; however, their presentations overlap and can impact their respective treatment options. For example, physical activity recommended for POTS may not be possible or safe for people with PEM, possibly due to dysfunctional oxygenation of body tissues.[15] Any physical activity prescribed for POTS must be tailored to avoid triggering PEM, with close monitoring of symptom thresholds and post-activity recovery times. Non-exertional strategies for POTS (like increased salt and fluid intake and compression garments) may also make additional energy demands on people with PEM. They must be incorporated into their "energy envelope" and pacing strategies (see Chapter 11).

Hypermobility syndromes, which include a range of conditions where joints move beyond their typical range, should also be considered, including connective tissue disorders (CTDs) such as Ehlers-Danlos Syndrome (EDS).[16,17] EDS is a group of 13 (at the time of publishing) heritable CTDs caused by genetic changes affecting connective tissue. Each has distinctive features; however, all show joint hypermobility, skin hyperextensibility, and tissue fragility. Disorders such as EDS can also affect blood vessels, and if present, the patient will require support from a complex specialist team to assess other associated risks, including the risk of vascular aneurysms.[16]

Joint hypermobility can impact activity prescription (see below) and participation in daily life. The Beighton hypermobility test[18] or the 5-point hypermobility screening questionnaire[19] can be performed easily and quickly in primary care to identify patients' possible hypermobility. The Beighton test measures joint hypermobility on a 9-point scale assessing the fifth fingers, thumbs, elbows, knees, and spine. A score greater than or equal to 6/9 in children (pre-puberty), 5/9 in adults and 4/9 in adults over 50 years is classified as a positive test[20] and indicates likely benefit from further specialist evaluation. These tests objectively measure whether the degree of movement of specific joints is within the expected range of movements relative to the general population.

MCAS frequently overlaps with POTS in patients with Long COVID.[1] Diagnosis can be challenging due to the current lack of consensus on diagnostic criteria and objective testing. People with MCAS[21] experience a range of symptoms, including itchy skin, nasal congestion, gastrointestinal problems, brain fog, joint pain, weakness or numbness, swelling, flushing, shortness of breath, and can experience severe manifestations with low BP and anaphylaxis. The main symptom driver is histamine release from mast cells, which can act as a vasodilator, thus causing symptom overlap with Long COVID and POTS due to postural symptoms. MCAS often responds favourably to antihistamines, and, where applicable, patients should be referred to an immunologist or allergy specialist for assessment and management.

For people who menstruate, hormonal fluctuation across the cycle can impact symptoms.[22] For example, oestrogen can decrease connective tissue stiffness, increase joint laxity, and worsen pain. Symptoms may be exacerbated during the luteal phase, between ovulation and the onset of menstruation. Progesterone increases in the luteal phase and may exacerbate POTS symptoms due to its vasodilatory effects.[22] Some people may benefit from exploring correlations between symptoms and cycle phases to help plan activities and allow for more efficient pacing.

16.5 BEST PRACTICE IN POTS MANAGEMENT

Both pharmacological and non-pharmacological interventions are effective for POTS. Management strategies focus on meeting one or more of the following aims (Figure 16.3).

16.5.1 Pharmacological Interventions

Pharmacological interventions are often required alongside non-pharmacological interventions and generally focus on increasing blood volume, vasoconstriction (narrowing blood vessels) with increased venous return and cardiac output through rate control. Once non-pharmacological strategies are trialled, repeating the NASA Lean test can help assess the severity of residual deficits and inform shared decision-making around medication options.

16.5.1.1 Increasing Blood Volume

Fludrocortisone is an aldosterone analogue and is frequently used to manage POTS symptoms. It works by retaining salt, resulting in increased blood volume. Side

---

Increasing Blood Volume

- To counteract the hypovolaemic state increasing blood volume through salt consumption, coupled with water as well as salt retaining medications can increase total blood volume.

Increasing Venous Return

- Venous return is the amount of blood that is being returned to the heart from the body. This is reduced in untreated POTS resulting in less blood being pumped out. Venous return can be increased by increasing the blood volume or by reducing blood pooling via compression.

Increasing Stroke Volume

- Stroke volume is the amount of blood that the heart pumps out with each beat. A larger stroke volume can counteract gravity better and improve cerebral perfusion. Stroke volume can be increased by increasing venous return or by slowing the heart with medications.

Figure 16.3 Aims of POTS Management.

effects include headache, which can prompt discontinuation, and hypokalaemia, which can occur following initiation.[23] Desmopressin is an alternative option with fewer side effects but can cause hyponatraemia.[23]

16.5.1.2 Increasing Venous Return

Midodrine is an alpha$_1$-adrenergic receptor antagonist that causes peripheral vasoconstriction and increases venous return.[23] Midodrine can provide effective symptom relief and is particularly useful in people with low BP. However, it has several side effects that limit tolerability and a short half-life that requires frequent dosing.[23] One expected and unavoidable side effect is a sensation of skin crawling due to piloerection. Other side effects include urinary retention, hypertension, including paradoxical supine hypertension, dry mouth, and anxiety. Midodrine is contraindicated in severe renal disease and can cause bradycardia due to the vagal reflex; therefore, monitoring is warranted. It can also interact with commonly used medications, including antihistamines and tricyclic antidepressants: these are not absolute contraindications, but use should be monitored carefully.[24]

Pyridostigmine is also used with some success.[23] It is a peripheral acetylcholinesterase inhibitor that increases synaptic acetylcholine. It is thought to act by increasing sympathetic vasoconstriction or decreasing vagal tone. Its most frequently reported side-effect is diarrhoea, which can also be a symptom of Long COVID. Pyridostigmine has few relevant drug interactions but does have a short half-life and requires frequent dosing. It may also cause bradycardia, so HR monitoring is recommended.

16.5.1.3 Increasing Stroke Volume

Rate control with ivabradine can be an effective treatment with few side effects.[23] It works by slowing HR, allowing increased filling time and, therefore, increased stroke volume, that is, the amount of blood pumped each heartbeat. There are some pharmacological interactions to be aware of, for example, calcium channel blockers and some COVID-19 antivirals, and it is contraindicated in pregnancy and breastfeeding. Ivabradine is usually used in heart failure and is not recommended in people with resting HR <70 bpm in these circumstances. However, clinical experience demonstrates it is well tolerated in otherwise healthy young people with resting HR 60–69 when awake. Beta-blockers are frequently recommended in guidelines but may not provide symptom relief as effectively as ivabradine.[23] They are, however, a safe alternative in pregnancy and can double up as an antihypertensive in patients with high BP.

Medications used for other conditions may also help manage symptoms but are less commonly prescribed. These include clonidine,[23] methyldopa,[23] guanfacine,[25] and amphetamines including modafinil.[26]

16.5.2 Non-pharmacological Interventions

16.5.2.1 Diet and Hydration

Optimal hydration and diet are essential.[1] A target of 8,000–10,000 mg of salt daily increases thirst and water retention. Patients should be educated on drinking 2–3 litres daily and having regular access to water. Most people with POTS do not experience hypertension, but a few do. Increased salt intake warrants medical monitoring to detect the development of hypertension.

Smaller, frequent meals or snacks are recommended instead of larger, carbohydrate-heavy meals. This approach manages nutrition while minimising the diversion of blood to the digestive tract.[1] Dietitians can offer expert advice on dietary management (see Chapter 15).

16.5.1.2 Supervised and Safe Physical Activity

Increasing cardiovascular fitness through physical activity can improve cardiac output but must be managed and supervised carefully to ensure safety. Physiotherapists and exercise physiologists have specific expertise in this area; however, other multidisciplinary team members can also promote physical activity (see Chapter 11).

BOX 16.4   PROVIDING SAFE AND SUPERVISED PHYSICAL ACTIVITY INTERVENTIONS FOR POTS

While estimates vary, up to 90% of people with Long COVID experience PEM[27] and up to 79% have POTS.[2] All people with Long COVID should be screened for PEM using a validated tool such as the DePaul Symptoms Questionnaire-Post Exertional Malaise short form.[28] Graded Exercise Therapy, involving predetermined incremental increases in physical activity, is not recommended for people with Long COVID and PEM.[29] The CDC, UK NICE, and WHO all caution against using this intervention. The best practice for people with POTS and PEM is based on pacing and adapted physical activity protocols (see Chapter 11).

An individualised approach to physical activity is recommended for people with POTS and PEM because it directly addresses their unique physiological challenges, including exercise intolerance, autonomic dysregulation, and PEM risks. By personally tailoring the intensity, type, and progression of exercise, the approach minimises symptom exacerbation while enabling gradual improvement. The following best practice principles ensure these patients participate in physical activity safely and supportedly.[30]

- An **individually tailored approach** prevents symptom exacerbation, and supervision and monitoring by appropriately trained health professionals ensure the activity is performed safely.[30] For people with POTS, this approach often begins with an initial consultation to collaboratively design an activity plan, followed by periodic in-person or virtual supervision.[31]
- **Focus on function** because, for many people, the goal is not achieving peak fitness but improving participation in daily life. To understand the impact of POTS on their patient, health professionals must engage with and evaluate contextual influences such as occupation, hobbies, and lifestyle choices. These are unique to individuals and were manageable before they developed Long COVID but are now challenging to perform without symptom exacerbation.
- **Gradual progression** helps to recondition the autonomic system without overwhelming it.[30] Start with manageable activities (e.g., increasing bed incline) to build a foundation for later participation in higher-intensity activities. Some patients may eventually be able to engage with POTS specific protocols for higher intensity physical activity.[32] Recumbent or floor-based activities minimise their BP impact, as does starting with endurance activities before progressing to resistance activities.[33]
- Core and proximal **strengthening activities** to improve stability and reduce strain during activity are particularly effective for people with mitochondrial dysfunction, decreased skeletal muscle activity, and joint instability (especially in cases of comorbid hypermobility).[30] Distal strengthening exercises in the lower limbs may also help build muscle strength, stamina, and contraction, which can increase cardiac output.
- **Adapting physical activity to address comorbidities** enables a holistic approach to intervention.[30] Example adaptations include:
  - EDS – An emphasis on joint stability and co-contraction to protect hyper-mobile joints
  - ME/CFS – Integrated pacing and rest to accommodate energy limitations
  - MCAS – Modification for exercise induced triggers (e.g., heat sensitivity)
- Many people with Long COVID who experience POTS and/or PEM have severe symptoms that leave them confined to their homes or bed bound.

Home-based, remote-delivery approaches support accessibility and provide a safe starting point for physical activity.[30] Remote delivery eliminates the burden of travelling to appointments, allowing patients to focus their limited energy on meaningful activity.

16.5.2.3 Compression Garments

Medical grade compression of at least 20–30 mmHg can support BP management by preventing blood pooling, allowing better circulation and decreasing POTS symptoms.[1] Compression garments come in many forms, including socks, stockings, leggings, underwear, and sleeves. Compression of the abdomen and lower limbs is effective for POTS[34]; however, many also report benefits from compression of other body parts.

Few medical contraindications exist for the use of compression; these include poor skin integrity, severe peripheral neuropathy and arterial insufficiency.[35] For people with severe fatigue, compression garments require significant energy to put on. Furthermore, people experiencing heat sensitivity or gastrointestinal issues may be unable to tolerate full length compression. Focusing on options that are better tolerated, such as abdominal with an abdominal binder, compression shorts or undergarments, is a pragmatic option. If a patient struggles with donning and doffing compression garments, refer to an occupational therapist for dressing training and/or the prescription of assistive aids (see Chapter 12).

16.5.2.4 Head Up Sleeping

Sleeping with the bed head elevated by 10–15 centimetres (4–6 inches) increases blood volume on waking and improves orthostatic tolerance by activating the renin-angiotensin system due to orthostatic pressure.[36] Whole bed elevation using bed blocks under the legs of the head of the bed is necessary, rather than increasing pillow numbers. This intervention is effective for patients with severe morning orthostatic intolerance, severe weakness and/or PEM, which limits their ability to participate in physical activities.

16.5.3 Patient Education

Empower people with Long COVID by providing information about pacing, PEM, and POTS to develop realistic and shared expectations mutually. All patient education must affirm that intolerance of physical activity is a physiological (and not a purely psychological) issue.

Many health professionals have experience providing patient education but may require additional training and expertise to deploy these skills for POTS. Topics of education may include but are not limited to, pathophysiology, objective and subjective assessment, physical activity, pacing, sleep hygiene, optimisation of participation in daily life, vocational rehabilitation, and other non-pharmacological strategies. All multidisciplinary team members must provide consistent advice within their scope of practice (see Chapter 10).

The key purpose of patient education for people experiencing POTS is to enhance understanding of their personal triggers, symptoms, functional profile, barriers to activity and participation, and management strategies. Identifying and managing the four primary triggers for POTS symptoms is a key strategy for supporting the patient's recovery journey. These triggers are (1) prolonged periods of sitting or standing, (2) dehydration, (3) heat, and (4) large meals or alcohol and caffeine intake. Providing this education and information supports self-determination and the development of self-management strategies for people with Long COVID (see Chapter 20).

However, living with POTS is not a linear journey. Setbacks, exacerbations, and relapses are very common, particularly in the early stages of recovery. This chapter's personalised and supportive approaches will help patients meet these challenges. Responding to setbacks by making individualised adjustments to interventions and acknowledging their impact on mental health and wellbeing will ensure coordinated and consistent care. Being present, reflecting, showing belief, empathy, and hope can enable people with Long COVID to regain control of their health and wellbeing. Psychologists and social workers can also provide specialist support for people experiencing psychosocial challenges associated with their POTS symptoms (see Chapter 14).

BOX 16.5   PRACTICE POINT

Reflect on your approach to managing dysautonomia. How do you currently prioritise interventions, monitor treatment impacts, and involve your Long COVID patient in decision-making? Is there anything you would change after reading this chapter?

BOX 16.6 RAEYA'S STORY

Raeya has lived experience with ME/CFS, Orthostatic Intolerance (OI), and POTS. Her ME/CFS diagnosis took 12 months, but her OI and POTS diagnoses took 8 years. Raeya awoke each morning with severe dizziness, headache, myalgia, and fatigue, and upon postural changes, experienced significant HR increases and a drop in BP. Raeya thought dizziness was normal and that everyone experienced it.

When a clinician finally asked, "Do you get dizzy when you stand up?" and she answered, "Yes, doesn't everyone?" she was told, " That's not actually normal." Her journey to diagnosis began.

Raeya would rise from 12 to 14 hours of sleep, jump straight in the shower to "wake up," and then have to spend the rest of her day resting and recovering. What she did not realise was that the prolonged sleep, the prolonged standing in the shower, and the lack of food and hydration (due to nausea) were all exacerbating her OI & POTS, debilitating her further and perpetuating her struggles with fatigue. After receiving her diagnosis and further answers, she recognised her OI and POTS, along with hypermobility-related needs.

This knowledge helped Raeya understand how best to manage her symptoms, which built on what she already knew about fatigue management. Raeya started to implement more pacing, manage her orthostatic challenges, increase her fluid intake, light snacking rather than big meals, and wear compression. Raeya saw a significant reduction in her symptoms and did not require pharmaceutical intervention.

Once her symptoms and fatigue were better managed, Raeya started physical activity interventions, which made the most significant change to her symptom experience. Raeya completed daily floor-based supine exercises and brief sessions (3 minutes) on her exercise bike. Over the next six months, she slowly built up to kneeling, then seated, then standing-based strength activities, and riding the exercise bike for up to 30 minutes a day. From there, Raeya was able to better tolerate upright activity and left the house more often as her capacity and stamina increased and her PEM decreased.

16.6 CONCLUSION

POTS is a complex condition that manifests with a core set of symptoms, as well as a variety of others, and has the potential to impact patients in all aspects of their lives severely. Both non-pharmacological and pharmacological management have roles to offer in improving symptom control. Collaborative working as part of the multidisciplinary team is essential for effectively managing POTS and COVID-19. The team members involved may vary on a case-by-case basis; however, all interventions must be founded on shared decision-making with patients. Ensuring patient-centred care is essential to engagement in rehabilitation and quality of life. The priorities of each patient are unique and should form the basis for each individualised management plan.

REFERENCES

1 Fedorowski A. Postural orthostatic tachycardia syndrome: Clinical presentation, aetiology and management. J Intern Med. 2019 Apr;285(4):352–66. doi:10.1111/joim.12852.

2 Seeley MC, et al. High incidence of autonomic dysfunction and postural orthostatic tachycardia syndrome in patients with Long COVID: Implications for management and health care planning. Am J Med. 2023. doi:10.1016/j.amjmed.2023.06.010.

3 Jammoul M, et al. Investigating the possible mechanisms of autonomic dysfunction post-COVID-19. Auton Neurosci. 2023;245:103071. doi:10.1016/j.autneu.2022.103071

4 Marques KC, et al. Cardiovascular autonomic dysfunction in "Long COVID": Pathophysiology, heart rate variability, and inflammatory markers. Front Cardiovasc Med. 2023;10:1256512. doi:10.3389/fcvm.2023.1256512.

5 Giunta S, et al. Long-COVID-19 autonomic dysfunction: An integrated view in the framework of inflammaging. Mechanisms of Ageing and Development. 2024;218:11915. doi:10.1016/j.mad.2024.111915

6 Wirth KJ, et al. Myalgic Encephalomyelitis/Chronic Fatigue Syndrome (ME/CFS) and comorbidities: Linked by vascular pathomechanisms and vasoactive mediators? Medicina (Kaunas). 2023;59(5):978. doi:10.3390/medicina59050978

7 Cantrell C, et al. Post-COVID postural orthostatic tachycardia syndrome (POTS): A new phenomenon. Front Neurol. 2024;15:1297964. doi:10.3389/fneur.2024.1297964

8 Narasimhan B, et al. Postural orthostatic tachycardia syndrome in COVID-19: A contemporary review of mechanisms, clinical course and management. Vasc Health Risk Manag. 2023;19:303–17. doi:10.2147/VHRM.S380270

9 Mar PL, et al. Postural orthostatic tachycardia syndrome: Mechanisms and new therapies. Annu Rev Med. 2020 Jan 27;71:235–48. doi:10.1146/annurev-med-041818-011630.

10 Sheldon RS, et al. 2015 Heart Rhythm Society expert consensus statement on the diagnosis and treatment of postural tachycardia syndrome, inappropriate sinus tachycardia, and vasovagal syncope. Heart Rhythm. 2015;12(6):e41–63. doi:10.1016/j.hrthm.2015.03.029

11 Spahic JM, et al. Malmö POTS symptom score: Assessing symptom burden in postural ortho-static tachycardia syndrome. J Intern Med. 2023 Jan;293(1):91–99. doi:10.1111/joim.13566.

12 Sletten DM, et al. COMPASS 31: A refined and abbreviated composite autonomic symptom score. Mayo Clin Proc. 2012;87(12):1196–201. doi:10.1016/j.mayocp.2012.10.013

13 Committee on the Diagnostic Criteria for Myalgic Encephalomyelitis/Chronic Fatigue Syndrome; Board on the Health of Select Populations; Institute of Medicine. Beyond myalgic encephalomyelitis/Chronic fatigue syndrome: Redefining an illness. Washington (DC): National Academies Press (US); 2015.

14 Chu L, et al. Deconstructing post-exertional malaise in myalgic encephalomyelitis/chronic fatigue syndrome: A patient-centred, cross-sectional survey. PLoS One. 2018;13(6):e0197811. doi:10.1371/journal.pone.0197811

15 Kahn PA, et al. Differential cardiopulmonary haemodynamic phenotypes in PASC-related exercise intolerance. ERJ Open Res. 2024;10(1):00714–2023. doi:10.1183/23120541.00714-2023

16 Roma M, et al. Postural tachycardia syndrome and other forms of orthostatic intolerance in Ehlers-Danlos syndrome. Auton Neurosci. 2018 Dec;215:89–96. doi:10.1016/j.autneu.2018.02.006

17 Bettini EA, et al. Association between pain sensitivity, central sensitisation, and functional disability in adolescents with joint hypermobility. J Pediatr Nursing. 2018;42:34–38. doi:10.1016/j.pedn.2018.06.007e/pii/S0882596318300010

18 Nicholson LL, et al. Hypermobility syndromes in children and adolescents: Assessment, diagnosis and multidisciplinary management. Aust J Gen Pract. 2022;51(6):409–14. doi:10.31128/AJGP-03-21-5870

19 Glans M, et al. Self-rated joint hypermobility: The five-part questionnaire evaluated in a Swedish non-clinical adult population. BMC Musculoskelet Disord. 2020;21:174. doi:10.1186/s12891-020-3067-1

20 Hakim AJ, et al. A simple questionnaire to detect hypermobility: An adjunct to the assessment of patients with diffuse musculoskeletal pain. Int J Clin Pract. 2003;57(3):163–66.

21 Frier M. Mast cell activation syndrome. Clinic Rev Allerg Immunol. 2018;54:353–65. doi:10.1007/s12016-015-8487-6

22 Goff A, et al. Menstrual cycle variability in symptoms of postural orthostatic tachycardia syndrome (POTS). Heart Lung and Circ. 2022;31: S213. doi:10.1016/j.hlc.2022.06.352

23 Raj SR, et al. Diagnosis and management of postural orthostatic tachycardia syndrome. CMAJ. 2022. 194;10:e378–85. doi:10.1503/cmaj.211373

24 Therapeutic Goods Administration (TGA). Australian Product Information – Midodrine ANS (Midodrine Hydrochloride) tablets [Internet]. Canberra: TGA; 2021 Jul 16[cited 2025 Feb 7]. Available at: https://www.tga.gov.au/sites/default/files/auspar-midodrine-hydrochloride-210716-pi-03.pdf.

25 Okamoto LE, et al. Hyperadrenergic postural tachycardia syndrome: Clinical biomarkers and response to guanfacine. Hypertension. 2024;81(11):2248–50. doi:10.1161/HYPERTENSIONAHA.124.23035

26 Kpaeyeh AG, et al. Hemodynamic profiles and tolerability of modafinil in the treatment of POTS: A randomised, placebo-controlled trial. J Clin Psychopharmacol. 2014;34(6):738–41. doi:10.1097/JCP.0000000000000221

27 Vernon SD, et al. Post-exertional malaise among people with Long COVID compared to myalgic encephalomyelitis/chronic fatigue syndrome (ME/CFS). Work. 2023;74(4):1179–86. doi:10.3233/WOR-220581

28 Cotler J, et al. A brief questionnaire to assess post-exertional malaise. Diagnostics. 2018;8(3):66. doi:10.3390/diagnostics8030066

29 van Rhijn-Brouwer FCCC, et al. Graded exercise therapy should not be recommended for patients with post-exertional malaise. Nat Rev Cardiol. 2024;21(6):430–31. doi:10.1038/s41569-024-00992-5

30 Trimble KZ, et al. Exercise in postural orthostatic tachycardia syndrome: Focus on individualised exercise approach. J Clin Med. 2024;13(22):6747. doi:10.3390/jcm13226747

31 Wheatley-Guy CM, et al. Semi-supervised exercise training program more effective for individuals with postural orthostatic tachycardia syndrome in randomised controlled trial. Clin Auton Res. 2023;33(5):659–72. doi:10.1007/s10286-023-00970-w.

32 Gonçalves Leite Rocco P, et al. Exercise interventions in the management of postural orthostatic tachycardia syndrome: A scoping review. J Multidisc Healthcare. 2024;17:5867–85. doi:10.2147/JMDH.S495088

33 Peebles KC, et al. The use and effectiveness of exercise for managing postural orthostatic tachycardia syndrome in young adults with joint hypermobility and related conditions: A scoping review. Auton Neurosci. 2024;252:103156. doi:10.1016/j.autneu.2024.103156

34 Smith EC, et al. Splanchnic venous compression enhances the effects of ß-blockade in the treatment of postural tachycardia syndrome. J Am Heart Assoc. 2020;9:e016196. doi:10.1161/JAHA.120.016196

35 Rabe E, et al. Risks and contraindications of medical compression treatment; A critical reappraisal. An international consensus statement. Phlebology 2020;35(7):447–60. doi:10.1177/0268355520909066

36 van Lieshout JJ, et al. Fludrocortisone and sleeping in the head-up position limit the postural decrease in cardiac output in autonomic failure. Clin Auton Res. 2000;10(1):35–42. doi:10.1007/BF02291388.

SECTION FIVE
MODELS OF CARE FOR LONG COVID

Chapter 17

Hospital-Based Models of Care for Long COVID

Steven Faux, Louis Irving, Nada Hamad, and Joanne Wrench

BOX 17.1   LEARNING OUTCOMES

By the end of this chapter, readers should be able to:

- Describe inpatient and outpatient hospital services that support Long COVID recovery.
- Understand the management of acute COVID-19 and how it may lead to the prevention of Long COVID.
- Understand different models of hospital-based Long COVID care and when they are applicable.
- Outline the role of multidisciplinary team (MDT) clinics operating with specialist rehabilitation physicians.

17.1 INTRODUCTION

Long COVID treatment and management can occur across the whole of the healthcare sector. Regardless of setting, it is important to recognise the often invisible burden of Long COVID and to approach each person's care with empathy and respect. Lived experience must be validated for care needs to be met, especially for people from vulnerable minorities, First Nations, and underserved populations.

This chapter describes the role of hospitals and the associated acute, subacute, and clinic-based services they provide. Hospital settings provide coordinated, expert care for people with Long COVID, integrating the skills of medical specialists, allied health professionals, and nurses to address the holistic needs of patients.

DOI: 10.4324/9781003528104-22

They are also able to provide continuity of care from the acute and subacute phases through to community care following discharge. For example, respiratory physicians may provide care during an acute COVID-19 admission and then follow patients up as an outpatient or within Long COVID hospital clinics. Likewise, rehabilitation specialists support patients following prolonged COVID-19 related Intensive Care Unit (ICU) or inpatient stays and can support the role of early rehabilitation, subacute rehabilitation, and outpatient care via Long COVID clinics. Patients treated during acute COVID-19 admissions also have access to general or pulmonary rehabilitation outpatient services.

There is no "one size fits all" approach to Long COVID care as patient populations vary depending on the local context. It is, therefore, critical that services adapt to local community needs and teams proactively communicate with patients and their families, to address concerns about their recovery trajectory and offer clear, compassionate guidance. This chapter should be read in conjunction with the other models of care presented in this book (see Chapters 18 and 19). These models complement each other and may be more relevant or applicable in different local contexts, or for the same patient at different points in their Long COVID journey. Further information on ICU treatment can be found in Chapter 22.

17.2 ACUTE HOSPITAL CARE

17.2.1 Acute Hospital Respiratory Care

Acute respiratory care for severe COVID-19 pneumonia/pneumonitis includes specific antivirals, steroids, titrated supplemental oxygen, and in some situations invasive or non-invasive ventilatory support.

Recovery can be quick, even in someone with life-threatening acute COVID-19, with a rapid reduction in supplemental oxygen needs, an increase in activity, and discharge from inpatient care. However, for some, particularly if they required ventilatory support, or if there are pre-existing respiratory or cardiac comorbidities, recovery is prolonged, over weeks, and months. Prolonged recovery is particularly true for people who experience complications, for example, Acute Lung Injury, Acute Respiratory Distress Syndrome, bacterial pneumonia, pulmonary emboli, or exacerbations of pre-existing interstitial lung disease or airways disease.

Respiratory care during the acute phase involves titration of supplemental oxygen, management of any underlying airways disease (asthma, Chronic Obstructive Pulmonary Disease) that may have been exacerbated by COVID-19, and awareness that bacterial bronchitis and pneumonia are common complications following COVID-19 infection. Hospital acquired infections are frequent, and one of many reasons to press for timely discharge from inpatient care. As the person improves, supplemental oxygen may not be required at rest, but if significant lung damage is yet to resolve or is permanent, it may be required with exercise, or during sleep, necessitating domiciliary supplemental oxygen. Mucous hypersecretion can also occur following acute COVID-19 and should be managed by strategies like coughing following a full inspiration and supervised or guided physical activity.

Ward-based allied health professionals such as physiotherapists, occupational therapists, social workers, and psychologists also provide care for people with acute COVID-19, including addressing respiratory functioning, mobility, cognition, participation in daily life, and psychosocial impacts.

17.2.2 In-Reach and Early Rehabilitation

In-reach rehabilitation is the process of providing multidisciplinary team (MDT) rehabilitation to patients while they are still being treated by acute care physicians or surgeons in an acute ward.[1] It operates in addition to ward-based allied health and is an integrated service within the rehabilitation medicine department of the hospital. In-reach rehabilitation has been shown to be cost effective, shorten length of stay and improve patient outcomes.[1,2] However, randomised controlled studies have indicated a need for careful targeting of patients for in-reach rehabilitation[3] based on levels of functional impairment and other factors during acute injury or illness such as COVID-19. This model was applied in many hospitals during the initial years of the COVID-19 pandemic.[4] For example, in one hospital in New South Wales, Australia, a subacute rehabilitation ward operated for 3 months during 2021 for patients who were no longer in need of respiratory support but still requiring acute medical and rehabilitation care.[5]

Individuals recovering from an ICU admission also benefit from a rehabilitation consultation while in the ICU, which can empower them to regain function, be discharged early and address the long-term impacts of critical illness.[6] Addressing emotional and psychological needs is critical, and trauma-informed care practices like active listening and validation can help reduce anxiety and distress. Current guidelines recommend an MDT approach rather than just a physical approach for early rehabilitation to be successful.[5] This approach includes delirium prevention, family information provision and access to an MDT rehabilitation service. The ideal form of follow-up service for those in ICU with or without Long COVID is yet to be defined, so early rehabilitation is provided from a pragmatic and preventative approach. A study by Chou et al.[7] identified a number of distinct aftercare trajectories following hospitalisation for acute COVID-19, including community-based rehabilitation (through allied health services), day admission and outpatient medical rehabilitation, inpatient rehabilitation in nursing facilities, and true inpatient MDT rehabilitation in rehabilitation wards and hospitals.

17.3 SUBACUTE MANAGEMENT OF SYMPTOMS

Subacute care for COVID-19 infection encompasses symptom management and treatment occurring between 6 and 12 weeks after initial infection, before a diagnosis of Long COVID. In this period, standard rehabilitation approaches to managing recovery and improving functional outcomes are provided. Many people receiving subacute rehabilitation will recover from their acute COVID-19 illness, although some will go on to develop Long COVID.

Respiratory symptoms are managed with standard MDT and/or pulmonary rehabilitation principles, focused on improving endurance, strengthening chest wall muscles and focusing on regaining functional independence, such as climbing stairs and independent personal care and daily living tasks. Understandably, for some individuals, feelings of anxiety – provoked by fear of reinfection, physical incapacity, or increased dependency – may intensify breathlessness and impact rehabilitation. This is particularly true when individuals experience re-infection and avoid activities that could trigger breathlessness, a phenomenon known as kinesophobia. In these situations, compassionate and tailored support from healthcare professionals, such as clinical psychologists, can help people explore and address their concerns, reframe fears, and develop strategies to build confidence. Specialised targeted interventions also play a critical role in holistic recovery, such as speech pathology interventions for people recovering from intubation and nutritional guidance from dietitians for those experiencing weight loss. Occupational therapists are also skilled and experienced in enabling these patients to improve their participation in daily activities and meaningful life roles.[8]

17.4 PREVENTATIVE STRATEGIES FOR LONG COVID IN ACUTE CARE

Evidence supports a variety of strategies (outlined in Box 17.2) for modifying or reducing risk factors for acute COVID-19, and their associated influence on lowering the incidence of Long COVID.[9]

BOX 17.2   EVIDENCE-BASED STRATEGIES FOR COVID-19 AND LONG COVID RISK REDUCTION

Vaccination: Staying up to date with vaccinations is an empowering step that can reduce the risk of severe infection, hospitalisation, and Long COVID. Evidence shows that vaccinated people have between a 15% and 75% reduction (with a mean of 40%) in the incidence of Long COVID.[10]

Healthy lifestyle practices: Practices like balanced nutrition, regular physical activity and smoking cessation may mitigate clinical risk factors associated with Long COVID.[9]

Chronic disease management: Similarly maintaining good control over co-morbidities such as diabetes, hypertension, and kidney disease may reduce risk.[9]

Antivirals for people at risk: For example, in Australia antivirals are available to anyone over 50 years, those over 18 years who are immunocompromised or those over 30 years who identified as First Nations people.[11] These medications have been shown to prevent hospitalisation for people with acute COVID-19 and reduce the risk of Long COVID by 14–26%.[12]

Early use of metformin may be beneficial: A randomised controlled study[13] reports introducing this treatment following acute COVID-19 led to a 40% reduction in emergency department presentations, hospitalisations, and death from COVID-19 compared to placebo. A review article suggested that this result is clinically meaningful as it decreases the risk of a Long COVID diagnosis by 42% compared to placebo.[14,15]

Evidence suggests that engaging in high-intensity exercise during an acute COVID-19 infection may contribute to prolonged fatigue for some individuals.[16] While the exact relationship between overexertion and the development of Long COVID is not yet fully understood,[17] it is clear that physical activity must be carefully personalised, monitored, and supervised with respect to the person's fatigue levels and overall health. This particularly applies to people who test and validate their "wellbeing" by pushing physical boundaries, and can lead to significant exacerbation and relapse of symptoms related to Post-Exertional Malaise (PEM). See Chapter 11 for further details about safe approaches to physical rehabilitation (including exercise prescription).

BOX 17.3   PRACTICE POINT

What opportunities do/did your patients with COVID-19 have during their admission (if they had one) that might support improved outcomes or reduce the risk of them experiencing Long COVID?

17.5 INTERNATIONAL APPROACHES TO MODELS OF CARE: WHERE DOES HOSPITAL CARE FIT?

Unfortunately, community-based rehabilitation remains out of reach for many people with Long COVID as it is frequently unfunded by public health systems. For example, in Australia, acute care is available at no cost under its universal healthcare system, but community-based care for chronic conditions often attracts additional out of pocket costs, which is a significant barrier for many. Hospitals have the expertise to bridge this gap, but funding to provide Long COVID–specific services is all but absent.

An Australian study reported there were 16 Long COVID clinics operating in Australia in 2023.[18] These clinics were mostly located in the private health sector (largely due to reluctance to fund public MDT clinics), with the expectation that people with Long COVID will primarily be managed in the community by their General Practitioner (GP). An Australian Federal Government inquiry on Long COVID recommended that outreach services (including telehealth) be funded for rural and regional areas and as a GP resource.[19] As of early 2025, this is yet to be actioned.

Community and hospital care is integrated into the National Health System (NHS) of the United Kingdom (UK), providing a flexible and bespoke solution to the management of all Long COVID severity levels. The NHS developed a tiered approach to manage Long COVID in 2021,[20] with Level 3 for mild symptoms supported by patient education websites and NHS and GP monitored Facebook groups. Level 2 was for people with persistent symptoms for whom self-management was insufficient and included GP referral to community allied health services or specialist care. Level 1 was for people with multisystem diseases and severe functional issues, who were managed in MDT clinics within major teaching hospitals (usually one or two per NHS trust). These clinics had the capacity to coordinate therapies and specialist treatment plans and to admit patients, organise sleep studies or commence complex hospital-based investigations such as magnetic resonance imaging, cognitive testing, and tilt-table testing.[21]

In the United States, a similar model of care exists with larger academic centres in major cities providing MDT clinics, and the bulk of Long COVID care provided by family doctors in primary care.[22] Most MDT clinics reside within departments of rehabilitation medicine (40%) and respiratory medicine (22%) and incorporate allied health.[22]

For most patients with mild or moderate Long COVID, rehabilitation can be provided in the community. However, for those with severe disease, limited access to primary care or complex care, there is clearly a need for hospital-based MDT centres.

BOX 17.4   PRACTICE POINT

What is the interface or relationship between your service and hospital-based services (or other hospital departments) that your patients with Long COVID may require? Are there formalised care pathways and processes?

17.6 HOSPITAL-BASED MDT CLINICS

MDT clinics must operate efficiently to maximise their impact, ensuring equitable access to care and meaningful outcomes for people with Long COVID. Tailored interventions should be prioritised based on individual needs and developed via shared decision-making with the patient (see Chapter 7). Managing multiple appointments can be overwhelming and MDT teams should coordinate services to focus on the most impactful interventions, streamlining care pathways to reduce the burden while supporting recovery goals, quality of life, and functional independence. It is, therefore, important to ensure the population serviced by the MDT is well defined and that staff are working at the top of their scope. Admission and discharge criteria from the clinic must be well defined and based upon shared patient and referrer expectations. For that reason, all communication to referrers and patients must be clear and accessible to support mutual understanding. In addition to direct patient care, Long COVID clinics provide a critical role in supporting the broader education and skill development of community providers (including GPs and allied health), who may have little experience of providing Long COVID care. This approach means not every patient will need the MDT clinic and may instead have access to Long COVID care via their existing health providers.

Admission criteria for MDT Long COVID clinics should be based on a clinical diagnosis of Long COVID that considers history of exposure to the COVID-19 (SARS-CoV-2) virus and persistent symptoms following exposure. A symptom and functional impairment workup should be completed, including a full history and examination, blood tests and/or medical imaging. On occasion, referral to a specialist might be required to evaluate alternative undiagnosed causes for symptoms, particularly if specialised tests are required (e.g., endoscopy, bronchoscopy). Once Long COVID is clinically diagnosed, the GP or a nurse practitioner may choose to initiate rehabilitation and other therapies in the community or refer to a Long COVID clinic. Ideally, GP and nurse practitioners should also have access to MDT clinics for secondary consultation. Screening questionnaires and outcome measures should be used on entry to the clinic so that improvement can be measured against a baseline inventory of symptoms and their severity (see Chapter 6), for example via the Yorkshire COVID-19 screening tool.[23]

The MDT team should include a doctor and nursing staff due to the varied presentations and frequent complex comorbidities. Ideally, the clinic's specialist physicians should include a rehabilitation physician and a respiratory or general physician given one of the common presentations involve pulmonary sequelae.[24] However, in rural and remote settings, finding appropriately qualified specialists is not always possible. Access to telehealth services in metropolitan areas provides an option for these patients (see Chapter 25).

Allied health professionals are crucial to the MDT clinic's diagnostic and symptom management function. The breadth of allied health disciplines available in clinics vary, but usually include physical therapists, psychologists, occupational therapists, and sometimes speech pathologists and dietitians. These professionals provide a range of assessments and interventions for the cognitive, physical and psychosocial impacts of Long COVID.

BOX 17.5   NADA'S STORY

I had a hard time learning to breathe again because I didn't realise that is what I needed to do. The hardest thing was facing the loss of my cognition which was so tightly linked to my identity. My cognition was also linked to my recovery because I found even following the number of appointments and instructions extremely challenging. It took a very competent psychologist to help me navigate my recovery.

17.7 CASE STUDY 1: THE ROYAL MELBOURNE HOSPITAL LONG COVID CLINIC

The Royal Melbourne Hospital Long COVID clinic was a respiratory medicine clinic. All patients were first seen by respiratory/general medicine physicians and then discussed by an MDT team. This team consisted of GPs, liaison psychiatry, clinical neuropsychology, physiotherapist, exercise physiologist, and clinical psychologist. The MDT also had access to cardiology, neurology, sleep medicine, rheumatology, other specialists, and allied health professions as required.

The clinic was established shortly after the first wave of COVID-19 in early 2020. Referrals consisted of people recovering from severe COVID-19 pneumonitis, and a second, novel group, who had mild acute COVID-19 but then experienced persisting symptoms. Our principles of management were to validate patient symptoms, listen to concerns, perform targeted investigations, treat contributing factors to symptoms (e.g., asthma, migraine, sleep disturbance, mood change), reassure, and, importantly, support through regular review.

This approach led to a rapid improvement and discharge of about a half of the initial referrals to this clinic. This left a group of people with Long COVID whose predominant symptoms and functional impairments were marked fatigue, brain fog, inability to work, frustration, and mood change. They are a complex group of patients who the team learnt required very individualised care.

Tailored approaches to fatigue management and deconditioning were important and included low level activity overseen by exercise physiologists and physiotherapists (being mindful of PEM), appropriate advice and medical certificates to enable time off work, followed by graded return to work. Postural Orthostatic Tachycardia Syndrome, sleep disturbance, depression, or systemic inflammatory conditions can also be significant contributors to fatigue.

The clinic and MDT discussions provided value by enabling the team to learn from patients over time, allowing them to identify recurring patterns specific to the types of patients referred to our clinic. These patterns differed from those observed in other hospital-based clinics because the majority were young, professional adults (often healthcare workers) who had contracted COVID-19 at work. It is important to take the referred population into account during service design, as a focus on this population group may lead to the minimisation or under-recognition of Long COVID in other populations.

17.8 CASE STUDY 2: THE ST VINCENTS HOSPITAL SYDNEY MODEL OF CARE

This model of care was introduced in March 2022 at St Vincents Hospital Sydney. It has seen over 1000 people with Long COVID and continues to have a waiting list of over 6 months. The clinic operates through a defined model of care that commences with referral from a GP, specialist, or nurse practitioner.[25] The referrer receives a request for blood and imaging results, while the patient is asked to complete the Yorkshire COVID-19 questionnaire[23] via an online platform.

Once received, the Clinical Nurse Consultant (CNC) reviews the documents and decides whether the patient has a suitable service provider closer to their residential postcode for onward referral. If not, the CNC evaluates the presenting symptoms and classifies the phenotype as (1) respiratory type, (2) respiratory plus other symptoms type, or (3) non-respiratory type. The respiratory physicians see all people with the respiratory phenotype, and some who experience respiratory and other symptoms. This provides access to specialist respiratory expertise and enables the rehabilitation physicians to deal with more general symptoms.

After triage, the person with Long COVID is offered initial face-to-face appointments with the CNC and a specialist physician. Observations and respiratory tests are completed as well as cardiac dysautonomia clinical testing (NASA lean testing) for people with cardiac symptoms. The nurse also provides information regarding expectations of the clinic appointment and documentation of outcome. The patient then has an extended consultation with the specialist who takes a history, completes a physical examination and explains the diagnosis, any further testing requirements and discusses a provisional treatment plan.

The specialist presents individual cases to a weekly MDT case conference, which is attended by a psychologist, physiotherapist, the CNC, three respiratory physicians, three rehabilitation physicians, as well as students and any interested GPs. The treatment plan is presented and added to or modified before referrers and the patient are notified of the outcome. Local cases that require physical therapy, psychology, or both are treated by MDT members, while others are linked in with services in their local community.

Occasionally patients have existing respiratory physicians, physiotherapists, or psychologists, so the MDT team contact their clinician to liaise. Patients are reviewed at three to six months to ensure that the intervention plan is being executed well and that goals are being met. Some patients recover more slowly and are followed up for longer until they show signs of improving in function and quality of life. Discharge from the clinic is defined as a return to work or usual activities, and improved control of symptoms.

17.9 CONCLUSION

Hospital settings provide a myriad of services for both the acute phase of COVID-19 infection and the longer-term consequences faced by many patients. This includes identifying and treating risk factors for the development of Long COVID and providing timely access to both acute and sub-acute rehabilitation programmes. MDT clinics based within hospitals can offer coordinated access to the medical, allied health, and nursing expertise required for effective rehabilitation and management of Long COVID. Hospital-based Long COVID clinics can also provide equitable access to care that may otherwise be financially prohibitive for many. Above all, services should ensure that patients feel safe, heard, and respected throughout their care journey.

REFERENCES

1 Wade D. Rehabilitation - a new approach. Part four: A new paradigm, and its implications. Clin Rehabil. 2016;30(2):109–18. doi:10.1177/0269215515601177.

2 Wu J, et al. Can in-reach multidisciplinary rehabilitation in the acute ward improve outcomes for critical care survivors? A pilot randomized controlled trial. J Rehabil Med. 2019;51(8):598–606. doi:10.2340/16501977-2579.

3 Wu J, et al. Targeted rehabilitation may improve patient flow and outcomes: Development and implementation of a novel Proactive Rehabilitation Screening (PReS) service. BMJ Open Qual. 2021;10(1). doi:10.1136/bmjoq-2020-001267.

4 Agostini F, et al. Rehabilitation setting during and after Covid-19: An overview on recommendations. J Rehabil Med. 2021;53(1):jrm00141. doi:10.2340/16501977-2776.

5 New South Wales Agency for Clinical Innovation (ACI). Multidisciplinary rehabilitation communication and referral for patients diagnosed with, or recovering from COVID-19 [Internet]. Sydney: ACI; [cited 2025 Feb 7]. https://aci.health.nsw.gov.au/__data/assets/pdf_file/0008/608678/ACI-Rehabilitation-communication-COVID-19-acute-care-allied.pdf.

6 Goodwin VA, et al. Rehabilitation to enable recovery from COVID-19: A rapid systematic review. Physiotherapy. 2021;111:4–22. doi:10.1016/j.physio.2021.01.007.

7 Chou R, et al. Long COVID definitions and models of care: A scoping review. Ann Intern Med. 2024;177(7):929–40. doi:10.7326/M24-0677.

8 Scott HM, et al. Occupational therapy practice for post-acute COVID-19 inpatients requiring rehabilitation. Aust Occup Ther J. 2024;71(6):940–55. doi:10.1111/1440-1630.12976.

9 Tsampasian V, et al. Risk factors associated with post-COVID-19 condition: A systematic review and meta-analysis. JAMA Intern Med. 2023;183(6):566–80. doi:10.1001/jamainternmed.2023.0750.

10 Al-Aly Z, et al. Solving the puzzle of Long Covid. Science. 2024;383(6685):830–32. doi:10.1126/science.adl0867.

11 Lopez D, et al. Supply of nirmatrelvir/ritonavir and molnupiravir for patients with COVID-19 in the first eight months since listing on the Australian Pharmaceutical Benefits Scheme: A retrospective observational study. Infect Dis Now. 2024;54(6):104953. doi:10.1016/j.idnow.2024.104953.

12 Al-Aly Z. Prevention of long COVID: Progress and challenges. Lancet Infect Dis. 2023;23(7):776–77. doi:10.1016/S1473-3099(23)00287-6.

13 Bramante CT, et al. Outpatient treatment of COVID-19 and incidence of post-COVID-19 condition over 10 months (COVID-OUT): A multicentre, randomised, quadruple-blind, parallel-group, phase 3 trial. Lancet Infect Dis. 2023;23(10):1119–29. doi:10.1016/S1473-3099(23)00299-2.

14 McCarthy M. Metformin as a potential treatment for COVID-19. Expert Opin Pharmacother. 2023;24(10):1199–203. doi:10.1080/14656566.2023.2215385.

15 Yong SJ, et al. Experimental drugs in randomized controlled trials for long-COVID: What's in the pipeline? A systematic and critical review. Expert Opin Investig Drugs. 2023;32(7):655–67. doi:10.1080/13543784.2023.2242773.

16 Thirupathi, A et al. Exercise and COVID-19: Exercise intensity reassures immunological benefits of post-COVID-19 condition. Front Physiol. 2023;14:1036925. doi:10.3389/fphys.2023.1036925.

17 Barker-Davies RM, et al. The Stanford Hall consensus statement for post-COVID-19 rehabilitation. Br J Sports Med. 2020;54(16):949–59. doi:10.1136/bjsports-2020-102596.

18 Luo S, et al. An overview of Long COVID support services in Australia and international clinical guidelines, with a proposed care model in a global context. Public Health Rev. 2023;44:1606084. doi:10.3389/phrs.2023.1606084.

19 Parliament of Australia. Sick and tired: Casting a long shadow. Inquiry into Long COVID and repeated COVID infections [Internet]. Canberra: Parliament of Australia; 2023 [cited 2025 Feb 7]. Available from: https://www.aph.gov.au/Parliamentary_Business/Committees/House/Health_Aged_Care_and_Sport/LongandrepeatedCOVID/Report.

20 Parkin A, et al. A multidisciplinary NHS COVID-19 service to manage post-COVID-19 syndrome in the community. J Prim Care Community Health. 2021;12:21501327211010994. doi:10.1177/21501327211010994.

21 Personal Communication between Bakerly N and Manoj S with Faux S, editor. 2024.

22 Barshikar S, et al. Integrated care models for long coronavirus disease. Phys Med Rehabil Clin N Am. 2023;34(3):689–700. doi:10.1016/j.pmr.2023.03.007.

23 O'Connor RJ, et al. The COVID-19 yorkshire rehabilitation scale (C19-YRS): Application and psychometric analysis in a post-COVID-19 syndrome cohort. J Med Virol. 2022;94(3):1027–34. doi:10.1002/jmv.27415.

24 Lewthwaite H, et al. Treatable traits for Long COVID. Respirology. 2023;28(11):1005–22. doi:10.1111/resp.14596.

25 St Vincents Lung Health. Post-acute & Long COVID clinic [Internet]. Melbourne: St Vincent's Hospital Lung Health; [cited 2025 Feb 7]. Available from: https://www.svhlunghealth.com.au/about-us/whats-new/post-acute-long-covid-clinic#:~:text=You%20will%20require%20a%20current,or%20two%20after%20COVID%2D19.

Chapter 18

Interdisciplinary Allied Health Models of Care for Long COVID

Approaches to Symptom Management and Recovery

Joanne Wrench, Leigh Seidel-Marks, and Karen Dickinson

BOX 18.1 LEARNING OBJECTIVES

By the end of this chapter, readers should be able to:

- Understand the benefits and challenges of different models of care in managing persistent symptoms and impacts related to Long COVID.
- Identify the key principles and components of effective allied health led interdisciplinary models of care for Long COVID rehabilitation.
- Consider practical strategies for implementing and scaling interdisciplinary care models for Long COVID.

18.1 INTRODUCTION

The broader healthcare system-level responses required to manage the long-term impacts of COVID-19 infection were recognised early in the pandemic, with multiple models of care developed internationally within the first year.[1-3] With severe acute disease, the focus was initially on hospitalised patients who were likely to face a lengthy recovery, particularly those admitted to the Intensive Care Unit (ICU). As such, early models understandably placed a strong emphasis on pulmonary rehabilitation and the multisystem impacts of severe acute infections such as post ICU syndrome.[2,4]

DOI: 10.4324/9781003528104-23

As the pandemic progressed, vaccine programmes took effect, the treatment improved, and COVID-19 variants evolved; fewer people needed acute hospitalisation, and with this, the focus on acute care shifted to community management. At the same time, evidence mounted that many people who were not hospitalised during their acute COVID-19 infection were also experiencing an array of sustained, often devastating symptoms, now termed Long COVID. Recommendations for interventions and care models for Long COVID were developed, primarily based on expert consensus due to the lack of evidence for efficacy. Chief among these recommendations was that Long COVID rehabilitation should use a multidisciplinary approach with physical, psychological, and social aspects of management.[5]

This chapter focuses on allied health interdisciplinary care models delivered within outpatient or community settings. We acknowledge that allied health interdisciplinary models are part of the broader system, which includes primary care and specialist medical models. The allied health service described cannot, and should not, operate without this broader system in place. For further information about other models of care, see Chapters 17 and 19.

18.2 MODELS OF CARE IN LONG COVID

BOX 18.2

Models of care are the organisational structures required to deliver care within a health system. They include consideration of processes, service management, and core care components (who provides care, to whom and in what form) with the aim of delivering high-quality, evidence-based care to improve patient outcomes.

A recent review of Long COVID models of care recommended several key principles, including: A core lead team, broad multidisciplinary expertise, a wide range of diagnostic services, patient-centred, individualised and equitable care, and capacity to meet demand.[6] Models were found to vary on several key components, including the healthcare disciplines involved, delivery methods, timing and length of service, and interventions offered. Given it takes, on average, 17 years for research evidence to be clinically translated,[7] the lack of consensus on the best way to deliver care for people experiencing Long COVID is not surprising.

18.3 A NOTE ON MULTIDISCIPLINARY AND INTERDISCIPLINARY REHABILITATION

Although the terms multidisciplinary and interdisciplinary are often used interchangeably, particularly in practice, they are conceptually different. We will use the term *interdisciplinary* to refer to an integrated and coordinated team comprising multiple disciplines (e.g., medical, nursing, allied health) who work on individual goals relevant to their specialty while collaborating on shared goals.[8] This requires interactive problem solving, strong communication and an understanding of other professionals' roles and responsibilities. Multidisciplinary teams likewise comprise numerous expert disciplines but tend to collaborate and work in parallel and independently within their expertise to meet a patient goal.

18.4 WHY IS AN INTERDISCIPLINARY MODEL OF CARE IMPORTANT IN LONG COVID?

18.4.1 Long COVID Is a Multisystem Disease

By nature, Long COVID impacts multiple body systems and has a diverse array of symptoms that require treatment by numerous healthcare professionals. Complicating this, many people have a non-linear course of illness and symptom profiles, and their impact, can vary over time. Therefore, models of care to address Long COVID require a flexible, multipronged approach that allows fluid access to a range of collaborating healthcare providers and scalable therapeutic options.

18.4.2 Efficacy of Interdisciplinary Care

There is abundant evidence for the efficacy of interdisciplinary care models across various health conditions, including chronic pain, pulmonary disease, Myalgic Encephalomyelitis/Chronic Fatigue Syndrome, and a range of other long-term, chronic conditions.[9–11] These rehabilitation programmes have been shown to improve patient quality of life and functional status, including supporting self-management of symptoms.

Interdisciplinary rehabilitation is generally reported to be feasible, safe, and acceptable to people living with Long COVID.[12,13] There is also emerging evidence of the efficacy of team-based rehabilitation in improving symptoms, quality of life, and understanding of the condition.[3,14] Harenwall et al.[3] found Long COVID patients had an improved quality of life following a structured 7-week course of allied health interdisciplinary rehabilitation focusing on sleep, activity management, stress management, nutrition, and breathing optimisation. Other studies have also reported improved physical and psychological functioning,[15,16] although many of these have small sample sizes, lack comparison groups, and included mainly people hospitalised during acute COVID-19 infection.

18.4.3 Coordinated Care Reduces Patient Burden and Improves Outcomes

I didn't know what different allied health disciplines would do, so I didn't know who to ask for help… [interdisciplinary services] take some of that burden of knowing who you need to see.

Karen

Patients with Long COVID have repeatedly advocated for a "one stop shop" for care.[17,18] Coordinated interdisciplinary clinics reduce the cognitive, physical, and psychological burden on patients who are otherwise required to advocate and manage multiple specialist appointments. They can also have financial benefits, requiring a single referral to see a team of healthcare professionals rather than repeated general practitioner (GP) visits for individual specialist appointments. Many people with Long COVID find themselves the purveyors of up-to-date knowledge and research as they search for treatments and symptom relief. Dedicated Long COVID clinics also have the advantage of centralising expertise, allowing access to clinicians with expertise and an interest in treating Long COVID.

BOX 18.3   KAREN'S HEALTHCARE JOURNEY

The last three years have seen me access care from a variety of different healthcare professionals and systems for my Long COVID (Figure 18.1).

Initially in 2022 I had weekly telehealth appointments with my GP. When it became clear my symptoms were not resolving, I requested a referral to an exercise physiologist and was also seen within a local pop-up respiratory clinic. This was the first of many self-directed requests for care. I was struggling with anxiety around my new health condition and sought a referral to a psychologist for support, which was very helpful. This was all self-funded and neither the exercise physiologist nor psychologists had experience in Long COVID.

I spent a lot of time early in my diagnosis researching Long COVID and was very well informed and able to seek out independent referrals from my GP. This included a Long COVID interdisciplinary clinic that provided allied health support. This helped me better understand the chronic nature of Long COVID and I learnt all manner of skills and coping mechanisms, such as pacing, energy preservation, prioritisation, meditation, and setting new goals for a meaningful life with my family. The Long COVID clinic's occupational therapist, exercise physiologist, and neuropsychologist support was unparalleled and enhanced my capability to understand Long COVID and advocate for growth in my life. This clinic also gave me a greater sense of legitimacy and agency when it came to further specialist treatment and telling my "story."

The allied health clinic unfortunately closed, and I continued to get support from my GP, private psychologist, and private OT. I also sought support from medical specialists including a rheumatologist for joint, muscle and nerve pain and then a neurologist for migraines and fatigue (after an acute vestibular migraine).

I know I'm privileged. I have a science degree and a high level of health literacy. I am able to engage actively in managing my health and am well supported by family and friends. I've read extensively and have suggested treatments, including novel pharmacological options, to my doctors who then support my access. I live in a large city and have been able to financially access this level of care, though even with this, the ongoing out-of-pocket expenditure for appointments has taken a financial toll. The mental and physical load on patients to manage their symptoms, medications and appointments cannot be understated, especially given that fatigue, post-exertional malaise, and cognitive dysfunction are continual symptoms for some sufferers.

Long COVID still impacts all aspects of my life, but I am grateful to my whole team who have helped me learn how to manage and control the extent of my symptoms so I can lead a meaningful life.

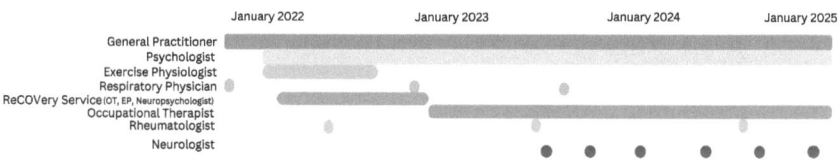

Figure 18.1 A visual journey of Karen's health service utilisation over three years.

BOX 18.4   PRACTICE POINT

Patients move through a system of care, sometimes accessing multiple services simultaneously. Reflect on Karen's lived experience. In three years, she has accessed multiple "models" for her Long COVID symptoms – primary care, interdisciplinary allied health services, private individual medical specialists, and allied health practitioners. Her experience highlights that these models and their components do not operate in isolation. Consider how your healthcare role fits into this system. How do you decide which care is appropriate and helpful at which point in a patient's journey?

18.5 AN ALLIED HEALTH INTERDISCIPLINARY MODEL OF CARE FOR LONG COVID

These practitioners are interested in Long COVID, and they know about the reality of Long COVID.... They will be across the latest approaches, medicines and the latest developments.

Karen

Without a "cure" for Long COVID, symptom management approaches that improve quality of life and participation in daily activities are essential. This is ideally suited to allied health teams, who collaborate and use shared decision-making approaches to provide symptom relief and support return to, or establishment of, new, life roles. Allied health teams should also function as an integrated source of therapeutic intervention and rehabilitation rather than assessment only and a source for referrals to other specialists.[17]

Allied health-led approaches are part of the Long COVID management system, which includes GPs and medical specialist clinics, all of which have a critical role in providing care. The purpose of calling teams "allied health led" is to acknowledge that this workforce therapeutically supplies symptom management approaches. Allied health-led models do not indicate an absence of medical specialists, nor should they limit medical assessments or collaboration. In fact, they often include physicians in their teams (e.g., Rehabilitation Physicians) and should remain well connected to a range of other medical specialists and the patient's GP to ensure appropriate medical management.[13]

Allied health-led models also require careful triaging to ensure appropriate referrals and linkages to other teams for additional assessments and tests (e.g.,

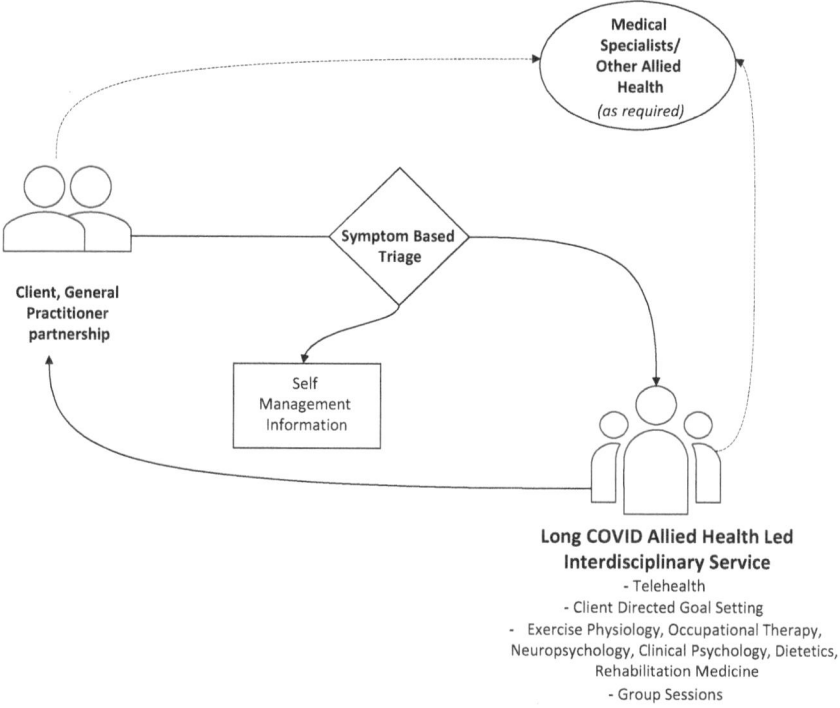

Figure 18.2 The interconnectedness of Interdisciplinary Allied Health clinics with the broader health system.

Respiratory Medicine, Sleep and Hypertension Clinics). Integration with the broader health system is critical to the success of allied health models, with the interface with the GP particularly crucial given their role in many healthcare systems as care coordinators (see Figure 18.2).

18.5.1 Principles of Allied Health-Led Care Models

All Long COVID models must engage with local social, funding and health system factors that may vary geographically (e.g., metropolitan versus regional or rural areas). Whilst models differ in how they are operationalised, we suggest that broad overarching guiding principles can be applied across settings to support the delivery of consistent, timely best practice care. These guiding principles are expanded upon in Box 18.5 and include: (1) collaborative and centralised care, (2) cutting-edge evidence-based care, (3) equitable and timely access, (4) interventions tailored to individual needs, for example, a stepped care approach, (5) integrated care within existing healthcare systems that reduces duplication, and (6) research aligned services that support evaluation of intervention efficacy.

BOX 18.5   PRINCIPLES OF ALLIED HEALTH INTERDISCIPLINARY MODELS OF CARE FOR LONG COVID

Collaborative and centralised: Removing the need for people to retell their Long COVID experience, prior interventions or advocate for specialist input. Reduced referral duplication and waitlisting, with more streamlined coordinated interventions.

Evidence informed: There is no "gold standard" of treatment for Long COVID, and research evidence is growing. Dedicated teams are better positioned to remain abreast of developments, reducing the burden on patients to research options themselves.

Equity of access: Centralising care using a hub and spoke model opens specialist care across geographical boundaries, removing the burden of travelling to attend multiple appointments.

Stepped care: With limited resources available, effective triage and scalable models, including self-management pathways and group interventions, promote service access to those with the greatest need and prevent excessive waitlists for intervention.

Integrated within the existing health system: The care should complement and leverage existing services. This supports access to specialist interventions and avoids duplication and burden on the system.

Evidence generating: Services should contribute to the knowledge and research base on the efficacy of interventions.

BOX 18.6   PRACTICE POINT

Do you think the six principles of allied health interdisciplinary care listed in Box 18.2 apply to other models of care? How does your service translate these principles into everyday practice?

18.5.2 Practical Considerations for Allied Health-Led Models

To effectively apply these principles, allied health-led models must carefully consider the practical components of service delivery –*who* is delivering *what* to *whom* and *where* this occurs. Early models had a focus on patients with severe respiratory impacts (*whom*) by delivering physiotherapy-led *(who)* pulmonary rehabilitation (*what*) within hospital contexts (*where*). With the overwhelming demand for services and expanding symptom profiles, models quickly became about stratifying "need" based on symptom presentation, for example, tiered models of the National Health Service in the United Kingdom, with access to multidisciplinary rehabilitation reserved for those with the most severe and multifaceted symptoms.[1] Whilst there is no one-size-fits-all approach to Long COVID interdisciplinary care, Box 18.6 identifies the key components of these models. An example of their operationalisation is provided in the following case study.

BOX 18.6   COMPONENTS OF ALLIED HEALTH MODELS OF CARE FOR LONG COVID

Clinical Setting: *Is the clinic based within a hospital or community setting?*
Many interdisciplinary clinics are in tertiary hospitals, which supports access to specialist staffing and resources required to implement larger-scale rehabilitation models. They also provide easy access to specialist medical care that may not form part of the core treatment team but is occasionally required. Positioning services within such settings also provides opportunities for research alignment.

Clinic Eligibility: *What are the referral criteria, and who is your target clinical population?*
This includes effective triage assessment for waitlist management and suitability for rehabilitation to ensure responsible use of clinical resources. Self-management options for those with less severe symptoms and group education sessions to support scalability are recommended.

Interdisciplinary Team: *Who are the key members of the interdisciplinary team, and which disciplines might you consult outside the team?*
A base level team should include allied health with specialty skills to support the most common symptoms of Long COVID, for example, cognitive changes, fatigue, and psychological sequelae. As such, many clinics include exercise physiology, occupational therapy, clinical

---

psychology, neuropsychology, and dietetics.[11,12] Linkages with other allied clinicians, such as speech pathology and social work, may occur outside the "core" clinical team. In addition to the GP, specialist medical teams may also be engaged and scaled up and down as necessary, including specialists in neurology, rheumatology, respiratory medicine, and cardiology.

Team Leadership: *How is the team structured, and who is "leading" it?*
Coordinated care requires leadership with dedicated time to support effective service functioning. This role is not limited to a specific discipline in allied health-led models. Instead, it recognises that a particular skill set in leadership, service planning and people management supports effective team functioning.

Delivery Modality: *Is the service delivered in person, via telehealth, or in combination?*
Virtual care models became the predominant care method in Long COVID, and many early concerns around access have not been realised.[2] In fact, telehealth has remarkably low fail-to-attend rates and can help people living with fatigue and cognitive impairments access appointments more efficiently. Face-to-face options may be required for specific assessments and interventions or to ensure equity of access for some communities, including culturally and linguistically diverse communities and those with limited access or knowledge of technology.

Clinical Interventions: *What are the core interventions offered, and will they be individual or in group settings?*
Despite the individual presentation of Long COVID, the commonality of reported symptoms presents an opportunity for virtual group education supporting service scalability, timely access to care and peer support.

Timeframe for Service: *Is the rehabilitation programme time limited?*
Most Long COVID rehabilitation programmes have set timeframes, often up to 12 weeks, to ensure patient flow and access to care within limited resources. Setting clear expectations around the length of intervention, setting realistic goals, and considering step-down care pathways are essential early in the programme. As with other chronic health conditions, options for re-referral as required should be considered to account for fluctuation in symptoms.

18.6 CASE STUDY: THE RECOVERY SERVICE AT AUSTIN HEALTH

In 2022, Austin Health, a large tertiary hospital in Melbourne, Australia, piloted an interdisciplinary allied health led rehabilitation service for people living with persistent symptoms following COIVID-19 infection based on the National Institute for Health and Care Excellence (NICE) recommendations for management. Using a continuous improvement approach, the service evolved by incorporating learnings from the research literature and partnerships with our patients to provide up-to-date, evidence-informed care.

The service-assisted 280 people in nine months, providing a stepped model of care based on self-reported symptom impact (Figure 18.3). The length of service was

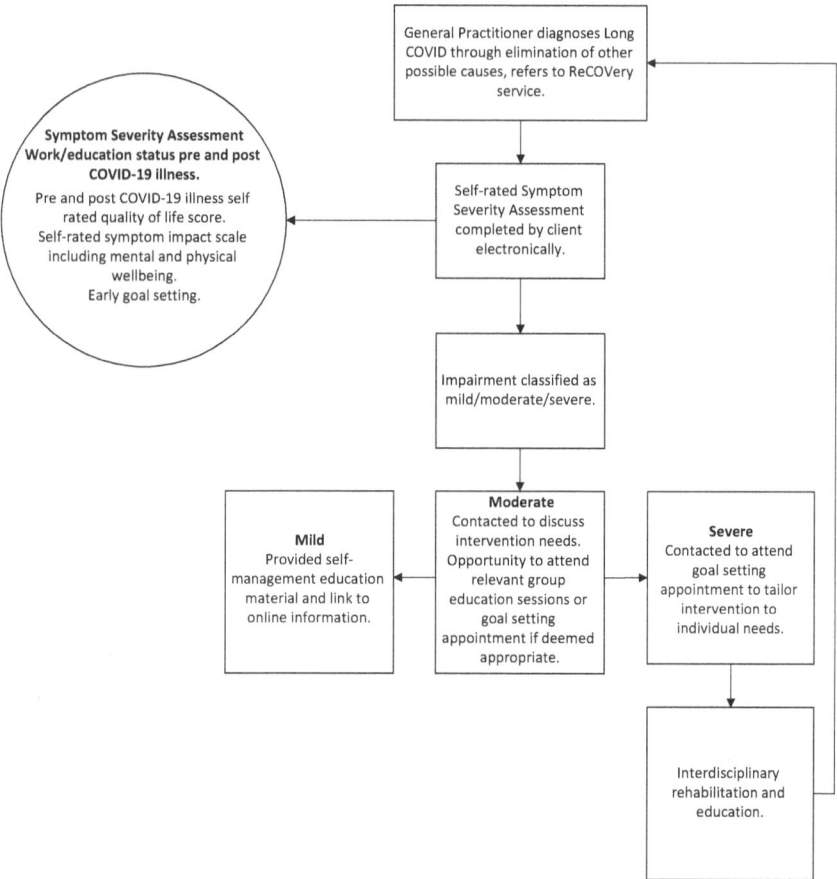

Figure 18.3   An example of triaging Long COVID interdisciplinary allied health clinics based on the ReCOvery programme.

initially set at 12 weeks but was individually negotiated, with some people requiring more protracted intervention and others less.

Patients favoured the flexibility of telehealth interventions, which negated the need to attend the healthcare services by providing care to people in the comfort of their own homes. Face-to-face appointments were reserved for specific circumstances, such as client requests or assessments that telehealth cannot provide (e.g., some aspects of neuropsychology assessment). Scalability was enhanced by adopting group education sessions about commonly reported symptoms (fatigue, brain fog, olfactory impairment and living with Long COVID) facilitated by relevant disciplines. Group sessions were also offered by telehealth, which provided education and the opportunity for social connection and shared empathy.

The service included exercise physiology, occupational therapy, neuropsychology, clinical psychology, dietetics, speech pathology, and rehabilitation medicine, which exemplified interdisciplinary therapeutic collaboration. Collaboration was further enhanced by weekly meetings to discuss patient management and relevant research updates via a monthly journal club, ensuring service resources were used effectively. The centralisation of documentation within medical records further strengthened the visibility of interventions within the ReCOVery service and the broader healthcare service, preventing patients from retelling their stories and justifying their diagnoses when presenting for care elsewhere within the organisation.

A senior dietitian led this service; however, this role could be filled by any allied health professional with leadership capability and sound knowledge of the role of other disciplines. Leadership responsibilities included planning and coordinating clinic processes to ensure service access and scalability, joint mentoring of health professionals with the relevant discipline department supervisor through monthly meetings, advocacy both within and external to the organisation and analysis and reporting of activity data. Liaising with health professionals and people with Long COVID regarding service eligibility and responding to feedback was also key to the role.

Communication with patients was shared across the team, with each person allocated a central contact person to facilitate communication of key information between them and the rehabilitation team in addition to individual discipline contact. This reduced confusion for the person with Long COVID and health professionals by reducing conflicting information and promoting relationship building and trust.

A community of practice was established with external health professionals (GP and Physiotherapist) also providing care to patients with Long COVID, meeting regularly to discuss therapeutic interventions and share learnings. This also offered an opportunity to refer between services to support patient access. Collaboration with other service providers enhanced broader advocacy for this novel condition and alignment in clinical approaches despite the minimal evidence available. Partnerships were also forged with Sleep Medicine and the Hypertension Clinic to support streamlined assessment and management of sleep disturbance and Postural Orthostatic Tachycardia Syndrome.

GP and specialist medicine referrals were accepted, as were Austin Health staff self-referrals (acknowledgement of the pandemic's impact on healthcare workers) at the rate of one referral per day. Whilst limited to the hospital catchment area, the telehealth modality lends itself to a hub and spoke model to support people beyond health service catchment areas, which can address equity issues faced by those living regionally or without access to specialised services (as demonstrated in Chapter 26). More information regarding the Pilot and service data can be found in Wrench and Seidel Marks.[13]

18.7 CONCLUSION

The long-term impacts of COVID-19 infection require a comprehensive and adaptable approach to care and symptom relief. Interdisciplinary allied health-led models offer a coordinated approach that supports symptom management, recovery, and participation in valued daily activities and life roles in collaboration with medical specialists and primary care. This chapter has highlighted the need to base models on a clear set of principles, regardless of individual differences in the health system or social context. As research into mechanisms and treatments for Long COVID continues to evolve, so will the associated models of care. As such, any model should be, in the first instance, adaptive, flexible, and closely aligned with emerging research evidence.

REFERENCES

1 Parkin A, et al. A multidisciplinary NHS COVID-19 service to manage post-COVID-19 syndrome in the community. J Prim Care Community Health. 2021;12. doi:10.1177/2150132 7211010994.

2 Brigham E, et al. The Johns Hopkins post-acute COVID-19 team (PACT): A multidisciplinary, collaborative, ambulatory framework supporting COVID-19 survivors. Am J Med. 2021; 134(4):462–67.e1. doi:10.1016/j.amjmed.2020.12.009.

3 Harenwall S, et al. Post-Covid-19 syndrome: Improvements in health-related quality of life following psychology-led interdisciplinary virtual rehabilitation. J Prim Care Community Health. 2021;12:21501319211067674. doi:10.1177/21501319211067674.

4 Lutchmansingh DD, et al. A clinic blueprint for post-coronavirus disease 2019 recovery: Learning from the past, looking to the future. Chest. 2021;159(3):949–58. doi:10.1016/j.chest.2020.10.067.

5 National Institute for Health and Care Excellence (NICE). COVID-19 rapid guideline: Chapter 5 – Management [Internet]. London: NICE; 2020 [cited 2025 Feb 7]. Available from: https://www.nice.org.uk/guidance/ng188/chapter/5-Management#multidisciplinary-rehabilitation.

6 Chou R, et al. Long COVID definitions and models of care: A scoping review. Ann Intern Med. 2024;177(7):929–40. doi:10.7326/M24-0677.

7 Morris ZS, et al. The answer is 17 years, what is the question: Understanding time lags in translational research. J R Soc Med. 2011;104(12):510–20. doi:10.1258/jrsm.2011.110180.

8 Choi BC, et al. Multidisciplinarity, interdisciplinarity and transdisciplinarity in health research, services, education and policy: 1. Definitions, objectives, and evidence of effectiveness. Clin Invest Med. 2006;29(6):351–64.

9 Zaina F, et al. A systematic review of clinical practice guidelines for persons with non-specific low back pain with and without radiculopathy: Identification of best evidence for rehabilitation to develop the WHO's package of interventions for rehabilitation. Arch Phys Med Rehabil. 2023;104(11):1913–27. doi:10.1016/j.apmr.2023.02.022.

10 Lamper C, et al. Interdisciplinary care networks in rehabilitation care for patients with chronic musculoskeletal pain: A systematic review. J Clin Med. 2021;10(9). doi:10.3390/jcm10092041.

11 COPD Working Group. Pulmonary rehabilitation for patients with chronic pulmonary disease (COPD): An evidence-based analysis. Ont Health Technol Assess Ser. 2012;12(6):1–75.

12 D'Souza AN, et al. Feasibility of an allied health led, workplace delivered Long COVID service for hospital staff: A mixed-methods study. Aust Health Rev. 2024;48(6): 729–38 doi:10.1071/AH24146.

13 Wrench JM, et al. An allied health model of care for Long COVID rehabilitation. Med J Aust. 2024;221 Suppl 9:S5–S9. doi:10.5694/mja2.52457

14 Raunkiaer M, et al. Experiences of improvement of everyday life following a rehabilitation programme for people with long-term cognitive effects of COVID-19: Qualitative study. J Clin Nurs. 2024;33(1):137–48. doi:10.1111/jocn.16739.

15 Compagno S, et al. Physical and psychological reconditioning in Long COVID syndrome: Results of an out-of-hospital exercise and psychological - based rehabilitation program. Int J Cardiol Heart Vasc. 2022;41:101080. doi:10.1016/j.ijcha.2022.101080.

16 Nopp S, et al. Outpatient pulmonary rehabilitation in patients with Long COVID improves exercise capacity, functional status, dyspnea, fatigue, and quality of life. Respiration. 2022;101(6):593–601. doi:10.1159/000522118.

17 Laestadius LI, et al. "The dream is that there's one place you go": A qualitative study of women's experiences seeking care from Long COVID clinics in the USA. BMC Med. 2024;22(1):243. doi:10.1186/s12916-024-03465-1.

18 Ladds E, et al. Persistent symptoms after COVID-19: Qualitative study of 114 "long Covid" patients and draft quality principles for services. BMC Health Serv Res. 2020;20(1):1144. doi:10.1186/s12913-020-06001-y.

Chapter 19

Community and Primary Care for People with Long COVID

Emma Tippett, Bernard Shiu, Brìghde Collins, and Anonymous[1]

BOX 19.1   LEARNING OBJECTIVES

By the end of this chapter, readers should be able to:

- Understand the complexities and varied symptoms of Long COVID.
- Examine the role of community-based care models like General Practitioner (GP)-led clinics and telehealth.
- Identify barriers to effective care and strategies to overcome them.
- Explore collaborative approaches to improve outcomes and align care with international evidence.

19.1 INTRODUCTION

Long COVID has emerged as a considerable health issue, impacting a significant number of individuals who have recovered from an acute COVID-19 infection.[1,2] Estimating its prevalence is challenging due to evolving pandemic factors such as variant mutations and vaccination rates. While estimates vary, it is a significant public health concern, with studies suggesting a prevalence between 7.5% and 41%.[3–4]

Primary care providers bear the responsibility for managing this poorly understood condition, often relying on outdated guidelines amid evolving information. The absence of clear diagnostic criteria or biomarkers adds uncertainty, while the broad symptom spectrum – such as fatigue, cognitive impairments, and sensory sensitivities – necessitates complex, multisystem consultations that strain already overburdened practices.

DOI: 10.4324/9781003528104-24

This chapter explores community-based strategies for managing Long COVID, drawing on the experiences of two Australian clinics: a General Practitioner (GP)-led face-to-face multidisciplinary clinic and a telehealth-based service. These models demonstrate practical approaches to developing care pathways, integrating patient-centred strategies within the Australian healthcare context, and leveraging international evidence to address the challenges of this multifaceted condition.

19.2 MODELS OF DELIVERY

19.2.1 Face-to-face General Practitioner–Led Long COVID Clinic

One option is the creation of specialised Long COVID clinics led by GPs. This model embodies a multidisciplinary approach, integrating GPs with specialised expertise in managing COVID and chronic diseases, along with non-GP specialists in fields such as cardiology, respiratory, and psychiatry, as well as allied health such as exercise physiologists, social workers, occupational therapists, and psychologists.

The development of a dedicated, face-to-face, Long COVID clinic allows easy referral pathways, instantaneous sharing of clinical details and progress, development of comprehensive care plans, and technical support from peers dedicated to the same field.

19.2.2 Telehealth Model of Care

As is often the case, individuals in regional and remote areas face significant hurdles in accessing medical care. A telehealth approach eliminates geographical barriers, delivering specialist care to areas lacking Long COVID services and enabling treatment to occur within the patient's home, thereby alleviating the challenges of leaving the house for those with severe energy deficits or undertaking long-distance travel for care.

Providing care through telehealth does come with certain limitations that require attention. Long COVID is well-suited for telehealth delivery due to the typically normal examination findings; however, it heavily depends on the referrer closely monitoring the patient for any evident signs or potential disease mimickers. Should any concerns arise during a telehealth consultation that would typically be addressed through a physical examination, the patient may need to attend in person, return to their GP for a focused clinical assessment or undergo investigations to definitively exclude the issue. Delivering care via telehealth from metropolitan hubs so restricts clinicians' local awareness of available allied health, investigative, and specialist services. To overcome this challenge, it is essential to establish a network of clinicians and allied health providers who are well-versed in Long COVID, whether in specific locations or those also offering telehealth services.

BOX 19.2 BRÌGHDE'S EXPERIENCE OF TELEHEALTH SERVICES

I have had Long Covid for over two years… [and] as someone living in a rural community, approximately 1.5 hours drive from Melbourne, being able to access the clinic via telehealth has been invaluable. Even now, when I am much improved from the first year of my illness, travelling to Melbourne and back in a day is virtually impossible. If I absolutely must go to Melbourne, I need to book into a hotel overnight, alone, to avoid overstimulation and rest in a dark quiet room for 12+ hours before the return journey the next day, and even then, my energy that week is severely impacted.

… Telehealth was such an unexpected boon –…[attending] appointments from the comfort of my home (where I could finish the appointment and be resting minutes later, if needed). If I were given the option in those early days, I would have pushed myself to attend in-person because I felt a huge sense of societal pressure to (over)perform and also because I was in denial about just how incapacitated I was, and how long I would be unwell. A fit active person who does everything all the time does not easily accept overnight incapacitation, particularly when that incapacity is not physically obvious.

Brighde

19.2.3 The Benefits of a Dedicated Long COVID Service

Evidence and patient-led treatment trials are emerging rapidly in the field of Long COVID, likely more so than in any other disease in history. Keeping abreast of new evidence and trends can easily become overwhelming. Multidisciplinary case discussion meetings enable contributions from various professions with diverse perspectives, helping to stay updated on new and emerging findings. In the absence of a dedicated Long COVID service, connecting with colleagues who share similar interests to exchange experiences can be an effective alternative. This includes building a referral network of multidisciplinary allied health and medical professionals with an interest or focus in Long COVID.

19.3 MANAGEMENT OF PEOPLE WITH LONG COVID IN COMMUNITY SETTINGS

GPs may feel underqualified to manage Long COVID due to its complex symptoms and evolving understanding. However, they can enhance patients' quality of life by addressing symptoms individually, tailoring treatment plans, and leveraging available resources such as allied health referrals, lifestyle adjustments, and supportive therapies. A structured, patient-centred approach enables GPs to effectively manage this multifaceted condition and support recovery.

Effectively managing specific symptoms like cardiac dysautonomia, pain, and unrefreshing sleep can greatly enhance an individual's overall quality of life. The upcoming section is designed to guide and enable primary care providers in the management of patients with Long COVID. The main care approaches focus on the following seven areas.

19.3.1 Evidence-Based Symptom Management

Treat individual symptoms based on the symptom and its severity. This includes the use of evidence-based pharmacological interventions, such as bronchodilators for appropriate respiratory symptoms.[5] Medications considered include those for cardiac dysautonomia, mood stabilisation, and sleep support, as well as other widely available medications based on individual symptom and comorbidity profiles, in consultation with specialists and allied health clinicians.

19.3.2 Clinical Care

As with all chronic conditions, it is important to rule out other diagnoses or conditions that may contribute to the patient's symptoms. This may involve comprehensive assessments, including laboratory tests and imaging studies. However, over-investigation is not in the patient's interest, as it can lead to unnecessary anxiety, additional costs, and potential harm. A balanced approach that prioritises the patient's wellbeing while ensuring thorough evaluation is essential for effective management.

19.3.4 Patient Education

Patient education, engagement, and empowerment are essential in helping patients participate in self-management. Comprehensive Long COVID education involves validation of the patient's experience, discussions on pacing, disease progression, and risk mitigation. Lifestyle modifications, including physical activity, dietary habits, smoking cessation, alcohol consumption, and stress management can improve the general wellbeing of individuals with Long COVID. This can be supported by developing a patient education library of curated or freely available self-education resources.[6]

19.3.5 Early Rehabilitation Programmes

Early physical, cognitive and psychological rehabilitation employs a multifaceted approach that encompasses exercise, physical training (such as re-breathing exercises), cognitive and mental health assessment and intervention, and psychosocial support. This comprehensive intervention addresses the physical, physiological, and psychological aspects of Long COVID-related dysfunction.[5,7,8,9]

Key components of rehabilitation include the early introduction of tailored exercise programmes to improve muscle strength, endurance, and overall fitness specific to the consumer's post-exertional malaise (PEM) threshold.[10] Aerobic and strength training have also been reported to enhance exercise capacity and help patients regain functional independence. The risk of graded exercise therapy (GET) in Long COVID patients, particularly those experiencing PEM, has been a topic of concern (see Chapter 11). Studies have shown that GET can exacerbate symptoms in individuals with Long COVID who experience PEM. The hallmark of PEM is a worsening of symptoms following even minor physical, mental, or emotional exertion. This response is unpredictable and often disproportionate to the activity level.[10,11] Patients are typically advised to pace themselves on a day-to-day basis (see Chapter 12), educating them on lung health and breathing techniques to self-manage their symptoms, take an active role in their recovery,[12–16] and adhere to treatment plans.[7]

19.3.6 Psychological and Cognitive Support

Long COVID often carries a significant psychological burden and can impact cognitive functions. Two guidelines[1,12] recommend specific management to improve cognitive function as part of treatment. This requires referral to a neuropsychologist or occupational therapist with expertise in formal cognitive assessment and rehabilitation. However, access to these services is often limited and inadequate.

While Long COVID is not a psychological condition, interventions may support the associated psychological impacts of the condition. The potential benefits of various psychological therapies, including cognitive-behavioural therapy, mindfulness-based interventions, and supportive counselling, have been reported.[2,6,17,18] Psychosocial support, including counselling and stress management, alleviates anxiety and depression, which may also exacerbate respiratory symptoms. Furthermore, psychological therapy has demonstrated potential benefits in helping individuals cope with the uncertainty and frustration that often accompanies the prolonged course of Long COVID, providing patients with tools and strategies to manage their symptoms, enhance resilience, and improve their overall sense of control over their health.[19]

19.3.7 Psychosocial Wellbeing

Other supports that can improve the wellbeing of someone with Long COVID include social workers who provide social care and logistical support, such as addressing work or domestic issues or assisting with welfare support or social security benefits. For sufferers navigating legal matters such as income protection or other workplace insurance, experienced lawyers can offer valuable assistance in navigating the cognitively burdensome administrative processes.

19.3.8 Comorbidity Management

Studies also emphasise the role of the GP and primary care in managing underlying medical conditions or background social issues, both of which have the potential to exacerbate symptoms.[20]

19.4 BARRIERS TO EFFECTIVE LONG COVID CARE IN PRIMARY HEALTH SETTINGS

19.4.1 Access to Care

Access to Long COVID care is hindered by limited provider awareness and inadequate geographical availability of specialised clinics. Many healthcare practitioners struggle to recognise the often vague and wide-ranging symptoms, leading to misdiagnosis or insufficient care plans. Patients have frequently faced disbelief about their symptoms, with some being misdiagnosed as having anxiety or psychosomatic issues, leaving them feeling marginalised and unsupported, which can worsen their condition.

Fragmented care across specialties further complicates access, forcing patients to navigate multiple referrals without a cohesive treatment plan. This disjointed approach not only disrupts the patient experience but also hampers effective interdisciplinary collaboration, which is essential for managing complex conditions like Long COVID.

19.4.2 Cost to the Patient

Long COVID is a truly multisystem disorder. In terms of complexity, there is no doubt that Long COVID is one of the most time-consuming conditions encountered in a clinical consult. Access to the multidisciplinary care required to manage Long COVID, particularly outside of the public health system, often incurs significant out-of-pocket expenses for the patient at each step. Furthermore, often medications used to manage Long COVID and Postural Orthostatic Tachycardia Syndrome (POTS) are not government subsidised, and the costs to the patient, whose income is often affected by their disease, can be considerable. This financial burden can exacerbate the already significant emotional and psychological toll that Long COVID takes on individuals, leading to increased anxiety and stress about their health and financial stability.

19.4.3 Physical Barriers

Attending face-to-face appointments can be an insurmountable hurdle for some people with Long COVID. Many patients may experience debilitating fatigue or cognitive difficulties that prevent them from traveling and may also experience sensory overload in the environment of a busy clinic. This can lead to missed appointments and a lack of continuity in care. Assessing these burdens and adapting to the patient's needs – such as employing telehealth or considering their sleep requirements and scheduling later appointments – can improve outcomes and reduce the physical toll of treatment.

19.4.4 Care Delivery

Caring for individuals with Long COVID is challenged by systemic barriers. Consultations are complex, multisystem evaluations often accompanied by psychosocial stress, requiring significant time and resources. However, these lengthy consultations are poorly supported by public health funding or insurance, creating financial strain for both clinicians and patients already burdened by the illness and its associated costs. Inadequate funding for essential services limits access to comprehensive care, making it difficult for healthcare providers to deliver the support Long COVID patients need. This highlights the urgent need for better resource allocation and funding structures to address these challenges effectively.

BOX 19.3   PRACTICE POINT

Reflect on the barriers to accessing care in Long COVID outlined above. What might you do differently in your practice to support access to primary care or rehabilitation for people with Long COVID?

19.5 IMPLICATIONS FOR THE HEALTH SYSTEM

To enable smooth implementation, several key, deep-rooted systematic challenges must be urgently addressed by health systems.

19.5.1 Variability in Care

There is significant variability in the quality and level of Long COVID care across remote, regional, and metropolitan areas across the globe, which may lead to inequities in access and disparities in patient outcomes. The options for referral back to tertiary hospitals for cases necessitating tertiary care have been limited and, when available, are generally restricted to metropolitan cities.[21]

19.5.2 Lack of Standardised, Widely Adopted Clinical Protocols

Standardised clinical guidelines and protocols for Long COVID care have yet to be widely adopted in practice to ensure consistent care.[21] Although in Australia, the National Clinical Task Force led the way during the COVID pandemic,[5] the current lack of ongoing funding from the federal government jeopardises its ability to provide up-to-date, evidence-based recommendations in the long term.

19.5.3 Limited Treatment Options

The absence of specific pharmacological treatments for Long COVID symptoms across different body systems poses a significant challenge. Research into potential therapeutic interventions is ongoing, but to date, has not yielded significant new or effective therapeutic agents for Long COVID.

19.5.4 Workforce Challenges

The demand for specialised healthcare professionals in Long COVID clinics places an additional burden on an already overstretched healthcare workforce. This becomes particularly challenging when some healthcare professionals are also suffering from Long COVID themselves.[22,23] Recruitment and education/ training of clinicians with expertise in Long COVID management need to be better coordinated.

19.5.5 Access to Care Technology

The use of modern technology to better screen and detect patients is still in its infancy. This affects Long COVID diagnosis, particularly in differentiating Long COVID from similar conditions such as Chronic Fatigue Syndrome/Myalgic Encephalomyelitis or POTS.[24] Further research and development will enable cross-specialty collaboration for treatment advancement. For example, telehealth options for managing Long COVID should be more widely utilised to improve access to care in remote or underserved areas.[25,26]

19.5.6 Patient Education and Support

There is a need to develop centralised, up-to-date educational materials for Long COVID patients to help them understand their condition and empower them to self-manage symptoms. Both physical and mental health support should be enhanced within Long COVID clinics to address the multifaceted impact of this condition.[27]

These barriers can be addressed by developing a structured strategy for caring for patients with Long COVID. This may include structured consultations focusing on one symptom or issue at a time, with planned regular check-ups to stay on top of emerging issues. Group support, pre-developed education packages, and resources for self-management can also play a crucial role in empowering patients to navigate their recovery journey effectively. Assessing these burdens and adapting care to meet patient needs – by employing telehealth or considering their sleep requirements, for instance – can improve outcomes and reduce the physical toll of treatment.

19.6 TWO CASE STUDIES OF SUCCESSFUL MODELS OF LONG COVID CARE IN AUSTRALIA

19.6.1 Geelong Long COVID Clinic

The Geelong Long COVID Clinic, established in June 2022 in Victoria, Australia, provides care for individuals with Long COVID through GP, healthcare provider, and self-referrals. Its multidisciplinary team – including respiratory specialists, physiotherapists, psychologists, dietitians, and social workers – collaborates to create personalised treatment plans based on evidence-based guidelines, such as those from the National Clinical Evidence Task Force.

From June 2022 to August 2024, the clinic treated over 400 patients, predominantly adults aged 40–70, with 68% being female. Referrals came mainly from GPs (49.3%) and hospitals (34.0%), reflecting a shift toward primary care-led management. Patients were primarily from Western Victoria and Melbourne, with a smaller percentage from rural areas and only 2.5% under 18 years old. The clinic's model emphasises collaboration with hospital specialists and allied health clinicians to address diverse patient needs.

BOX 19.4   PATIENT EXPERIENCE OF THE GEELONG LONG COVID CLINIC

I accessed the Geelong Long COVID Clinic on a colleague's recommendation after 18 months of persistent symptoms from early pandemic COVID. The clinic's validation, treatments (low dose naltrexone & Intuniv), and strategies from the occupational therapist and exercise physiologist significantly improved my symptoms, including fatigue, cognitive changes, and POTS, which had restricted my life. For the first time, I felt hope. The clinic's skilled practitioners and collaborative approach made managing my condition possible. Their generous communication and resources also enhanced understanding for me, my family, GP, and pharmacist.

Anonymous

19.7.2 Clinic Nineteen

Clinic Nineteen, established in 2022 in Melbourne, Australia, addresses the gap in public Long COVID clinics by offering MBS-subsidised telehealth appointments with non-GP specialists. This model has provided care to over 900 patients across Australia, alleviating the financial and physical burdens of travel while attracting healthcare professionals who might otherwise be unable to commit to regular clinic roles.

Recognising the need for paediatric care, the clinic integrated paediatric physicians early on. Clinicians share resources and consistent medical approaches to manage the diverse symptoms of Long COVID effectively. With the potential to expand into allied health services, the clinic has also built a referral network of professionals. Rising demand and growing wait times highlight the need for additional resources to meet patient and provider needs.

19.8 CONCLUSION

International guidelines emphasise the importance of a multidisciplinary approach to managing Long COVID, involving collaboration between specialists such as hospital physicians, physiotherapists, occupational therapists, and mental health professionals. This model allows for a comprehensive assessment of physical, cognitive, and psychological symptoms, enabling tailored treatment plans. Regular assessments are crucial for tracking progress and adjusting treatment as needed, while ongoing support is essential given the fluctuating nature of Long COVID symptoms.[28,29]

Addressing lifestyle factors, including physical activity, stress management, and pacing, is also vital. These modifications can improve long-term outcomes, as recommended by various guidelines.[5,18] However, the evidence supporting new pharmacological treatments for Long COVID remains limited and inconsistent. Prescribing decisions should be individualised, carefully considering the potential risks and benefits of specific treatments.[17] Patient education and engagement are key to successful Long COVID management. Studies show that informed patients, actively involved in their care, are more likely to adhere to treatment plans and achieve better outcomes.[5,7,13,14,18] Involving patients in decision-making enhances satisfaction and helps them navigate both the medical and psychological aspects of the condition.

In conclusion, effective management of Long COVID requires a holistic, patient-centred approach. This includes multidisciplinary care, regular assessments, lifestyle modifications, and patient engagement. While new pharmacological options are still under investigation, a focus on individualised care can significantly improve outcomes for Long COVID patients.

NOTE

1   Lived Experience Author who has chosen to remain anonymous.

REFERENCES

1   Crook H, et al. Long COVID-mechanisms, risk factors, and management [published correction appears in BMJ. 2021 Aug 3;374:n1944. doi: 10.1136/bmj.n1944]. BMJ. 2021;374:n1648. doi:10.1136/bmj.n1648.

2   Byambasuren O, et al. Effect of COVID-19 vaccination on Long COVID: Systematic review. BMJ Med. 2023;2(1):e000385. doi:10.1136/bmjmed-2022-000385.

3   Nittas V, et al. Long COVID through a public health lens: An umbrella review. Public Health Rev. 2022;43:1604501. doi:10.3389/phrs.2022.1604501.

4 Holmes A, et al. Persistent symptoms after COVID-19: An Australian stratified random health survey on Long COVID. Med J Aust. 2024;221(9):S12–17. doi:10.5694/mja2.52473.

5 Australian National COVID-19 Clinical Evidence Taskforce and Australian Living Evidence Collaboration. Caring for people with COVID-19 [Intenet]. Melbourne: Living Evidence; [cited 2025 Feb 7]. Available from: https://livingevidence.org.au/living-guidelines/covid-19/.

6 Royal Australian College of General Practitioners (RACGP). Post-COVID-19 community of practice resources [Internet]. Melbourne: RACGP; [cited 2025 Feb 7]. Available from: https://www.racgp.org.au/the-racgp/faculties/vic/post-covid-19-community-of-practice.

7 World Health Organization (WHO). Clinical management of COVID-19: Living guideline [Internet]. Geneva: WHO; 2023 [cited 2025 Feb 7]. Available from: https://www.who.int/publications/i/item/WHO-2019-nCoV-clinical-2023.2.

8 Maley JH, et al. Multidisciplinary collaborative consensus guidance statement on the assessment and treatment of breathing discomfort and respiratory sequelae in patients with post-acute sequelae of SARS-CoV-2 infection (PASC). PM&R. 2022;14(1):77–95. doi:10.1002/pmrj.12744.

9 Estebanez-Pérez MJ, et al. The effectiveness of a four-week digital physiotherapy intervention to improve functional capacity and adherence to intervention in patients with Long COVID-19. Int J Environ Res Public Health. 2022;19(15):9566. doi:10.3390/ijerph19159566.

10 Gloeckl R, et al. Practical recommendations for exercise training in patients with Long COVID with or without post-exertional malaise: A best practice proposal. Sports Med Open. 2024;10(1):47. doi:10.1186/s40798-024-00695-8

11 National Institute for Health and Care Excellence (NICE). Myalgic encephalomyelitis (or encephlopathy)/Chronic fatigue syndrome: Diagnosis and management [Internet]. London: NICE; 2022 [cited 2025 Feb 7]. Available from: https://www.nice.org.uk/guidance/ng206.

12 Fine JS, et al. Multidisciplinary collaborative consensus guidance statement on the assessment and treatment of cognitive symptoms in patients with post-acute sequelae of SARS-CoV-2 infection (PASC). PM&R. 2022;14(1):96–111. doi:10.1002/pmrj.12745.

13 Royal Australian College of General Practitioners (RACGP). Caring for patients with post-COVID-19 conditions: Introduction [Internet]. Melbourne: RACGP; [cited 2025 Feb 7]. Available from: https://www.racgp.org.au/clinical-resources/covid-19-resources/clinical-care/caring-for-patients-with-post-covid-19-conditions/introduction

14 Singh SJ, et al. Respiratory sequelae of COVID-19: Pulmonary and extrapulmonary origins, and approaches to clinical care and rehabilitation. Lancet Respir Med. 2023;11(8):709–25. doi:10.1016/S2213-2600(23)00159-5.

15 Okan F, et al. Evaluating the efficiency of breathing exercises via telemedicine in post-COVID-19 patients: Randomized controlled study. Clin Nurs Res. 2022;31(5):771–81. doi:10.1177/10547738221097241.

16 Phillip K, et al. An online breathing and wellbeing programme (ENO Breathe) for people with persistent symptoms following COVID-19: A parallel-group, single-blind, randomised controlled trial. Lancet Respir Med. 2022;10(9):851–62. doi:10.1016/S2213-2600(22)00125-4.

17 Whiteson JH, et al. Multi-disciplinary collaborative consensus guidance statement on the assessment and treatment of cardiovascular complications in patients with post-acute sequelae of SARS-CoV-2 infection (PASC). PM&R. 2022;14(7):855–78. doi:10.1002/pmrj.12859.

18 Yelin D, et al. ESCMID rapid guidelines for assessment and management of Long COVID. Clin Microbiol Infect. 2022;28(7):955–72. doi:10.1016/j.cmi.2022.02.018.

19 Kuut TA, et al. Efficacy of cognitive behavioural therapy targeting severe fatigue following COVID-19: Results of a randomized controlled trial. Clin Infect Dis. 2023;77(5):687–95. doi:10.1093/cid/ciad257.

20 Agency for Healthcare Research and Quality (AHRQ). Models of care for post-COVID-19 condition (long COVID): A technical brief [Internet]. Rockville, MD: AHRQ; 2023 [cited 2025 Feb 7]. Available from: https://effectivehealthcare.ahrq.gov/products/long-covid-models-care/tech-brief.

21 Greenhalgh T, et al. What is quality in Long COVID care? Lessons from a national quality improvement collaborative and multi-site ethnography. BMC Med. 2024;22(1):159. doi:10.1186/s12916-024-03371-6

22 British Medical Association (BMA). Over-exposed and under-protected: The long-term impact of COVID-19 on doctors [Internet]. Patient Safety Learning Hub; 2023 Jul 4 [cited 2025 Feb 7]. Available from: https://www.pslhub.org/learn/coronavirus-covid19/patient-recovery/bma-over-exposed-and-under-protected-the-long-term-impact-of-covid-19-on-doctors-4-july-2023-r9710.

23 Office for National Statistics (ONS). Prevalence of ongoing symptoms following coronavirus (COVID-19) infection in the UK [Internet]. London: ONS; 2023 Feb 2 [cited 2025 Feb 7]. Available from: https://www.ons.gov.uk/peoplepopulationandcommunity/healthandsocialcare/conditionsanddiseases/bulletins/prevalenceofongoingsymptomsfollowingcoronaviruscovid19infectionintheuk/2february2023.

24 Seeley MC, et al. High incidence of autonomic dysfunction and postural orthostatic tachycardia syndrome in patients with Long COVID: Implications for management and health care planning. Am J Med 2023;S0002–9343(23)00402-3. doi:10.1016/j.amjmed.2023.06.010

25 Romaszko-Wojtowicz A, et al. Telemonitoring in Long-COVID patients—preliminary findings. Int J Environ Res Public Health. 2022;19(9):5268. doi:10.3390/ijerph19095268

26 Rinn R, et al. Digital interventions for treating post-COVID or Long-COVID symptoms: Scoping review. J Med Internet Res. 2023;25:e45711. doi:10.2196/45711

27 NSW Agency for Clinical Innovation (ACI). Post-acute sequelae of COVID-19 [Internet]. Sydney: ACI; [cited 2025 Feb 7]. Available from: https://aci.health.nsw.gov.au/statewide-programs/critical-intelligence-unit/post-acute-sequelae.

28 Dillen H, et al. Clinical effectiveness of rehabilitation in ambulatory care for patients with persisting symptoms after COVID-19: A systematic review. BMC Infect Dis. 2023;23(1):419. doi:10.1186/s12879-023-08374-x.

29 Jimeno-Almazán A, et al. Rehabilitation for post-COVID-19 condition through a supervised exercise intervention: A randomized controlled trial. Scand J Med Sci Sports. 2022;32(12):1791–1801. doi:10.1111/sms.14240.

Chapter 20

Self-Determination and Self-Management for People with Long COVID

Thomas Ponissi, Tanya Ward, and Danielle Hitch

BOX 20.1   LEARNING OBJECTIVES

By the end of this chapter, readers should be able to:

- Understand the relevance of self-determination and self-management principles to people with Long COVID.
- Identify barriers to self-determination and empowerment, along with strategies to address them.
- Apply key concepts such as shared decision-making, personalised care plans, and symptom monitoring to support self-management during rehabilitation.
- Recognise the potential value of innovative tools in supporting equity, autonomy, and effective self-management.

20.1 INTRODUCTION

People with Long COVID, like everyone else, have a fundamental right to self-determination. Human rights conventions emphasise the principle of autonomy, which is the freedom to make independent decisions about one's life, health, and wellbeing.[1] This principle is crucial for managing Long COVID, a complex condition with highly variable symptoms and impacts.

Self-determination enables people to customise care and management strategies to their unique needs and circumstances. Supports based on self-determination are linked to improved health outcomes for people with various health conditions.[2–5] Active involvement in healthcare decisions helps people with

DOI: 10.4324/9781003528104-25

Long COVID meaningfully navigate the challenges of their condition. Promoting self-determination also tackles systemic barriers, such as delayed care and social stigma, by empowering them to advocate for their needs and preferences.

Self-management strategies employed by people with Long COVID are an expression of self-determination. They take meaningful steps towards recovery and wellbeing by exercising control, such as deciding when to rest, what treatments to pursue, or how to use support networks. Self-determination also enhances healthcare engagement, as respected and empowered patients are more likely to practise self-management and use health services. Self-determination honours the dignity and expertise of people with Long COVID while underpinning effective self-management.

BOX 20.2   PRACTICE POINT

Rehabilitation health professionals are ethically and professionally obligated to uphold patients' human rights. Reflect on your practice. Do you ask patients about strategies they have independently developed? Do you incorporate these into intervention plans?

20.2 WHAT IS SELF-DETERMINATION?

Self-determination is the intentional actions people take to control what happens in their lives and to maintain their health and wellbeing.[6] Self-determination involves behaviours and skills enabling people to take control of their lives,[7] which can be learnt or developed over time. It encompasses how people make decisions, solve problems, and manage their lives in ways that reflect their beliefs, values, and goals. Empowerment refers to activities and supports that help people with Long COVID gain greater control over their health and wellbeing by enhancing their knowledge, shared understandings and decision-making, and improving health service access.[8]

Self-determination underpins empowerment, mutually beneficial relationships, knowledge and skills, and shared social power.[9] Many people with Long COVID feel disempowered due to the condition's impact, personal circumstances, and broader societal and structural factors. There are many theories for self-determination and empowerment in healthcare, mainly originating from disability research and advocacy. While not everyone considers Long COVID a disability, these frameworks illustrate how these concepts function in practice.

20.2.1 Causal Agency Theory

Causal Agency Theory developed from positive psychology and strengths-based approaches to disability, providing a framework for understanding self-determination.[10] The three core components of self-determined actions it describes are highly context-dependent and may act as supports or barriers for people with Long COVID in exercising self-determination (see Figure 20.1).

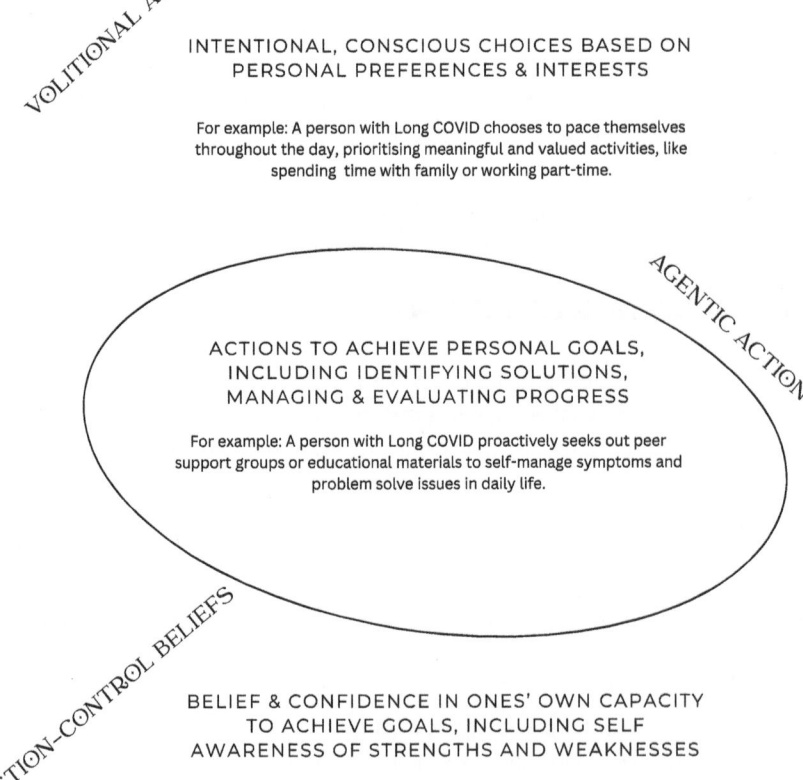

Figure 20.1 Essential components of Causal Agency Theory.[10]

BOX 20.3 PRACTICE POINT

How might this theory support self-determination for people with Long COVID? Identify one rehabilitation strategy or intervention for each component. How else can you support their self-determination?

20.2.2 Empowerment

A recent synthesis of the literature[11] highlighted barriers to fostering patient empowerment across healthcare. Persistent power imbalances and paternalistic attitudes undermine equitable decision-making. Patient participation is often tokenistic and superficial, reinforcing feelings of powerlessness and coercion. Stigma and discrimination, compounded by poor communication, further impede patients' ability to navigate healthcare systems. Empowerment strategies frequently focus on patient behaviour change rather than health professionals' responsibility to address power imbalances, for example, by providing motivational interviewing or patient education. Recommended strategies for overcoming these barriers include participatory practices (such as shared decision-making and service co-design), education for health professionals about addressing power dynamics (e.g., reflection on conflicting values/beliefs and shifting from authoritarian to collaborative language), and tailored strategies that respect patients' autonomy and expertise.

BOX 20.4 PRACTICE POINT

Select a barrier to patient empowerment that affects your rehabilitation practice. What changes can health professionals make to mitigate its impact, and who would need to implement them?

Peer support models exemplify self-determination as an example of patient-led support. Peer support may be offered as part of rehabilitation services (i.e., through the employment of lived experience workers) or exist independently in the community. Research demonstrates they can empower people with Long COVID in a meaningful and authentic way[12] by validating lived experiences, reducing isolation, fostering autonomy through shared knowledge and mutual support, and promoting advocacy. When supported by quality training, internal and external supervision and wellbeing options, and mechanisms for feedback and evaluation, they address both personal needs and systemic challenges. Figure 20.2 outlines key features when designing or partnering with peer support providers for people with Long COVID.

20.3 SELF-MANAGEMENT STRATEGIES

People with Long COVID employ diverse self-management strategies tailored to their specific symptoms, personal circumstances, and lived experiences.

> *My thoughts on Long COVID self-management and self-determination are specific to my lived experience. My symptoms mainly affect the brain and involved depleted energy and cognitive function. Strict self-management has helped me get back to a close approximation of my pre-infection life. However, my approach may not suit someone whose symptoms affect areas like the lungs or ear, nose, and throat.*
>
> Thomas

There are some general principles that are broadly relevant for people with Long COVID. Many strategies align with those commonly used by people with chronic health conditions,[13] while others reflect the condition's unique characteristics.

Self-management strategies do not exist in a vacuum – effective self-management relies on integrating patient preferences and innovations into structured rehabilitation interventions.[13] Health professionals should identify and engage with strategies already used by people with Long COVID to ensure sustainable implementation.[14] They should also use their expertise to identify and address unintentionally harmful or ineffective strategies, working with patients to adopt more effective approaches. Interventions that disrupt existing roles and routines are unlikely to be integrated into daily life. In other words, everyone must be on the same page for rehabilitation for Long COVID to be relevant and practical.

20.3.1 Develop Knowledge about Long COVID

Knowledge underpins effective self-management by empowering people with Long COVID to make informed health decisions. As discussed in Chapter 4, those with Long COVID were the first to identify the condition and are experts in its daily impacts. Health professionals, however, also bring valuable knowledge about its causes, symptoms, triggers, progression, complications, and treatment.

Flexible & Inclusive Approaches to Peer Support

Designed to meet the diverse needs of people with Long COVID, whose lived experience varies widely.
- Varied Modes of Delivery: Online forums, face to face groups, social media groups, hybrid models.
- Individually Tailored: Allowing choice about level of involvement, frequency and form of meetings, and type of support offered.
- Accessible: Accomodating of varying levels of fatigue and brain fog
- Trauma-Informed: Providing psychologically, physically and culturally safe spaces which promote trust and understanding, prevent re-traumatisation, and support strength-building and skill development.
- Founded on Lived Experience: Providing validation, shared understanding and practical insights

Addressing Structural Inequities

Factors like socio-economic disadvantage, racism, sexism and ableism are barriers to accessing peer support.
- Inclusivity: Proactive approaches to engaging with marginalised groups (such as people with disablity and culturally and linguistically diverse communities).
- Culturally Sensitive Support: Incorporating culturally relevant practices and participation by people from these communities in peer support design and delivery.
- Equitable Resource Allocation: Prioritising funding and resources on the basis of need for individuals and disadvantaged groups.
- Reducing Access Barriers: Mitigating the effects of travel costs, internet access issues, limited digital literacy or implicit bias held by facilitators.

Co-Design

People with Long COVID and the broader community should be involved in designing and delivering peer support programs to ensure they are relevant and useful.
- Collaborative Development: Co-designing with people with lived experience of Long COVID, to ensure supports are effective and respectful.
- Power Sharing: Addressing power imbalances between health professionals and patients by ensuring both groups have an equal say in decision making.
- Iterative Feedback: Incorporating participant feedback into program redesign and evolution to ensure continuous improvement and responsiveness.
- Avoiding Over-Professionalisation: Maintaining a balance between formal structure and grassroots authenticity to avoid replicating hierarchical healthcare dynamics.
- Engaging with Intersectionality: Considering and reflecting on the complex effects of multiple aspects of identity for people with Long COVID (i.e. race, gender, age, socio-economic status).

Figure 20.2 Recommended features and characteristics for peer support models.[12]

Patients attend rehabilitation to benefit from the professional expertise of the multidisciplinary team, which they may draw upon to anticipate and proactively respond to setbacks and challenges.

In the absence of diagnostic criteria, many people with Long COVID learn about their condition through online communities, which offer crucial support and validation.[15] Online information varies in quality and credibility, so patients may need direction or support to find reliable sources.[16] Self-management programmes by health professionals often include education on Long COVID, but it is essential to acknowledge that knowledge development is a mutual process. Studies show the health workforce has generally limited knowledge about Long COVID.[17–19] Developing knowledge about Long COVID is a process of mutual, iterative learning between people with Long COVID and health professionals across multiple services and sectors.[20]

> *I figured a lot of this stuff out as I went along, through trial and error, under the guidance of my GP (and eventually my specialist), as well by engaging an online support group.*
>
> Thomas

The general public requires education about Long COVID to address systemic inequities faced by people with this condition. Repeated stigma and discrimination profoundly harm the health and wellbeing of people with Long COVID and typically stem from misconceptions and unfounded assumptions.

> *Once, when I mentioned I had Long COVID, an acquaintance stepped back in concern thinking I was infectious. Another time, when I disclosed my chronic illness in job applications, the person said they wouldn't hire someone with Long COVID, because they were in the "too hard basket". I see this social stigma and lack of understanding around the condition as a form of ableism. But my experience of chronic illness is a strength and a sign of perseverance, not to mention a simple truth that I want to be honest about it. The armchair medical advice I have been given without requesting or consenting to it is endlessly frustrating; many of these 'recommendations' have been unproven or potentially harmful practices.*
>
> Thomas

Underestimating people with Long COVID's knowledge of their condition can harm therapeutic alliances. Understanding the extent and nature of their invaluable lived experience is essential to ensure Long COVID education is appropriately targeted and relevant.

The implication underneath this advice is that I ought to be doing more to get better — as though I haven't been giving recovery any serious thought. There is a fine line between offering support and inappropriately intervening - I certainly don't have all the answers, but I think people without Long COVID (or a similar condition) should do less talking and more listening when it comes to the lived experience of chronic illness and disability.

Thomas

20.3.2 Shared Decision-Making

Shared decision-making leads to people with Long COVID and health professionals combining their expertise to decide on assessments, interventions, and supports. Long used in chronic disease management, this practice improves patient satisfaction and trust in health professionals.[21] It is particularly relevant when interdisciplinary communication is required, uncertainty is high, and patient risk tolerance varies.[22,23] People with Long COVID may accept, decline, or set limits on health professional recommendations through this process.

I have navigated decisions about my care and treatment for Long COVID by choosing not to pursue any potential treatment that wasn't under the supervision of my General Practitioner or Long COVID specialist.

Thomas

For shared decision-making, people with Long COVID and health professionals should access, understand, and discuss evidence-based information about treatment options, benefits, harms, side effects, potential outcomes, uncertainties, and patient values and needs. This information facilitates informed consent but can also be overwhelming. A common tool for shared decision-making is decision aids, which are resources that provide information about treatment options under consideration.[24] The International Decision Aid Standards Collaboration identified their features, as shown in Figure 20.3.

BOX 20.5   PRACTICE POINT

Create a one-page decision aid for an intervention you offer to people with Long COVID. Ensure the information is concise, accessible, and supported by evidence.

Patient Decision Aids ...

- ✓ Describe the condition related to the decision
- ✓ Describe the decision that needs to be considered
- ✓ List all potential options
- ✓ Describes the benefits and advantages of the options
- ✓ Describes the harms, side effects and disadvantages of the options
- ✓ Help patients clarify their perceptions and preferences for outcomes by prompting them to envision their effects

Figure 20.3 Features of patient decision aids in shared decision-making.[25]

20.3.3 Monitoring and Managing Signs and Symptoms

People with Long COVID can benefit from tools and techniques to track symptoms and activate action plans in response to health fluctuations. Proactive monitoring can prevent complications, reduce the need for health services, and promote long-term stability.

Symptom monitoring is essential to pacing, a self-management strategy for preventing relapse by managing energy use (see Chapters 11 and 12). Effective pacing requires people with Long COVID to stop the activity before complete depletion, relying on moment-to-moment awareness of energy levels. Symptom monitoring helps them respond to current symptoms and plan for future issues.

> *Instead of waiting to reach 20% (or run out entirely), I start slowing down around 40–50%. If I have a big commitment on Monday, I may need to rest on Sunday, even if I feel well enough to be active. I am very mindful of 'energy hangovers'; if I expend lots of energy one day, my reserves are even more depleted than usual the next, and I will need to carve out extra time to recover. I embrace rest as not just restorative, but as preparative too.*
>
> Thomas

Symptoms can be monitored using various tools, depending on personal preference. Hard copy symptom diaries are accessible and convenient but require effort to collate data and identify trends. Increasingly, people with Long COVID are adopting digital diaries or tools that summarise data in real time and provide early warnings of deterioration.[26] Wearable devices, such as smartwatches, also offer passive, unobtrusive monitoring of physiological metrics.[27]

20.3.4 Managing the Impact of Long COVID on Daily Life

Self-management strategies are integral to addressing address more than just symptoms. Long COVID significantly affects all aspects of daily life (see Chapter 12), and effective self-management approaches can positively influence quality of life. A holistic approach is essential, as a single self-management strategy, like pacing, often supports participation in multiple activities.

Some self-management strategies require additional resources, such as hiring a cleaner for housework. People with Long COVID may not be eligible for the same financial support as others with a disability; for instance, they are currently ineligible for National Disability Insurance Scheme support in Australia. The financial impact of Long COVID is well documented, highlighting a phenomenon known as the "disability tax" where people's additional healthcare needs incur higher costs than the general population. Therefore, recommendations for self-management strategies must consider the financial circumstances of these patients, who may also benefit from support to navigate the complex processes of applying for welfare payments.

> *I had to quit my job, and request special consideration from university, due to my symptoms, and am only now capable of returning to work after two years. Specialist appointments and my medication are expensive, and this experience has been extremely financially draining. I have been fortunate to live at home and have a strong support network. I do not know how less-privileged people can be expected to live with, let alone recover from, Long COVID without financial support.*
>
> Thomas

Setting boundaries is integral to self-management for people with Long COVID. Prioritising personal needs may conflict with others who lack lived experience of chronic conditions or disabilities, contributing to marginalisation. However, sticking to self-care plans allows people to maintain their health and wellbeing and supports a return to participating in all areas of daily life in the longer term.

> *I had to implement strategies that appear strange or excessive to some people. It is challenging to resist the social pressure to abandon self-management practices; I don't know how many events I've left early or*

simply not attended so that I could go to bed at a reasonable hour, despite pleas to stay out and be "more fun". This isn't easy, but it truly pays off in the long run. Setting boundaries is an act of self-respect; after all, you are the one who will ultimately experience symptom exacerbation, so you need to put yourself first or you will suffer the consequences.

Thomas

Some people with Long COVID practice acceptance, which is a challenging process of coming to terms with the limitations, challenges, and impact of this condition on their lives. The uncertainty associated with Long COVID can be one of the most challenging issues to navigate.[28] Acceptance is not the same as passivity or giving up hope – it can empower people to adapt to their "new normal" and live a meaningful life with Long COVID. Feelings of acceptance can fluctuate over time, impacting the person's ability to use self-management strategies and accept assistance from others.

I recognise it's my current reality, and instead of resisting I adjust to it. It doesn't stop me from self-managing my symptoms, or having hope for a full recovery, or mourning what I have lost; all these things are important, and necessary. Because I accept that I have Long COVID, I also accept I need special supports and care. Despite this being my 'new normal', I possess the same dignity as before.

Thomas

20.3.5 Health Promoting Lifestyle Choices

Lifestyle measures such as improved diet, regular physical activity, and stress management are part of self-management for many people with Long COVID. These habits reduce risk factors for conditions linked to Long COVID, prevent deterioration, and enhance long-term health outcomes. Evidence indicates that programmes supporting people with Long COVID in adopting healthy lifestyles can improve symptoms and quality of life.[29–31] Health professionals play a key role in motivating and supporting patients choosing to adopt these changes through education, goal setting, and ongoing support. Their guidance ensures these measures are implemented safely; see Chapters 11 and 15 for detailed advice on exercise and diet.

Long COVID has highlighted the importance of taking care of myself all the time. I eat better, giving more thought to what my body needs and what I should consume. Now I am recovering (and able to), I regularly exercise to

*build my strength and endurance. However, for over 18 months, I experienced
extreme post exertional malaise after any exercise beyond moderate walking.*

Thomas

Sleep hygiene strategies are a vital, yet often overlooked, aspect of
self-management for people with Long COVID. Sleep supports immune function,
cognitive performance, mental health, and overall wellbeing.[32] Approximately
half of people with Long COVID report sleep issues, including insomnia, repeated
waking, poor sleep quality, and excessive daytime sleepiness.[33] Effective strategies
include maintaining consistent sleep and wake times, regular exercise, avoiding
caffeine and alcohol late in the day, limiting fluid intake at night, ensuring a
well-ventilated room, avoiding digital screens for at least two hours before
bedtime, and following a consistent pre-sleep routine.[34]

20.3.6 Formulating a Personalised Self-Management Care Plan

The strategies and approaches can be combined into a structured, personalised
care plan created collaboratively by the person with Long COVID, their health
professionals, family, kinship, and carers. These plans aim to improve health
and wellbeing by preventing relapses, maintaining progress, and ensuring the
multidisciplinary team works towards shared goals. Plans may include the person's
symptom profile and its impact, collaboratively setting goals, triggers and early
warning signs, treatment preferences, self-management and support-seeking
strategies, daily or weekly schedules, rehabilitation interventions, and review
dates.[35,36]

*I believe that each person who develops Long COVID should be actively
supported to develop a holistic, long-term treatment plan, focusing on both
physical and mental health.*

Thomas

Family, kinship, friends, and carers play a vital role in self-management and
should be included, if willing, in care plans with the consent of the person
with Long COVID. Research shows their involvement improves outcomes,
enhances communication with health professionals, and supports sustainable
implementation.[37] While essential for children and young people, their involvement
is relevant to all ages, as explained here,

*During a period of weakness, I asked my best friend to help me cook soup
to freeze for easy, healthy meals. I've found many people are willing to help*

but don't know how. Clearly articulating my needs to friends or family has lightened my load, however it also made me feel vulnerable, and I'm still processing this emotionally — but this is the reality of chronic illness and not something to be ashamed of.

Thomas

20.4 CASE STUDY: SUPPORTING SELF-MANAGEMENT WITH THE COVID CHECK-IN

The COVID Check-In (CCI) is an online self-management platform co-designed by health professionals and people with Long COVID in Australia. Developed within the DisCOVeRY model of care (see Chapter 10), it met a need identified by people with lived experience around finding local support. They wanted a tool to access this information independently without waiting for it to be provided by health services and to monitor their progress.

The CCI begins with a checklist of daily activities rather than focusing on symptoms. This reflects feedback from our co-design process that the limitations Long COVID imposes on daily life are what it "means" for patients. Users prioritise activities by personal importance and complete a symptom checklist for each, capturing the nuanced relationship between function and symptoms. An algorithm then generates a personalised and prioritised list of activities and symptoms. Early user testing and the complexity of Long COVID led to users being instructed to focus on their top three priorities to avoid overwhelm.

The final CCI section allows patients to set personal goals using the Goal Attainment Scale,[38] which are securely saved and can be revisited throughout recovery. The platform generates a personalised directory of local services and supports aligned with their goals to facilitate tailored care planning. It provides credible health information relevant to the person's symptoms to enhance their knowledge (Figure 20.4). For instance, if mobility improvement is a priority, general information about mobility, tips for improving mobility and local physiotherapy services are provided. People with Long COVID receive all algorithm-generated information, while an abbreviated version is available for their care team in response to feedback about the time pressures faced by rehabilitation health professionals. Both these reports can facilitate shared decision-making, goal setting, and adjustment during rehabilitation sessions.

The CCI is undergoing extensive user testing with people with Long COVID to ensure accessibility and relevance and will be released as a free online platform. It

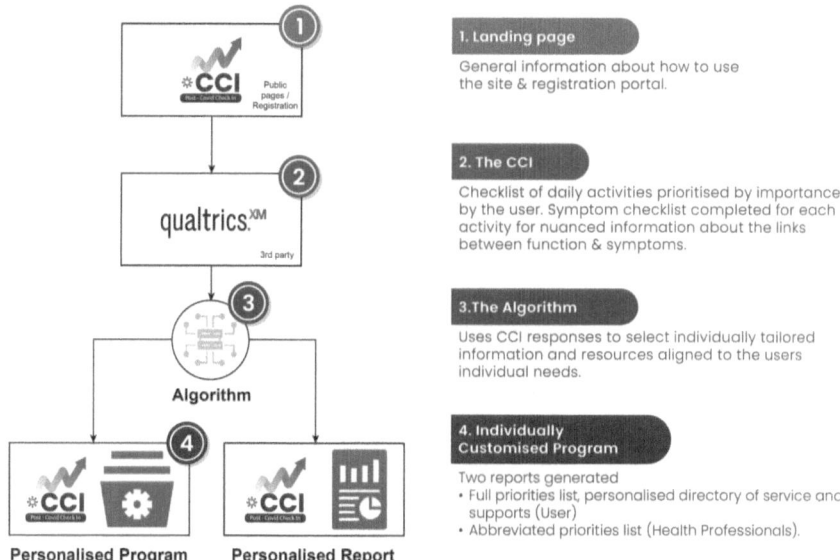

Figure 20.4 The COVID Check-In (CCI).

links to existing and newly developed resources rigorously assessed for accuracy and credibility. Quality reports for all resources, video instructions, and case studies will be freely accessible to users.

The CCI is an example of how technology, lived experience, and clinical expertise can combine to enhance self-management for people with Long COVID. By offering tools for prioritisation, goal setting, and tailored support, the CCI embodies the principles of self-determination and personalised care explored in this chapter. It is, therefore, a case study in innovation that promotes equity and autonomy for people with Long COVID.

20.5 CONCLUSION

In conclusion, self-determination and self-management are crucial to supporting the health and wellbeing of people with Long COVID. This chapter highlights how empowering people through shared decision-making, personalised care plans, and self-management interventions improves outcomes and quality of life. Effective care is underpinned by autonomy, equity, mutual respect, and integrating lived experience with professional knowledge. Therefore, prioritising self-determination and self-management is an ethical imperative and pathway to sustainable recovery. Innovations like the CCI demonstrate how co-designed tools can offer practical support that equitably addresses the unique challenges of people with Long COVID.

20.6 ACKNOWLEDGEMENTS

The authors gratefully acknowledge the contributions of Eric O, Chatpakorn Prasertsung, and Jane Willcox in the development of the CCI to date.

REFERENCES

1 United Nations (UN). Convention on the Rights of Persons with Disabilities (CRPD) [Internet]. Adopted 13 December 2006, entered into force 3 May 2008. New York: UN; [cited 2025 Feb 7]. Available from: https://www.un.org/development/desa/disabilities/convention-on-the-rights-of-persons-with-disabilities.html.

2 Wu R, et al. Effect of self-determination theory on knowledge, treatment adherence, and self-management of patients with maintenance hemodialysis. Contrast Media Mol Imaging. 2022;1416404. doi:10.1155/2022/1416404.

3 Knox L, et al. Using self-determination theory to predict self-management and HRQoL in moderate-to-severe COPD. Health Psychol Behav Med. 2021;9:527–46. doi:10.1080/21642850.2021.1938073.

4 Shackleford JL, et al. Applying the self-determination theory to health-related quality of life for adolescents with congenital heart disease. J Pediatr Nurs. 2019;46:62–71. doi:10.1016/j.pedn.2019.02.037

5 Simonsen SM, et al. About me as a person not only the disease - piloting Guided Self-Determination in an outpatient endometriosis setting. Scand J Caring Sci. 2020 Dec;34(4):1017–27. doi:10.1111/scs.12810.

6 Shogren KA, et al. Theoretical underpinnings and approaches to self-determination. In: Self-Determination and Causal Agency Theory. Wehmeyer ML, Shogren KL, Little TD, Lopez SJ, editors. Dordrecht: Springer; 2017. p. 13–25.

7 Vicente E, et al. Self-determination in people with intellectual disability: The mediating role of opportunities. Int J Environ Res Public Health. 2020;17(17):6201. doi:10.3390/ijerph17176201.

8 Jayakarani R, et al. Defining empowerment: Perspectives from international development organisations. Dev Pract. 2012;22(2):202–15. doi:10.1080/09614524.2012.640987.

9 Alghamdi MS, et al. Empowerment in the healthcare context: Concept analysis. Saudi J Nurs Health Care. 2022;5(9):176–81. doi:10.36348/sjnhc.2022.v05i09.001.

10 Shogren KA, et al. : Causal agency theory: Autonomy-supportive environments and interventions. In: Self-Determination and Causal Agency Theory. Wehmeyer ML, Shogren KL, Little TD, Lopez SJ, editors. Dordrecht: Springer; 2017. p. 53–67.

11 Halvorsen K, et al. Empowerment in healthcare: A thematic synthesis and critical discussion of concept analyses of empowerment. Patient Educ Couns. 2020;103(7):1263–71. doi:10.1016/j.pec.2020.02.017.

12 Mullard JCR, et al. Towards evidence-based and inclusive models of peer support for Long COVID: A hermeneutic systematic review. Soc Sci Med. 2023;320:115669. doi:10.1016/j.socscimed.2023.115669.

13 Lawn S, et al. Supporting self-management of chronic health conditions: Common approaches. Patient Educ Couns. 2010;80(2):205–11. doi:10.1016/j.pec.2009.10.006.

14 Wainwright TW, et al. Beyond acute care: Why collaborative self-management should be an essential part of rehabilitation pathways for COVID-19 patients. J Rehabil Med. 2020;52(5):jrm00055. doi:10.2340/16501977-2685.

15 Russell D, et al. Support amid uncertainty: Long COVID illness experiences and the role of online communities. SSM Qual Res Health. 2022;2:100177. doi:10.1016/j.ssmqr.2022.100177.

16 Wiederhold BK. The path forward: Self-management strategies for Long COVID. Cyberpsychol Behav Soc Netw. 2023;27(2):97–99. doi:10.1089/cyber.2023.29305.editorial.

17 Ojha S, et al. A quantitative evaluation of knowledge, perception, awareness, and preparedness of "Long COVID" among healthcare professionals and students in India. J Radiol Nurs. 2023;43(1):83–88. doi:10.1016/j.jradnu.2023.10.005.

18 Cruickshank M, et al. What is the impact of long-term COVID-19 on workers in healthcare settings? A rapid systematic review of current evidence. PLOS ONE. 2024;19(3):e0299743. doi:10.1371/journal.pone.0299743.

19 Thomas J, et al. A qualitative study of the general practice experience of diagnosing and managing Long COVID: Challenges and practical recommendations. Aust J Gen Pract. 2024;53(10):732–76. doi:10.31128/AJGP-10-23-6983.

20 Gustavson AM, et al. A learning health system approach to Long COVID care. Fed Pract. 2022 Jul;39(7):310–14. doi:10.12788/fp.0288.

21 Hoffmann TC, et al. Shared decision making: What do clinicians need to know and why should they bother? Med J Aust. 2014;201(1):35–39. doi:10.5694/mja14.00002.

22 Bingaman L. The art of shared decision making. JAAPA. 2023 Feb 1;36(2):31–34. doi:10.1097/01.JAA.0000902888.46676.73.

23 Said CM, et al. Co-designing resources for rehabilitation via telehealth for people with moderate to severe disability post stroke. Physiotherapy. 2024:109–17. doi:10.1016/j.physio.2024.02.006.

24 Wieringa TH, et al. Decision aids that facilitate elements of shared decision making in chronic illnesses: A systematic review. Syst Rev. 2019 May 20;8(1):121. doi:10.1186/s13643-019-1034-4.

25 Barry MJ, et al. What can we learn from rapidly developed patient decision aids produced during the COVID-19 pandemic? BMJ. 2022;378:e071530. doi:10.1136/bmj-2022-071530.

26 Hausberger A, et al. Long COVID diary: A user centered approach for the design of a mobile application supporting Long COVID patients. Int Conf Health Inform. 2022;5:769–76. doi:10.5220/0010972300003123

27 Khondakar KR, et al. Role of wearable sensing technology to manage Long COVID. Biosensors. 2022;13(1):62. doi:10.3390/bios13010062.

28 O'Mahoney L, et al. The prevalence and long-term health effects of Long Covid among hospitalised and non-hospitalised populations: A systematic review and meta-analysis. EClinicalMedicine. 2022;55:101762. doi:10.1016/j.eclinm.2022.101762

29 Navas-Otero A, et al. A lifestyle adjustments program in Long COVID-19 improves symptomatic severity and quality of life. A randomised control trial. Patient Educ Couns. 2024;122:108180. doi:10.1016/j.pec.2024.108180.

30 Storz MA. Lifestyle adjustments in Long-COVID management: Potential benefits of plant-based diets. Curr Nutr Rep. 2021 Dec;10(4):352–63. doi:10.1007/s13668-021-00369-x.

31 Leggat F, et al. An exploration of the experiences and self-generated strategies used when navigating everyday life with Long COVID. BMC Public Health. 2024; 24(1):789. doi:10.1186/s12889-024-18267-6.

32 Khosla S, et al. Sleep assessment in Long COVID clinics: A necessary tool for effective management. Neurol Clin Pract. 2023;13(1):e200079. doi:10.1212/CPJ.0000000000200079.

33 Chinvararak C, et al. Prevalence of sleep disturbances in patients with Long COVID assessed by standardised questionnaires and diagnostic criteria: A systematic review and meta-analysis. J Psychosom Res. 2023;175:111535. doi:10.1016/j.jpsychores.2023.111535.

34 Faux S. Long COVID: Expert advice, from diagnosis to treatment and recovery. Sydney: Murdoch Books; 2024.

35 Flinders Human Behaviour & Health Research Unit. The flinders chronic condition management program information paper. Adelaide (AU): Flinders University; 2017. [cited 2025 Feb 7]. Available from: https://www.flindersprogram.com.au/wp-content/uploads/Flinders-Program-Information-Paper.pdf.

36 Mak WW, et al. Brief Wellness Recovery Action Planning (WRAP®) as a mental health self-management tool for community adults in Hong Kong: A randomised controlled trial. J Ment Health. 2022;33:236–43. doi:10.1080/09638237.2022.2069723.

37 Alghtanie YA, et al. Family members involvement in patient care: Are they invited? World Fam Med J. 2022;20(12):144–49. doi:10.5742/MEWFM.2022.95251484.

38 Kiresuk TJ, et al. Goal attainment scaling: A general method for evaluating comprehensive community mental health programs. Community Ment Health J. 1968;4(6):443–53. doi:10.1007/BF01530764.

Chapter 21

Health Economics and the Broader Healthcare System for Long COVID

Mary Rose Angeles, Karen Dickinson, Danielle Hitch, and Martin Hensher

---

BOX 21.1   LEARNING OBJECTIVES

By the end of this chapter, readers should be able to:

- Examine how Long COVID affects quality of life and participation in employment.
- Describe the impact of Long COVID on the economy as a whole (macroeconomics).
- Analyse how economic evidence informs funding and policy decisions.
- Reflect on the economic impact of this condition on individuals with Long COVID.

21.1 INTRODUCTION

The emergence of Long COVID as a chronic condition following acute COVID-19 infection has significant economic consequences. At a personal level, people with Long COVID report substantial impacts on work, posing risks to their economic wellbeing. On a larger scale, these individual impacts affect national and global economies through reduced labour force participation and productivity. Healthcare needs of those with Long COVID also create new financial and resource burdens for healthcare systems and patients, influencing health financing and resource allocation.

This chapter explores Long COVID through the lens of health economics, which examines the use of money and resources in healthcare. It summarises current

DOI: 10.4324/9781003528104-26

evidence, identifies key areas for further study, and encourages readers to reflect on its relevance to their practice. Key topics include the effects of Long COVID on health-related quality of life (QoL), work and employment, macroeconomic implications, healthcare utilisation, treatment costs, access to services, and economic evaluations. Lived experiences are also highlighted to emphasise the impacts on people with Long COVID.

21.2 IMPACT OF LONG COVID ON QOL

Evidence shows Long COVID significantly affects wellbeing, daily activities, and work capacity.[1–10] Most studies, primarily observational, assess Long COVID cases or COVID-19 patients followed for six months to two years post-infection.[1–8] The EQ-5D is the most used QoL measure, with the Work and Social Adjustment Scale (WSAS) and adapted Work Ability Index (WAI) questions also applied.

21.2.1 EQ-5D

The EQ-5D measures QoL by describing and valuing health, widely used globally in health and health economics research for decades.[11] User guides and health economic weights are freely available for EQ-5D-3L, EQ-5D-5L, and EQ-5D-Y (youth). It has five questions on mobility, self-care, usual activities, pain/discomfort, and anxiety/depression, with response options ranging from no problems (1) to extreme problems (5). Responses form a five-digit code describing the patient's health state (e.g., 21133 = slight mobility issues, moderate pain, and anxiety/depression). The measure ends with a visual analogue scale where patients rate their health from "worst imaginable" to "best imaginable." EQ-5D scores range from 0 (death-equivalent health) to 1 (perfect health).

Four UK studies involving over 3,500 Long COVID patients found their mean EQ-5D-5L scores (0.49–0.64) were worse than those with chronic conditions like diabetes mellitus, chronic obstructive pneumonia disease, heart failure, multiple sclerosis, end-stage renal disease, and similar to advanced cancers.[2–5] A Canadian study[7] (n = 1,135) found higher EQ-5D-5L scores but reported lower health-related QoL for people with Long COVID compared to those who never developed post-COVID-19 condition (PCC) or have recovered from PCC. Other European studies, despite smaller sample sizes, also reported comparable EQ-5D-5L scores.[6,8] Studies from the United Kingdom[9,10] reported a 10% EQ-5D-5L score drop two to seven months after COVID-19 infection, with Intensive Care Unit (ICU) survivors having the lowest scores.

21.2.2 Work and Social Adjustment Scale

The WSAS[12] is a brief, self-reported tool designed to measure the impact of a condition or problem on daily functioning. It assesses five domains: work, home management, social activities, private leisure activities, and close relationships. Respondents rate the degree of impairment in each area on a scale from 0 (not impaired) to 8 (severely impaired), resulting in a total score ranging from 0 to 40, with higher scores indicating greater functional impairment.

Two UK studies[2,5] including people with Long COVID involved in the Living with Covid Recovery intervention (digital health intervention) reported worse functional impairment, indicated by mean WSAS scores ranging from 19.1–20.6.[2,5] There were small functional improvements over time, but the authors noted that it was deemed unlikely to be clinically significant.[2]

21.2.3 Work Ability Index

WAI[13] assesses a person's capacity to work in relation to the demands of their job and their overall health. It evaluates factors such as current work ability compared to lifetime best, work demands, health conditions, and mental resources. Scores are calculated to provide an overall indication of work ability, and are categorised as poor (7–27), moderate (27–37), good (37–43), and excellent (44–49).

A study of 11,710 adults with COVID-19[1] utilised a single question from the WAI: "What percentage of your original work capacity (before your positive corona test) have you regained today?" Participants rated their recovery from 0% (no capacity regained) to 100% (fully recovered), with mean recovery rated as 89.5% at 6–12 months post-infection. This indicates an overall health loss of 11.5% and a working capacity loss of 10.7%.[1]

BOX 21.2   PRACTICE POINT

What health-related QoL measures, if any, do you use with patients? How is this information used in your practice? If none, review the EQ-5D and consider its role in your rehabilitation service.

21.3 IMPACT OF LONG COVID ON EMPLOYMENT

21.3.1 Changes in Employment Status, Occupation, or Work Hours

Employment disruption is frequently reported in studies of people with Long COVID,[2,4,10,14–28] as summarised in Figure 21.1.[1] Outcomes such as occupational changes and reduced hours vary significantly, likely reflecting local economic contexts. However, the evidence consistently highlights the negative impact Long

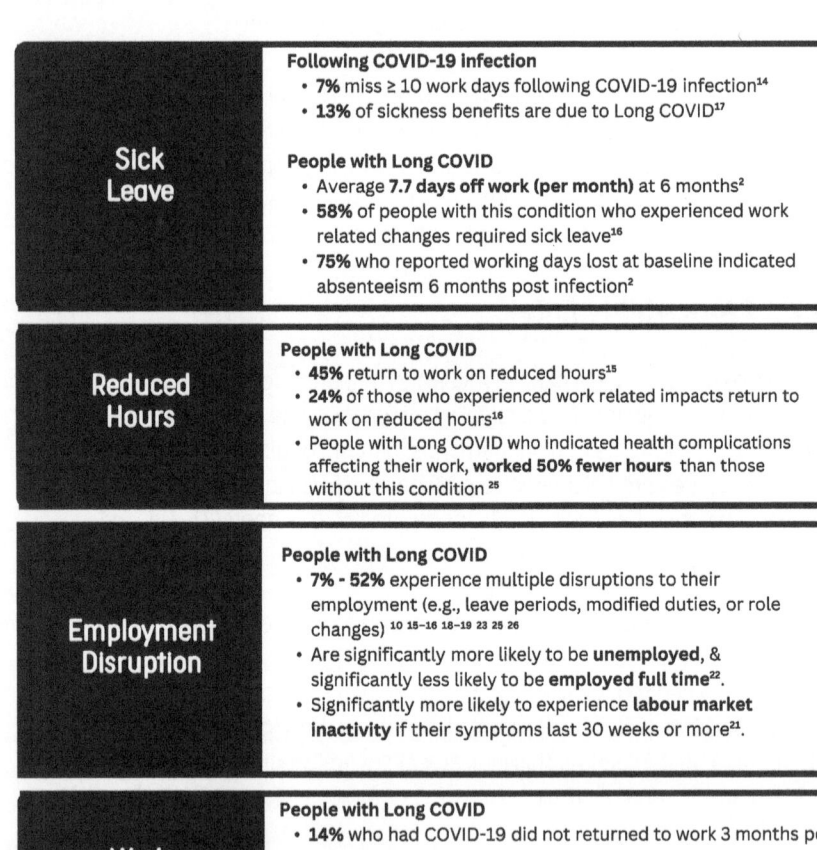

Sick Leave

Following COVID-19 infection
- **7%** miss ≥ 10 work days following COVID-19 infection[14]
- **13%** of sickness benefits are due to Long COVID[17]

People with Long COVID
- Average **7.7 days off work (per month)** at 6 months[2]
- **58%** of people with this condition who experienced work related changes required sick leave[16]
- **75%** who reported working days lost at baseline indicated absenteeism 6 months post infection[2]

Reduced Hours

People with Long COVID
- **45%** return to work on reduced hours[15]
- **24%** of those who experienced work related impacts return to work on reduced hours[16]
- People with Long COVID who indicated health complications affecting their work, **worked 50% fewer hours** than those without this condition [25]

Employment Disruption

People with Long COVID
- **7% - 52%** experience multiple disruptions to their employment (e.g., leave periods, modified duties, or role changes) [10 15–16 18–19 23 25 26]
- Are significantly more likely to be **unemployed**, & significantly less likely to be **employed full time**[22].
- Significantly more likely to experience **labour market inactivity** if their symptoms last 30 weeks or more[21].

Work Cessation

People with Long COVID
- **14%** who had COVID-19 did not returned to work 3 months post infection[14]
- **18%** not returned to work after 4.5 months and 12 months post infection[18 19]
- **2%-23%** did not return to work at follow-up period (3 up to 12 months)[14–16 19 23]

Figure 21.1 Summary of findings from international research on employment impacts from Long COVID.

COVID has on participation in productive activities. Notably, these disruptions incur substantial financial losses for around 40.5% of people with Long COVID.[16]

BOX 21.3   KAREN'S EXPERIENCE OF EMPLOYMENT DISRUPTION

Before developing Long COVID, Karen had a senior permanent position in the state public service. For a long time, she sought to return to work:

> I had an ongoing position in public service, and I had good access to paid leave. But I used that leave up very quickly. I had very empathetic workplace, and I was able to have…extended leave without pay. So, for a long time I held onto that job hoping I'd be well enough to return. I tried a staggered return to work a few times, but I failed because it was too much for me, both cognitively and physically. And recently, so only in the last couple of months, I actually resigned from work, taking my accrued leave as payout. I'd love to work again, but I'm not sure what my career looks like anymore. Long COVID has destroyed my career.
>
> Karen

BOX 21.4   PRACTICE POINT

Does your rehabilitation service offer employment or vocational interventions and assessments? These are usually delivered by occupational therapists; however, other disciplines may also contribute to work capacity assessments. What other services in your local community could Long COVID patients access for support in returning to work?

21.4 ECONOMIC IMPACT OF LONG COVID

Many studies[29–34] have estimated the economic impact of Long COVID across various countries from 2021 to 2024, typically indicating that it could represent losses of between 0.07% and 2.3%[29–34] of Gross Domestic Product (GDP). GDP refers to the total value of the goods and services produced by a country and provides a general indication of the size and state of its economy. As shown in Figure 21.2, Long COVID costs many nations around 0.5% of their GDP, although some report higher values. All values in the following discussion are shown in US$ 2024 value.

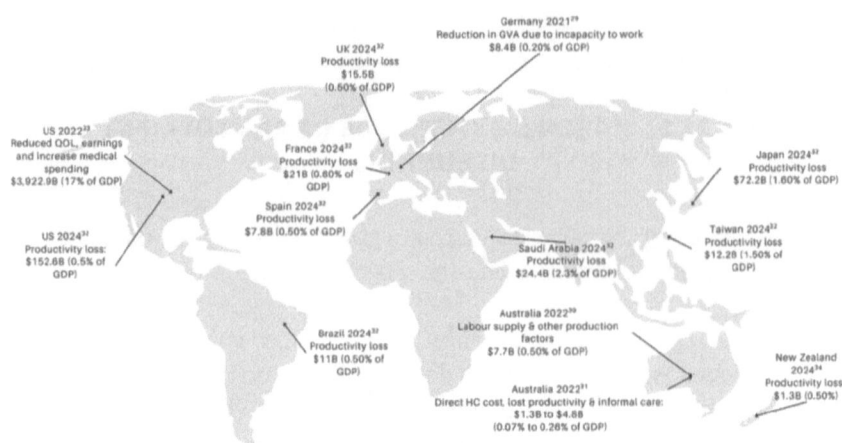

Figure 21.2 Gross Domestic Product (GDP) percentage and annual economic impact ($billion) by year[29–34].

Note: All values are shown in US$ 2024 value. UK = United Kingdom. US = United States of America

Differences in cost estimates arise from varying assumptions, methods, and cost ranges. A 17% cost of the 2019 U.S. GDP was estimated for 2022,[33,35] far higher than the 0.5% estimate for 2024.[32] The lower estimate only includes lost productivity,[32] while the higher accounts for reduced QoL, lower earnings, and higher medical costs.[33,35] Two modelling studies[30,31] estimated Long COVID costs for Australia between 0.07% and 0.26% of GDP. Some estimates are based on existing data, while others use modelling, which applies mathematical frameworks to predict outcomes under specific assumptions. Although comparisons are difficult, evidence consistently shows Long COVID imposes economic costs on the community.

Healthcare costs are critical for health professionals due to their impact on care funding. In the United States, healthcare needs contribute 14%–30% of total costs,[33,35,36] with reduced QoL projected to account for 59%.[33] An Australian study[37] estimated AUD$8.6 billion (US$6.1 billion) in annual costs from 2020 to early 2023 for COVID-19, while another study[31] estimated 2022 costs at AUD$1.7–$6.3 billion (US$1.3–$4.8 billion) based on Myalgic Encephalomyelitis/Chronic Fatigue Syndrome (ME/CFS) data. In the United Kingdom, healthcare costs reached £4.2–£9.3 billion (US$6.3–$13.9 billion), up to 2.7% of the 2022/23 health budget.[38] A German study reported US$0.5 billion in additional rehabilitation costs in 2021 alone.[29] These costs add more strain healthcare systems already struggling with resource constraints and funding pressures.[39]

BOX 21.5   KAREN'S EXPERIENCE OF INCOME LOSS

After using up her paid leave, Karen and her family relied solely on her husband's salary, which made them ineligible for social welfare. Fortunately, after a waiting period, Karen successfully claimed from her private income protection insurance.

> I didn't realise that income protection insurance only insures up to 75% of your salary. I'm so grateful we took out insurance when our kids were little, but I was still under-insured. I am getting a monthly payment from my insurance company, but it's probably at about 55, 60% of my normal income. So that gap we've had to just suck up. … I also didn't realise that payment doesn't cover super and you've got to pay tax out of it. [But] being insured has been a life saver for us.

Karen's extended leave without pay and reliance on income protection insurance has halted her superannuation contributions.

> Unpaid leave meant no superannuation contributions. I also can't afford to make voluntary contributions from my income protection insurance. So, my superannuation is appalling. Coupled with the impact of lower contributions when I took time off raising our kids, the continued impact on women is even greater… That's a real stress point for my future.

Karen highlighted financial impacts on her family, including higher costs from reduced bargain shopping and additional expenses for leisure activities, as she can no longer enjoy low-cost physical activities like cycling and walking.

> Long COVID has put huge limitations on our lives. Everything is so expensive and I have to consider the cost of our activities even more now. I don't have as much energy to search for the 'bargain' or pre-cook or prepare for activities. I'm more dependent on others to help me make things like holidays happen. Sometimes the easier activity is more expensive. I can't drive very far anymore. So, if I need to do things independently, then I need to Uber.

BOX 21.6   PRACTICE POINT

Consider how your practice could reduce costs for people with Long COVID while maintaining quality care. What interventions or information could your rehabilitation service provide to enhance financial wellbeing? Consider how the consequences of reduced GDP (like increased unemployment and reduced government revenue) impact on individuals with Long COVID, their families and the healthcare system.

21.5 HEALTHCARE UTILISATION

Long COVID patients have complex medical needs requiring ongoing treatment and diverse healthcare providers.[40] Studies[41–48] show increased use of primary care, telemedicine, urgent care, inpatient, and outpatient services among patients with Long COVID or those diagnosed with COVID-19 followed over six months. A review[46] of 41 studies found long-term higher healthcare use among Long COVID patients, with significantly increased resource use over ≥15 months. A COVID-19 diagnosis (not necessarily referring to Long COVID) was also linked to 4%–10% increased utilisation over six to eight months.

Studies from the United Kingdom[42,43] report that Long COVID patients have 49% higher healthcare utilisation,[42] twice the annual visits compared to controls,[42] and increased general physician[43] and outpatient care use.[43] Long COVID patients most often access primary and outpatient care. However, hospitalisation rates are also significantly higher, of which 53% were elective, and 42% were emergency care.[43] An Israeli study[48] found increased hospitalisation rates and a greater likelihood of requiring hospital care.

Three studies[44,45,47] reported increased healthcare utilisation within six months post COVID-19 diagnosis, with one estimating this incurred 212.9 additional medical visits per 1,000 patients during this period.[45] A US study[44] noted increased monthly healthcare visits post-COVID-19 diagnosis, with the largest increases observed in inpatient admissions, emergency care, and telemedicine. Acute care demands were particularly elevated for socially vulnerable neighbourhoods.[44] More blood, nervous, and mental health disorders, higher medication use, and medical costs, particularly among older and ICU-treated patients, but also among younger, non-hospitalised patients, have also been reported.[47]

Three studies[43–45] detail healthcare utilisation trajectories, showing usage peaking two to three months post-diagnosis, slightly declining but staying elevated.

A UK cohort study[43] found Long COVID patients' healthcare utilisation – including General Practitioner (GP) visits, outpatient care, hospital admissions, and ED attendances – peaked within two months and remained elevated for 2 years. A retrospective cohort study[44] reported visits spiking during the diagnosis month for non-hospitalised patients, before declining over five months but not returning to pre-diagnosis levels. Another study[45] found utilisation highest within three months and still elevated at four to six months.

21.6 HEALTHCARE COSTS

International research indicates an increase of approximately 40% in healthcare costs for Long COVID patients than controls, across primary care, hospitalisation, emergency visits, and outpatient services.[42,49] A UK study[42] estimated annual costs of £2,500 (US$4,158) per patient versus £1,500 (US$2,495) for controls. Other studies[46,50] found monthly costs were 7.6–13.1% higher over ≥15 months but then converged as symptoms resolved. However, people with a history of COVID-19 diagnoses (but not necessarily Long COVID) also recorded a 1.3- to 2.9-fold total healthcare cost increase over six months.[46] In the United Kingdom, additional primary care costs for Long COVID were estimated as £2.44 (US$4.06) per patient, totalling £23.4 million (US$38.9 million) nationally.[49] Most of these costs (60%) came from GP telephone consultations, with higher costs linked to older age, female gender, obesity, comorbidities, and frequent prior consultations.[49]

A US study[51] also reported increased medical costs for both children and adults with Long COVID over one to six months, particularly for hospitalised patients. A population-based cohort study[50] found 89% of Long COVID-related costs stemmed from hospital bills, with hospitalisation days being the largest expense. Similarly, an Israeli cohort study[48] reported healthcare costs for Long COVID patients rose from $2,435 (US$2,763) pre-infection to $2,810 (US$3,188) post-infection, compared to a 7.5% increase for those without Long COVID. Costs also remained elevated for an extended period relative to pre-diagnosis expenditures.[44] An Australian cost analysis[52] reported higher adjusted hospital admission costs for Long COVID patients per episode, while costs associated with COVID-19 patients were 1.5–1.8 times higher than controls over one to six months in the United States.[51]

21.7 CHALLENGES TO ACCESSING HEALTHCARE

Along with high healthcare utilisation, people with Long COVID face considerable financial challenges[53] and other barriers to care.[41,54] A UK analysis[53] linked Long COVID to worse financial wellbeing and higher benefit claims. A US survey[41] (n=18,117; 3.7% Long COVID) found these patients more likely to defer care, reduce prescriptions due to costs, and delay treatment due to transport issues. An internet survey[54] also showed people with Long COVID faced higher unmet healthcare needs than others, citing costs, provider availability, delays, transport, telehealth access, and insurance authorisation. Around a quarter of respondents to this survey reported having medical debt, compared to 16% without.[54]

BOX 21.7   DEFINITIONS

Incremental Cost Effectiveness Ratios (ICER): A metric comparing the value of two healthcare treatments by assessing their costs and resulting health outcomes. Lower ICERs indicate greater value for money and are compared to a predetermined "willingness to pay" threshold to assess cost-effectiveness.

Quality Adjusted Life Years (QALY): A metric evaluating interventions' impact on patients' QoL by comparing life expectancy (quantity) and health status (quality). It quantifies how interventions improve both life quality and quantity.

21.8 LONG COVID CARE COST ANALYSIS

Research on Long COVID costs and care models remains limited, with only three recent economic evaluation studies available.[55–57] One of these studies[55] investigated post-hospitalisation care pathways in the United Kingdom, including assessment, rehabilitation, and mental health support. The study reported that the intervention resulted to a higher QALYs (0.789 compared to 0.725 for minimal services) and concluded that the intervention is cost-effective with an ICER of £1,700 (US$2450) (95% UC: dominated to £24,800 (US$35,735)), which is well below the accepted WTP threshold (£20,000–£30,000).

Another UK study[56] compared an online home-based rehabilitation programme to usual care for 585 people with Long COVID, finding it incurred lower health and social care costs (but higher costs if intervention cost is included) over 12 months and had an 84% chance of being cost-effective. Finally, a Brazilian trial[57] added inspiratory muscle training to pulmonary rehabilitation for COVID-19 patients within three months of hospitalisation, thereby providing early intervention to potentially prevent Long COVID. Despite higher costs, the intervention was more effective than treatment as usual and 51.2% of outcomes were deemed cost-effective.

BOX 21.8 KAREN'S EXPERIENCE OF HEALTH CARE COSTS AND BURDEN

Karen has accessed various healthcare services and medications while living with Long COVID. These include public hospital Long COVID and Respiratory clinics (free), conventional and integrative GPs, specialist consultations partially covered by Medicare Benefits Schedule (MBS), medications partly subsidised by the Pharmaceutical Benefits Schedule (PBS), and additional psychological and medical support for her children due to family stresses from her condition. Most involve significant out-of-pocket gap payments.

There have been times when our out-of-pocket is in the thousands of dollars a month ...it's a huge amount of money.

Karen's family's healthcare spending exceeded the MBS Safety Net thresholds, triggering higher subsidies to alleviate these financial impacts.

I feel so grateful to be in Australia with universal access to healthcare and also the PBS for medication. It's amazing. If we didn't have that, I'd be ******.

Many of Karen's medications (including off-label uses) and supplements are not PBS subsidised, forcing tough choices between those clearly helping her:

There are times where I've weighed up: do I keep going with this medication given it costs hundreds of dollars a month, or do I stop? I know I'm fortunate that I can just afford it, but to make a wellbeing-based decision based on the cost of a medicine – that's not okay.

Karen and her family have private health insurance, which she has occasionally used to cover some costs:

We've got private health insurance, but it's basically useless. We get some rebate when we've reached the threshold of our mental healthcare plans, and we use the physio and massage extras. I've got the intellectual acumen to ask for things, and I'm patient enough to make claims for private prescription costs, but they've all been rejected. Having private health insurance has been basically pointless. We spent close to $6000 a year for family cover and it has not really helped economically at all for my long COVID.

A recurring theme for Karen was the administrative burdens of managing and accessing financial support, whether for the MBS / PBS Safety Net or insurance claims:

> The administrative burden of managing Long COVID is massive. Not only do I have to do more medical appointments and manage medications, but it is harder cognitively for me to get through the administration/paperwork of it all. For example, I'm pretty sure my family has hit our PBS threshold. My regular chemist said we were nearly at the threshold to get cheap prescriptions, but I go to different chemists and there's nowhere that holds all our records. At the end of the year, I really don't have the capacity to do the paperwork in addition to 'normal life'. The admin burden of the paperwork is too much for me, so I haven't bothered.

Karen recognises that her family was financially better prepared for the impact of her Long COVID than many, yet she reflects:

> You know Long Covid doesn't discriminate, and I was very well placed to manage it well. But it still had devastating impacts on us.

21.9 CONCLUSION

This chapter reviews the economic impacts of Long COVID, highlighting several key findings. People with Long COVID report significantly reduced health-related QoL, often comparable to or worse than that of other chronic conditions. Some are unable to return to work months after infection, while others reduce work hours or adjust roles. International research estimates Long COVID's economic costs at less than 1% of GDP – smaller than the most common chronic conditions (e.g., diabetes, asthma), but similar to significant conditions such as ME/CFS or multiple sclerosis. Reduced workforce participation is a primary driver of these costs, alongside increased healthcare expenditure. People with Long COVID utilise healthcare services more frequently and incur higher costs early in their illness trajectory, which declines over time. Many also face unmet healthcare needs and delayed care due to financial constraints.

Key gaps in our understanding remain. Most research focuses on people infected early in the pandemic, with limited data on later infections. Follow-up periods are often under a year, hindering understanding of long-term outcomes. There is also a limited cost-effectiveness evaluations due to insufficient evidence for effective treatments. However, rehabilitation health professionals can support people with Long COVID and their families with the severe financial hardships they experience, to ensure they don't have to bear the brunt of the illness's economic burden.

NOTE

1   Long COVID in this context refers to individuals who either self-report or with Long COVID identified by the study, as well as those who have had COVID-19 and continue to experience prolonged or persistent symptoms lasting beyond four weeks post-infection.

REFERENCES

1   Peter RS, et al. Post-acute sequelae of covid-19 six to 12 months after infection: Population based study. BMJ 2022;379:e071050. doi:10.1136/bmj-2022-071050.

2   Wang J, et al. Trajectories of functional limitations, health-related quality of life and societal costs in individuals with Long COVID: A population-based longitudinal cohort study. BMJ Open 2024;14:e088538. 20241113. doi:10.1136/bmjopen-2024-088538.

3   Carlile O, et al. Impact of Long COVID on health-related quality-of-life: An OpenSAFELY population cohort study using patient-reported outcome measures (OpenPROMPT). Lancet Reg Health Eur 2024;40. doi:10.1016/j.lanepe.2024.100908.

4   Sivan M, et al. National evaluation of outcomes in Long COVID services using digital PROM data from the ELAROS platform', LOng COvid Multidisciplinary consortium Optimising Treatments and services acrOss the NHS (LOCOMOTION) [Internet]. Leeds: LOCOMOTION; [cited 2025 Feb 7]. Available from: https://locomotion.leeds.ac.uk/news/national-evaluation-of-long-covid-services-outcomes/.

5   Walker S, et al. Impact of fatigue as the primary determinant of functional limitations among patients with post-COVID-19 syndrome: A cross-sectional observational study. BMJ Open 2023;13:e069217. doi:10.1136/bmjopen-2022-069217.

6   Moens M, et al. Health-related quality of life in persons post-COVID-19 infection in comparison to normative controls and chronic pain patients. Front Public Health 2022;10:991572. 20221020. doi:10.3389/fpubh.2022.991572.

7   Naik H, et al. Long-term health-related quality of life in working-age COVID-19 survivors: A cross-sectional study. Am J Med 2024. doi:https://doi.org/10.1016/j.amjmed.2024.05.016.

8   Vaes AW, et al. Recovery from COVID-19: A sprint or marathon? 6-month follow-up data from online Long COVID-19 support group members. ERJ Open Res 2021;7:20210524. doi:10.1183/23120541.00141-2021.

9   Sigfrid L, et al. Long COVID in adults discharged from UK hospitals after Covid-19: A prospective, multicentre cohort study using the ISARIC WHO Clinical Characterisation Protocol. Lancet Reg Health Eur 2021;8:100186. doi:10.1016/j.lanepe.2021.100186.

10   Evans RA, et al. Physical, cognitive, and mental health impacts of COVID-19 after hospitalisation (PHOSP-COVID): A UK multicentre, prospective cohort study. Lancet Respir Med 2022; 9(11):1271287. doi:10.1016/S2213-2600(21)00383-0.

11 Janssen MF, et al. Is EQ-5D-5L better than EQ-5D-3L? A head-to-head comparison of descriptive systems and value sets from seven countries. Pharmacoeconomics 2018;36:675–97. doi:10.1007/s40273-018-0623-8.

12 Mundt JC, et al. The work and social adjustment scale: A simple measure of impairment in functioning. Br J Psychiatry 2002;180:461–64. doi: 10.1192/bjp.180.5.461.

13 Ilmarinen J. The Work Ability Index (WAI). Occupat Med 2007;57:160. doi:10.1093/occmed/kqm008.

14 Venkatesh AK, et al. The association between prolonged SARS-CoV-2 symptoms and work outcomes. PLOS ONE 2024;19:e0300947. doi:10.1371/journal.pone.0300947.

15 Davis HE, et al. Characterizing Long COVID in an international cohort: 7 months of symptoms and their impact. eClinicalMedicine 2021;38:101019. doi:10.1016/j.eclinm.2021.101019.

16 Leitner M, et al. Characteristics and burden of acute COVID-19 and Long-COVID: Demographic, physical, mental health, and economic perspectives. PLOS ONE 2024;19:e0297207. doi:10.1371/journal.pone.0297207.

17 Westerlind E, et al. Patterns and predictors of sick leave after Covid-19 and Long Covid in a national Swedish cohort. BMC Public Health 2021;21:1023. doi:10.1186/s12889-021-11013-2.

18 The New York State Insurance Fund (NYSIF). Shining a light on Long COVID: An analysis of workers' compensation data [Internet]. New York: NYSIF; 2023. [cited 2025 Feb 7]. Available from: https://www.claimsjournal.com/app/uploads/2023/02/NYSIFLongCOVID-Study2023-1.pdf

19 Yelin D, et al. Patterns of Long COVID symptoms: A multi-center cross sectional study. J Clin Med 2022;11:20220209. doi:10.3390/jcm11040898.

20 Ayoubkhani D, et al. Self-reported Long COVID and labour market outcomes, UK, 2022 [Internet]. London: Office of National Statistics; 2022 [cited 2025 Feb 7]. Available from: https://www.ons.gov.uk/peoplepopulationandcommunity/healthandsocialcare/conditionsanddiseases/bulletins/selfreportedlongcovidandlabourmarketoutcomesuk2022/selfreportedlongcovidandlabourmarketoutcomesuk2022.

21 Ayoubkhani D, et al. Employment outcomes of people with Long COVID symptoms: Community-based cohort study. Eur J Public Health 2024;34:489–96. doi:10.1093/eurpub/ckae034.

22 Perlis RH, et al. Association of post–COVID-19 condition symptoms and employment status. JAMA Network Open 2023;6:e2256152. doi:10.1001/jamanetworkopen.2022.56152.

23 Kerksieck P, et al. Post COVID-19 condition, work ability and occupational changes in a population-based cohort. Lancet Reg Health Eur 2023;31:100671. doi:https://doi.org/10.1016/j.lanepe.2023.100671.

24 Dryden M, et al. Post-COVID-19 condition 3 months after hospitalisation with SARS-CoV-2 in South Africa: A prospective cohort study. Lancet Glob Health 2022;10:e1247–56. doi:10.1016/S2214-109X(22)00286-8.

25 Dasom I. Ham. Long-Haulers and Labor Market Outcomes. Institute working paper. No. 60, https://www.minneapolisfed.org/research/institute-working-papers/long-haulers-and-labor-market-outcomes

26 Kwon J, et al. Impact of Long COVID on productivity and informal caregiving. Eur J Health Econ 2024;25(7):1095–115. doi:10.1007/s10198-023-01653-z.

27 Buonsenso D, et al. Post-acute COVID-19 sequelae in a working population at one year follow-up: A wide range of impacts from an Italian sample. Int J Environ Res Public Health 2022;19(17):11093. doi:10.3390/ijerph191711093.

28 Mazer B et al. Functional limitations in individuals with Long COVID. Arch Phys Med Rehabil 2023;104:1378–84. doi:10.1016/j.apmr.2023.03.004.

29 Gandjour A. Long COVID: Costs for the German economy and health care and pension system. BMC Health Services Research 2023;23:641. doi:10.1186/s12913-023-09601-6.

30 Costantino V, et al. The public health and economic burden of Long COVID in Australia, 2022–24: A modelling study. Med J Aust 2024;221:217–23. doi:10.5694/mja2.52400.

31 Angeles MR, et al. The economic burden of Long COVID in Australia: More noise than signal? Med J Aust 2024;221(Suppl 9):s31–s39. doi:10.5694/mja2.52468.

32 Economist Impact. An incomplete picture: Understanding the burden of Long COVID [Internet]. London: The Economist Group; 2022 [cited 2025 Feb 7]. Available from: https://impact.economist.com/perspectives/sites/default/files/download/ei264_-_an_incomplete_picture_understanding_the_burden_of_long_covid_v8.pdf.

33 Cutler D. The economic cost of Long COVID: An update [Internet]. Cambridge, MA: Harvard Kennedy School; 2023 [cited 2025 Feb 7]. Available from: https://www.hks.harvard.edu/centers/mrcbg/programs/growthpolicy/economic-cost-long-covid-update-david-cutler.

34 Public Health Communication Centre (PHCC). Long COVID: High economic burden justifies further preventive efforts [Internet]. Wellington: PHCC; 2023 [cited 2025 Feb 7]. Available from:https://www.phcc.org.nz/briefing/long-covid-high-economic-burden-justifies-further-preventive-efforts.

35 Cutler DM. The costs of Long COVID. JAMA Health Forum 2022;3:e221809. doi:10.1001/jamahealthforum.2022.1809.

36 Mirin AA. A preliminary estimate of the economic impact of Long COVID in the United States. Fatigue: Biomedicine, Health & Behavior 2022;10:190–99. doi:10.1080/21641846.2022.2124064.

37 Merck Sharp & Dohme (MSD). A neglected burden: The ongoing economic costs of COVID-19 in Australia [Internet]. [Place unknown]: MSD; 2023 Aug [cited 2025 Feb 7]. Available from: https://www.covid19economicimpact.com/wp-content/uploads/sites/305/2023/08/White-Paper-AU-A-Neglected-Burden-The-Ongoing-Economic-Costs-of-COVID-19-in-Australia.pdf.

38 Cambridge Econometrics. The economic burden of Long COVID in the UK [Internet]. Cambridge: Cambridge Econometrics; 2024 Mar [cited 2025 Feb 7]. Available from: https://www.camecon.com/wp-content/uploads/2024/03/The-Economic-Burden-of-Long-Covid-in-the-UK_Cambridge-Econometrics_V1.1_March2024.pdf.

39 Paschoalotto MAC, et al. Health systems resilience: Is it time to revisit resilience after COVID-19? Soc Sci Med 2023;320:115716. doi:10.1016/j.socscimed.2023.115716.

40 Al-Aly Z, et al. Long COVID science, research and policy. Nat Med 2024;30(8):2148–64. doi:10.1038/s41591-024-03173-6.

41 Ford ND, et al. Health insurance and access to care in U.S. Working-age adults experiencing Long COVID. Am J Prev Med 2024;67(4):530–39. doi:10.1016/j.amepre.2024.05.007.

42 Lin L-Y, et al. Healthcare utilisation in people with Long COVID: An OpenSAFELY cohort study. BMC Medicine 2024;22:255. doi:10.1186/s12916-024-03477-x.

43 Mu Y, et al. Healthcare utilisation of 282,080 individuals with Long COVID over two years: A multiple matched control cohort analysis. J R Soc Med 2024;117(11):369–81. doi:10.2139/ssrn.4598962

44 Koumpias AM, et al. Long-haul COVID: Healthcare utilization and medical expenditures 6 months post-diagnosis. BMC Health Services Research 2022;22:1010. doi:10.1186/s12913-022-08387-3.

45 Tartof SY, et al. Health care utilization in the 6 months following SARS-CoV-2 infection. JAMA Network Open 2022;5:e2225657. doi:10.1001/jamanetworkopen.2022.25657.

46 Łukomska E, et al. Healthcare resource utilization (HCRU) and direct medical costs associated with long COVID or post-COVID conditions: Findings from a literature review [Preprint]. Preprints.org; 2024 Sep 2 [cited 2025 Feb 7]. Available from: https://www.preprints.org/manuscript/202409.0133/v1.

47 Scott A, et al. Substantial health and economic burden of COVID-19 during the year after acute illness among US adults at high risk of severe COVID-19. BMC Medicine 2024;22:46. doi:10.1186/s12916-023-03234-6.

48 Tene L, et al. Risk factors, health outcomes, healthcare services utilization, and direct medical costs of patients with Long COVID. Int J Infect Dis 2023;128:3–10. doi:10.1016/j.ijid.2022.12.002.

49 Tufts J, et al. The cost of primary care consultations associated with Long COVID in non-hospitalised adults: A retrospective cohort study using UK primary care data. BMC Prim Care 2023;24:245. doi:10.1186/s12875-023-02196-1.

50 Wolff Sagy Y, et al. Estimating the economic burden of Long-COVID: The additive cost of healthcare utilisation among COVID-19 recoverees in Israel. BMJ Glob Health 2023;8(7): e012588. doi:10.1136/bmjgh-2023-012588.

51 Pike J, et al. Direct medical costs associated with post-COVID-19 conditions among privately insured children and adults. Prev Chronic Dis 2023;20:e06. doi:10.5888/pcd20.220292.

52 Hitch D, et al. Hospital costs of COVID-19, post-COVID-19 condition and other viral pneumonias: A cost comparison analysis. Med J Aust 2024;221(Suppl 9): s23–s30. doi:10.5694/mja2.52465.

53 Rhead R, et al. Long COVID and financial outcomes: Evidence from four longitudinal population surveys. J Epiemiol Community Health 2024;78:458–65. doi:10.1136/jech-2023-221059.

54 Karpman M, et al. Health care access and affordability among US adults aged 18 to 64 years with self-reported post–COVID-19 condition. JAMA Network Open 2023;6:e237455. doi:10.1001/jamanetworkopen.2023.7455.

55 Nwankwo H, et al. Cost-effectiveness of an online supervised group physical and mental health rehabilitation programme for adults with post-COVID-19 condition after hospitalisation for COVID-19: The REGAIN RCT. BMC Health Services Research 2024;24:1326. doi:10.1186/s12913-024-11679-5.

56 Briggs AH, et al. Clinical and cost-effectiveness of diverse post-hospitalisation pathways for COVID-19: A UK evaluation utilising the PHOSP-COVID cohort. medRxiv 2024: 2024.2007.2015.24310151. doi:10.1101/2024.07.15.24310151.

57 Modesto GP, et al. Cost–utility analysis of supervised inspiratory muscle training added to post-COVID rehabilitation program in the public health system of Brazil. Int J Environ Res Public Health 2024;21:1434. doi:10.3390/ijerph21111434

SECTION SIX
KEY TOPICS IN LONG COVID REHABILITATION AND MANAGEMENT

Chapter 22

Intensive Care Unit Survivorship

Victoria Lai, Karlie Flannigan, and Gerard Flannigan

BOX 22.1   LEARNING OBJECTIVES

By the end of this chapter, readers should be able to:

- Identify the domains of post-ICU syndrome.
- Understand the guidelines and management strategies to improve outcomes following ICU admission.
- Understand the impact an ICU admission has on patients and their families and other close others.
- Describe the implications and similarities of an ICU admission for those with COVID-19 or other conditions.

22.1 INTRODUCTION

The Intensive Care Unit (ICU) is a complex and dynamic environment. Over the past decade, ICU admissions have increased significantly worldwide. While this trend was apparent before the COVID-19 pandemic, it intensified due to the surge of critically ill patients. At the peak, there were over 40,000 patients admitted to ICUs worldwide in one day in January 2021 for COVID-19.[1] Several factors have contributed more broadly to an overall rise in admissions, including an aging population and advances in medical care and surgical techniques. These improvements have led to more frail, elderly patients and those with comorbidities being admitted to ICUs, where previously they may not have been eligible or would not have survived the illness. Despite improved survival rates, with millions of patients discharged from ICUs each year, both patients and their families often face long-term challenges in recovery, which can persist for weeks, months, or even years.[2] This prolonged recovery process not only significantly burdens healthcare systems but also impacts the quality of life and meaningful survival for the patients

DOI: 10.4324/9781003528104-28

themselves. This is also seen in hospital admissions following acute COVID-19 infection, with or without an ICU admission.

As more patients survived an ICU admission, it became evident to healthcare professionals that outcomes beyond the doors of the ICU needed to be considered further than they had before. Previously, physical, cognitive, and mental health impairments were considered independently of each other. In 2010, the term "Post-Intensive Care Syndrome (PICS)" was coined by an international consensus group led by the Society of Critical Care Medicine. Since then, further research has emerged in these domains of overall health following an ICU admission.[3] During the COVID-19 pandemic, ICUs faced overwhelming, prolonged, and complex admissions worldwide. ICU professionals must work to mitigate PICS and ensure post-ICU healthcare providers address potential ongoing limitations, including the added effects of Long COVID, which can mimic or compound PICS symptoms.

22.2 UNDERSTANDING POST-INTENSIVE CARE SYNDROME

PICS refers to long-term disabilities persisting beyond critical illness in adults and children, categorised as new or worsening impairments in physical, cognitive, and mental functions compared to preadmission.[2] PICS also affects families, leading to psychological impacts such as stress, anxiety, and grief, termed PICS-Family (PICS-F).[4] Clinical presentations vary, resembling long COVID or COVID-19, with diverse symptoms across domains. PICS ultimately impacts quality of life, work, and daily activities. Although evidence is limited, the complexity and severity of COVID-19 cases suggest a similar recovery trajectory.

This understanding of PICS and PICS-F underscores the need for holistic approaches to ICU care, extending support not only to survivors but also to their families to address the wide-reaching impacts of critical illness. The effects of critical care admissions should also be considered for healthcare workers who have experienced illness themselves. One family member explained:

> As a health professional who has worked in many intensive care environments, I was surprised at how underprepared I was to see my loved one, my dad, critically unwell. I felt helpless and was desperate for the team to know how special he was, willing every conversation to include something positive for us to hold onto. To me, end-of-life support is the forgotten hero of critical care services.
>
> Anonymous

A healthcare professional shared how treating critical care patients while living with Long COVID affected them. They described being physically present at work but mentally detached, overwhelmed by compassion fatigue, guilt, and frustration with underperforming at work. They also feared that patients viewed discharge as recovery, while worse challenges might lie ahead.

As with many acquired conditions, there are risk factors that contribute towards the prevalence of PICs, some of which are modifiable during the ICU stay, which will be discussed in the management section of this chapter, and some of which are non-modifiable at the time of ICU admission (i.e., pre-existing conditions, female sex). Some risk factors span all domains due to the nature of care required in the ICU, such as mechanical ventilation, sedative medication, and pre-existing cognitive or mental health conditions.[5] Patients admitted to ICU with acute COVID-19 were often in acute respiratory failure, requiring significant respiratory support, such as mechanical ventilation or extracorporeal membrane oxygenation. Utilising prone positioning became a mainstay of treatment to improve oxygenation, which, due to the respiratory failure as well as the tolerance for this position, patients were often heavily sedated and paralysed.[6]

Cognitive impairment has been reported as prevalent as between 25% and 75% of patients following an ICU admission.[4] The commonly reported risk factors for this include delirium, previous cognitive impairments (i.e., older age, known cognitive deficit), hypoxia, or acquired brain injury. The risk factors associated with psychiatric or mental health changes are similar, with the highest risk factor being a history of psychiatric or mental health concerns.[5] While delirium is common in an ICU, it should be considered a risk factor for prolonged impairments in the psychological domain.

Psychological impairments can be challenging to identify, and as such, reporting ranges significantly between 1% and 62% of patients.[4] Anxiety is often reported, with one person describing it as "anxiety that pervaded every waking moment and tried to overwhelm her, particularly at night when the only distraction was the loud and constant beeping noises or the hiss of the ventilator." Anonymous

The physical domain of PICs is the easiest to identify for obvious reasons and is the most reported by patients, families and in research. The most discussed impairments relate to ICU-acquired weakness (ICUAW), in which patients have symmetrical and widespread weakness, including the limbs, trunk and respiratory muscles. ICUAW does not always follow a pattern and can be attributed to critical illness polyneuropathy, critical illness myopathy, or a combination of both.[7]

Diagnosis can be confirmed using electrophysiology, nerve conduction studies or muscle strength testing with the Medical Research Council (MRC) Sum Score. The MRC measures global muscle strength by calculating the summation of bilateral muscle strength testing in shoulder abduction, elbow flexion, wrist extension, hip flexion, knee extension, and ankle dorsiflexion. A score of <48 indicates significant weakness, and a score of <36 indicates severe weakness. This outcome measure has proven reliable and valid in assessing global muscle strength.[8] Risk factors for developing ICUAW commonly include prolonged mechanical ventilation, sepsis, multi-organ failure, sedative medication, neuromuscular blocking agents, steroid use, and immobility are frequently identified as the predominant risk factors.[7,9,10] Muscle wasting was found to occur quickly within the first week of a critical illness, worse in those with multi-organ failure.[11] ICUAW commonly require prolonged periods of rehabilitation and do not always return to their previous level of function. This impacts their ability to return to work, reduces their quality of life, and results in higher rates of complications, which can, in turn, result in high healthcare needs.

Environmental factors such as a prolonged ICU stay contribute towards PICS, some of which are mentioned above, such as the correlation between a prolonged stay and time on mechanical ventilation, ICU-associated infections (whether those were acquired during care or the reason for the admission), and the use of sedation. Effective management requires a multidisciplinary approach with regular assessments to identify and address concerns early, focusing on preventing and treating PICS.

22.3 MANAGEMENT AND INTERVENTIONS

Experts in ICU care developed the ICU-PAD to develop evidence-based guidelines on managing pain, agitation, and sedation/delirium in adult ICU patients (ICU PAD).[12] In 2013, these clinical practice guidelines were updated by the American College of Critical Care Medicine in collaboration with other groups with relevant expertise to develop the ABCDEF Bundle (see Table 22.1), which is an evidence-based guideline designed using aspects of the ICU PAD to coordinate multidisciplinary care to improve outcomes in critically ill patients.[13,14]

22.3.1 Assess and Manage Pain

Patients in ICU often experience pain, whether that be caused by the trauma or illness that resulted in their admission, surgery, or secondary issues such as infection, positioning, etc. Pain is a contributing factor to reduced mobility, and

Table 22.1 ABCDEF Bundle[10]

Guideline	Activity
A	Assess and manage pain
B	Both – spontaneous awakening trials and spontaneous breathing trials
C	Choice of analgesia and sedation
D	Delirium assessment, prevention, and management
E	Early mobility and exercise
F	Family engagement and empowerment

participation in activity increases delirium with prolonged medication use. The pain must be frequently assessed so it can be consistently managed, not only to alleviate suffering but to reduce the risk of developing PICS. Pain assessment can be challenging in patients who cannot rate their pain reliably on a visual analogue scale. Therefore, alternative assessments need to be carried out to identify the presence of pain. The Behavioural Pain Scale (BPS) and the Critical Pain Observational Tool (CPOT) are two commonly used tools validated within an ICU population who cannot communicate. The CPOT is more detailed than the BPS, but both consider facial expression, movement, and compliance with the mechanical ventilator as indicators of pain; scores of equal to/greater than 3 or 5, respectively, are deemed unacceptable and require a change in pain management.[13]

22.3.2 Both Spontaneous Awakening Trials and Spontaneous Breathing Trials

The combination of spontaneous awakening trials (SATs) and spontaneous breathing trials (SBTs) has been shown to reduce hospital and ICU length of stay, mechanical ventilation time, and one-year mortality rates. SATs are considered breaks in sedation, with the aim of having the least amount of sedation needed for the least amount of time. SBTs assess whether patients can be extubated from mechanical ventilation. Trials are conducted by reducing the ventilator support to the minimum amount required to overcome the challenge of breathing through a tube. Trials lasting between 30 and 120 minutes, monitoring agitation, respiratory, and cardiovascular measures.[15,16]

22.3.3 **Choice of Analgesia and Sedation**

The ABCDEF bundle prioritises adequate pain assessment and control before the use of sedative medications to reduce the need for sedation beyond what is necessary. Validated and reliable tools are recommended to be used for accurate assessment of sedation and agitation. The Richmond Agitation Sedation Scale (RASS) is an easy-to-use scale assessed at the bedside, with an ideal score between –2 and 0. The Riker Sedation Agitation Scale is an alternative, with an ideal score of 3–4.

22.3.4 **Delirium Assessment, Prevention, and Management**

Delirium is a significant ICU challenge, increasing the risk of PICS and complicating patient care, mobilisation, and psychological wellbeing. It may present as hyperactive, hypoactive, or mixed. Factors contributing to delirium include sedatives, hypoxaemia, sepsis, pain, immobility, and disrupted sleep patterns.[12] Associated with worse morbidity and mortality outcomes, frequent assessments are essential for ICU admission. The Confusion Assessment Method for the ICU (CAM-ICU)[17] is widely used and structured as a flow chart that assesses acute mental status changes, inattention, RASS score, and disorganised thinking.

Patients' lived experiences of ICU delirium are often disorienting and traumatic. Common descriptions include feeling abducted by aliens or perceiving medical procedures as assaults, with a sense of helplessness despite reassurance. These experiences contribute to lasting psychological impacts post-ICU.

22.3.5 **Early Mobility and Exercise**

Historically, patients in the ICU were kept in bed to provide rest, deep sedation, and stability. As the landscape of critical care has changed, as mentioned in the introduction to this chapter, so have the protocols and intensity of rehabilitation in the ICU.[18] The combined effects of the sequelae of bed rest and the complex nature of critical illness can result in profound weakness, lasting beyond the ICU or hospital stay.[11] Early activity, whether that includes mobilisation passive or active exercise, should start when the patient is able and stable to do so. Early mobilisation not only reduces morbidity and mortality[19] but has numerous other systemic and psychological benefits, positively impacting both short and long-term patient outcomes.[2] These benefits include reduced ICUAW by preserving muscle mass and strength[20] and improved functional outcomes,[21] reduced ICU and hospital length of stay,[22] fewer ventilator days,[23] and improved psychological wellbeing by reducing anxiety and delirium.[22] There is still work to be done in this space regarding defining "early mobilisation" and the exact dosage required.

There are barriers to mobilising patients in ICU across many units worldwide, such as medical instability, sedation, limited staff or resources within the unit, and the organisational culture in units that have not adopted mobilisation protocols or do not implement them frequently. This was apparent with patients in the ICU with COVID-19, where infection prevention and control measures, staffing resources, and patient stability limited early mobilisation. Implementing these protocols should be a multidisciplinary approach with clear protocols to determine when a patient is appropriate for mobilisation, the establishment of roles, and determinants of effectiveness and safety. In 2014, an "expert consensus and recommendations on safety criteria for active mobilisation of mechanically ventilated critically ill adults"[24] was published following a systematic review and a group discussion with multidisciplinary ICU experts. This study produced recommendations using a traffic light system (Green – low risk of an adverse event, Yellow – potential risk, Red – significant risk; with further information for each category) on respiratory, cardiovascular, neurological, and other (Surgical, i.e., fractures/ wounds; Medical, i.e., drains, active bleeding).

22.3.6 Family Engagement and Empowerment

Family engagement, added after the initial bundle development, is fundamental to a positive ICU experience and recovery.[13] ICU staff often interact meaningfully with families before engaging with patients who may be sedated or ventilated. Families advocate for patients, understand their wishes, and provide valuable insights, aiding communication and helping patients fill memory gaps from their ICU and rehabilitation journey. Davidson et al.[25] highlighted the importance of clear, consistent communication, and family involvement in improving outcomes. During the pandemic, these practices were challenged by restricted ICU access, with telehealth and video calls used where possible, though limited by staff availability and internet access issues.

BOX 22.2   KARLIE'S STORY

I was admitted to ICU in early 2020. There were no visitors, and staff contact was also limited. One nurse sat with me and the doctors often did telehealth consultations on an iPad. It wasn't normal then – Zoom and telehealth, it was all new. It felt like I was being "heard, but not seen." I also couldn't talk because of being so breathless. I couldn't always verbalise what was going on.

When they offered to Facetime with family – I thought – do I? Do I want them to see me like this? This might be their final memory of me. My family were confronted by what I looked like – grey, struggling to talk, tubes. On the positive side, I could see my family's faces – for the first time in over two weeks. We also used text messaging to stay connected because of my difficulty speaking.

22.3.7 Other Considerations

ICU follow-up clinics monitor and support patients with impairments post-ICU discharge. These clinics aim to identify symptoms early, provide tailored rehabilitation, and support patients and families through multidisciplinary teams. While the best follow-up method is unclear, many hospitals conduct phone screenings two to four weeks after discharge, followed by in-person appointments as needed.[26] Long COVID and PICS services benefit from offering varied follow-up options. Sleep disturbances are common and significant after ICU stays, linked to psychological trauma, delirium, anxiety, and disrupted ICU care routines that do not follow normal day-night cycles.[27]

BOX 22.3   KARLIE'S STORY

I worked in aged care – I knew first-hand the impacts of COVID-19, and I was infected early – before vaccinations when everyone was scared to go out. In the emergency department, I heard a person in the next cubical gasping for breath… this would be me soon.

On the ward I heard the Code called – I knew it was for me – it was my bed number. Normally, you expect doctors to come running to help– but with COVID staff had to go through infection control processes. You're left waiting. Even then staff stood metres away, fearful for themselves. A nurse held my hand. The first person to do this.

In ICU it was all bright lights and monitors. There was no sense of time. Only meals or a change of shift helped define what time of day it was. It's hard to know how long you've been there. I was aware of what is going on. I heard Codes for patients in the beds near me. I saw the curtains drawn. Then I'd see a trolley taken out later, and I knew….you look at your own monitors – how bad they are looking.

I understood social distancing, but you want someone to stop and look. The best thing was a nurse who asked "Would you like me to brush your hair?". Or when they held my hand. Things like that that make it more personal. Not so isolating. You have no control – I didn't get a choice in meals – just the same thing every day. I lost over 15 kilograms in ICU.

BOX 22.4   PRACTICE POINT

What impact might an ICU admission have on your patients? Reflect on how this could influence their presentation and rehabilitation.

22.4 CONCLUSION

This chapter highlights the long-term impacts of critical illness, sedation, and ICU admissions on function, health, quality of life, and healthcare costs. It remains unclear if ICU admissions for unrelated conditions in individuals with Long COVID results in higher PICS rates. Interventions should be tailored to the individual, considering Long COVID symptoms where applicable. The lived experiences of ICU survivors underscore the need for clear communication, even when patients seem unaware, family involvement, and creating a home-like environment. As one interviewee reflected, "I wondered if I would survive, before I even realised that I may never thrive again."

REFERENCES

1 Mathieu E, et al. Current COVID-19 patients in intensive care units (ICU) [Internet]. Oxford: Global Change Data Lab; [cited 2025 Feb 7]. Available from: https://ourworldindata.org/grapher/current-covid-patients-icu.

2 Needham DM, et al. Improving long-term outcomes after discharge from intensive care unit: Report from a stakeholders' conference. Crit Care Med. 2012;40(2):502–9. doi:10.1097/CCM.0b013e318232da75.

3 Hiser SL, et al. Post-Intensive Care Syndrome (PICS): Recent updates. J Intensive Care. 2023;11(1):23. doi:10.1186/s40560-023-00670-7.

4 Rawal G, et al. Post-intensive care syndrome: An overview. J Transl Int Med. 2017;5(2):90–92. doi:10.1515/jtim-2016-0016.

5 Rhodes A, et al. The psychiatric domain of post-intensive care syndrome: A review for the intensivist. J Intensive Care Med. 2024; Aug: 8850666241275582. doi:10.1177/08850666241275582.

6 Jackson A, et al. Prone positioning in mechanically ventilated COVID-19 patients: Timing of initiation and outcomes. J Clin Med. 2023;12(13):4226. doi:10.3390/jcm12134226.

7 Chen J, et al. Intensive care unit-acquired weakness: Recent insights. J Intensive Med. 2023;4(1):73–80. doi:10.1016/j.jointm.2023.07.002.

8 Turan Z, et al. Medical research council-sumscore: A tool for evaluating muscle weakness in patients with post-intensive care syndrome. Crit Care. 2020;24(1):562. doi:10.1186/s13054-020-03282-x.

9 Vanhorebeek I, et al. ICU-acquired weakness. Intensive Care Med. 2020;46(4):637–53. doi:10.1007/s00134-020-05944-4.

10 Deem S. Intensive-care-unit-acquired muscle weakness. Respir Care. 2006;51(9):1042–53. doi:10.1007/s00134-020-05944-4.

11 Puthucheary ZA, et al. Acute skeletal muscle wasting in critical illness [published correction appears in JAMA. 2014 Feb 12;311(6):625. Padhke, Rahul [corrected to Phadke, Rahul]]. JAMA. 2013;310(15):1591–1600. doi:10.1001/jama.2013.278481.

12 Barr J, et al. Clinical practice guidelines for the management of pain, agitation, and delirium in adult patients in the intensive care unit. Crit Care Med. 2013;41(1):263–306. doi:10.1097/CCM.0b013e3182783b72.

13 Marra A, et al. The ABCDEF bundle in critical care. Crit Care Clin. 2017;33(2):225–43. doi:10.1016/j.ccc.2016.12.005.

14 Leonard KM, et al. Preventing PICS with the ABCDEF Bundle. In: Haines KJ, McPeake J, Sevin CM, editors. Improving critical care survivorship: A guide to prevention, recovery, and reintegration. Cham: Springer International Publishing; 2021. p. 3–19.

15 Yang KL, et al. A prospective study of indexes predicting the outcome of trials of weaning from mechanical ventilation. N Engl J Med. 1991;324(21):1445–50. doi:10.1056/NEJM199105233242101.

16 Souza LC, et al. The rapid shallow breathing index as a predictor of successful mechanical ventilation weaning: Clinical utility when calculated from ventilator data. J Bras Pneumol. 2015;41(6):530–35. doi:10.1590/S1806-37132015000000077.

17 Devlin JW, et al. Clinical practice guidelines for the prevention and management of pain, agitation/sedation, delirium, immobility, and sleep disruption in adult patients in the ICU. Crit Care Med. 2018;46(9):e825–73. doi:10.1097/CCM.0000000000003299.

18 TEAM Study Investigators and the ANZICS Clinical Trials Group, et al. Early active mobilisation during mechanical ventilation in the ICU. N Engl J Med. 2022;387(19):1747–58. doi:10.1056/NEJMoa2209083.

19 Zomorodi M, et al. Developing a mobility protocol for early mobilisation of patients in a surgical/trauma ICU. Crit Care Res Pract. 2012;2012:964547. doi:10.1155/2012/964547.

20 Kayambu G, et al. Physical therapy for the critically ill in the ICU: A systematic review and meta-analysis. Crit Care Med. 2013;41(6):1543–54. doi:10.1097/CCM.0b013e31827ca637.

21 Needham DM, et al. Early physical medicine and rehabilitation for patients with acute respiratory failure: A quality improvement project. Arch Phys Med Rehabil. 2010;91(4):536–42. doi:10.1016/j.apmr.2010.01.002.

22 Schweickert WD, et al. Early physical and occupational therapy in mechanically ventilated, critically ill patients: A randomised controlled trial. Lancet. 2009;373(9678):1874–82. doi:10.1016/S0140-6736(09)60658-9.

23 Bailey P, et al. Early activity is feasible and safe in respiratory failure patients. Crit Care Med. 2007;35(1):139–45. doi:10.1097/01.CCM.0000251130.69568.87.

24 Hodgson CL, et al. Expert consensus and recommendations on safety criteria for active mobilisation of mechanically ventilated critically ill adults. Crit Care. 2014;18(6):658. doi:10.1186/s13054-014-0658-y.

25 Davidson JE, et al. Clinical practice guidelines for support of the family in the patient-centered intensive care unit: American College of Critical Care Medicine Task Force 2004–2005. Crit Care Med. 2007;35(2):605–22. doi:10.1097/01.CCM.0000254067.14607.EB.

26 Nakanishi N, et al. Post-intensive care syndrome follow-up system after hospital discharge: A narrative review. J Intensive Care. 2024;12(1):2. doi:10.1186/s40560-023-00716-w.

27 Altman MT, et al. Sleep disturbance after hospitalisation and critical illness: A systematic review. Ann Am Thorac Soc. 2017;14(9):1457–68. doi:10.1513/AnnalsATS.201702-148SR.

Chapter 23
Long COVID in Children and Young People

Michelle Scoullar, Henry Barker, and Emma Tippett

BOX 23.1   LEARNING OBJECTIVES

By the end of this chapter, readers should be able to:

- Understand the current definition of Long COVID in CYP.
- Describe the frequency of Long COVID in CYP, common symptoms and comorbidities.
- Identify initial management approaches for CYP with Long COVID.

23.1 INTRODUCTION

Long COVID can have debilitating effects on children and young people (CYP) that can lead to potentially lifelong implications depending on the severity of symptoms, functional impact, length of illness, and at what point in a child or adolescents' development Long COVID occurs.[1-4] In the absence of diagnostic biomarkers, the cornerstone of assessment and diagnosis centres around a detailed history to elicit symptoms and disentangle the timeline and potential causes. This is time-consuming and challenging, with unique considerations for children and adolescents.

Wide-ranging estimates of Long COVID in CYP have led to scepticism among some in the scientific and medical communities, exacerbating barriers to care and contributing to significant stigma for the patient and their guardians seeking care. This stigma further burdens affected CYP, impacting their self-esteem and mental health.[5] Long COVID affects more CYP than many clinicians realise, and even conservative estimates point to large numbers due to widespread transmission and low vaccination rates. Raising clinician and community awareness is essential for ensuring timely, person-centred, and age-appropriate care, including accurate diagnosis, initial management, and appropriate specialist referrals.

DOI: 10.4324/9781003528104-29

This chapter will focus on a practical approach to diagnosis and management of Long COVID in CYP, including both pharmaceutical and non-pharmaceutical management. Treatments will be discussed with a safety-focused, evidence-informed approach to including potentially effective treatments while ensuring risks are kept to a minimum.

BOX 23.2   DEFINITIONS OF LONG COVID FOR CHILDREN AND YOUNG PEOPLE

"Children and Young People" (CYP) in this chapter refers to people below 18 years.

"Young child(ren)" refers to under 12-year-olds or younger where specified.

"Adolescent(s)" or "young people" is used interchangeably for 12- to 17-year-olds.

WORLD HEALTH ORGANISATION PAEDIATRIC DEFINITION OF LONG COVID

The WHO definition of Long COVID will be used unless otherwise specified.

Post-COVID-19 condition in children and adolescents occurs in individuals with a history of confirmed or probable SARS-CoV-2 infection, when symptoms persist for at least 2 months and initially occurred within 3 months of acute COVID-19.[6]

Symptoms generally have an impact on everyday functioning... may be new onset following initial recovery from an acute COVID-19 episode or persist from the initial illness. They may also fluctuate or relapse over time. Workup may reveal additional diagnoses, but this does not exclude the diagnosis of post-COVID-19 condition.

BOX 23.3   TAKE HOME MESSAGES

- Long COVID can occur in 10–30% of CYP, it can occur with any infection and can lead to debilitating symptoms.
- Between 1% and 3% of all CYP may have Long COVID (around 6 million in the United States).[2]
- Much is now known about the biomedical basis of Long COVID.
- Timely diagnosis and treatment of Long COVID in CYP is critical to minimise impact on important developmental activities and maximise recovery.

23.2 KEY CONCEPTS IN LONG COVID, PATHOPHYSIOLOGY AND EPIDEMIOLOGY IN CYP

23.2.1 Mechanisms Driving Long COVID

Several mechanisms have been proposed for Long COVID (See Chapter 2) and include immune and inflammatory dysregulation, autoimmunity, endothelial and mitochondrial dysfunction, microbiota dysbiosis, abnormal neurological signalling, persistence of SARS-CoV-2, and reactivation of latent viruses.[7–11] These hypotheses are not mutually exclusive, and it may be that specific phenotypes of Long COVID are more or less likely to have a particular mechanism driving those symptoms.

23.2.2 Prevalence, Risk Factors, and Recovery of Long COVID in Children

Several important factors need to be kept in mind when examining studies of Long COVID in CYP including: the definition of Long COVID used, the method by which responses were collected, and whether reported data refers to incidence following acute infection, the prevalence of Long COVID at a single time-point, or the cumulative incidence of having ever had Long COVID. Importantly, almost all studies to date used online questionnaires and not clinician assessments. This is a particularly important consideration for CYP and could over- or under-estimate the presence of Long COVID.

Variations in definitions, diagnostic methods, and data collection approaches have resulted in diverse prevalence estimates for Long COVID in CYP (ranging from 4% to 65%), complicating meta-analysis in systematic reviews. More reliable estimates converge around 10–30% prevalence at two to three months post-infection, 10–20% at 6 months,[2,3,4,5,12] and 7–8% at two years post-infection.[13,14] Risk factors include age (12 years and older), multiple acute symptoms, hospital presentation or admission, comorbidities (e.g., allergy, asthma), and gender. Studies on very young children are limited, but persistent symptoms may occur in 5–10% of those under five.[15] While self-reported incident risk and symptoms appear to vary by gender, these differences appear more apparent in adolescents rather than in children. Protective factors like vaccination can roughly halve the risk of developing Long COVID, although this protection varies by age (younger children requiring 3 doses versus 1 or 2 in adolescents) and may wane over time.[13,16,17]

BOX 23.4   HENRY'S LONG COVID STORY

I spent a year confined to my bed, and further year and a half in the house, not because I was anti-social, but because I have Long COVID. I am currently 16, as of 1 month ago, and I often try not to reflect on the past couple of years, partly because there isn't much to reflect on besides pain. It started off with the worst possible headache and then falling like a drunk along the hallway, not able to walk properly. I can remember describing to my mum that I couldn't go to school because I felt like a giant had stepped on me. This was an understatement. I lost the ability to do the things I once loved, and instead, all I wanted to do was sleep, because in them I could run.

Now, two and a half years later I still can't run without regretting it. A week prior to writing this, I decided to jump off a [local] wharf …. I then did one of the stupider things of my life and decided to swim to shore, a distance of about 100 meters. I'm still feeling the effects now - crushing fatigue, headaches, muscle pain. What they call PEM [Post-Exertional Malaise]. For me, PEM is pretty much a constant in my life. I also have really red legs and feet from poor blood circulation. This is part of a condition called POTS that I have been diagnosed with.

School was really hard. I would try to go but never make it through a day. Sitting and listening, engaging in discussions and loud noise was impossible. The school tried but really didn't understand what I was going through. …

While I have seen massive improvement over the past seven or eight months – physically, mentally, and socially – I still can't ride my bike without losing the ability to walk and promptly vomiting…. As a 16-year-old boy who has spent the past couple of years in their bedroom … missed out on the supposed golden years of my life, I try not to think about it.

It is hard keeping friends because who can understand this condition. And I can't keep a conversation going without wanting to lay down. Pacing is really hard. It was really awful at the start telling doctors what was going on as I didn't know whether they believed me or not. … It was a huge relief to find doctors [and an exercise physiologist] who believed and listened to me…. They have treated me like a person who wants to understand as best as possible Long COVID…

…I couldn't have gotten to where I am now without the countless doctors I've seen and the people I'm surrounded by. Faith has helped me, and I am grateful for that. Luckily – or maybe unluckily – I've gotten to share this experience with my mum, who also suffers from this condition. We both wouldn't survive without sarcasm and laughing, … at our situation.

…if you, or maybe your child or relative, has Long COVID, know that you need to appreciate the good parts, however few or many there are.

BOX 23.5   PRACTICE POINT

Consider Henry's experiences of Long COVID and the health care system. How does his age and available support impact his experience of Long COVID symptoms? Consider a child or young person you may have seen with fatigue, what protective or risk factors existed in their school and support structures?

23.3 ASSESSMENT

23.3.1 History and Symptoms: The Importance of a Child-Centred, Developmentally Informed History

Establishing whether Long COVID is the underlying cause of symptoms hinges on understanding the timeline. It is critical to consider the timing of the COVID-19 infection, how it was diagnosed, and other significant illnesses or life events. Recalling whether symptoms appeared before or after COVID-19 infection may be easier when anchored to memorable events like birthdays, school terms, or holidays, helping clarify the timeline.

Long COVID studies in CYP have often been adapted from adult symptom sets potentially biasing our understanding of this condition in children. Children, especially younger children, often communicate through behaviours rather than necessarily articulating how they feel in words or using terminology that is reflective of the symptoms described in the literature. For example, a younger child may be observed by their guardians to only play with siblings or friends for shorter times than previously. They may respond "no" to a question about light-headedness or dizziness and instead explain this by saying that they "feel sick." Similarly, children more commonly complain of abdominal pain,[14] and this same term may be used to refer to any of nausea, bloating, pain, breathlessness, chest pain, palpitations, or exhaustion and fatigue. A detailed history, informed from several perspectives can help support and inform the interpretation of these changes.

Common Long COVID symptoms in CYP include fatigue, sleep disturbance, dizziness, headache, gastrointestinal symptoms, muscle and joint pain, and brain fog[2,4,5] with age-related symptom clustering.[18] However, a comprehensive understanding of the functional impact of symptoms is more valuable than simply listing them. It's also essential to assess what a CYP can do without worsening their symptoms. This includes exploring their capacity for activities such as walking, time spent outside the home, participation in family or social activities, engagement in school or work, and tolerance of sensory input, which can be undertaken through a symptom diary. Questionnaires and measurement tools can be useful but should not be overly relied upon, as many are not validated for CYP with Long COVID and may not account for cultural or linguistic differences. Discussing activities that precede prolonged rest helps identify post-exertional malaise (PEM), which can manifest 24–72 hours after exertion as increased fatigue or other symptoms (see Chapter 11).

23.3.2 Examination, Investigations, and Differential Diagnoses

Currently, no specific examination findings or biomarkers confirm the diagnosis of Long COVID. History and investigations remain important to identify treatable conditions or symptoms and ensure other diagnoses are not missed. Table 23.1 outlines potential comorbidities, differentials, and assessment components.

Few conditions could explain the wide variety of symptoms a CYP with suspected Long COVID experience, especially if they also have PEM. Without PEM, possible unifying causes of symptoms such as fatigue, low energy and brain fog include hypothyroid disease, specific nutritional deficiencies, primary sleep disorders and in some circumstances those with Attention Deficit Hyperactive Disorder (ADHD), anxiety or depression. Key areas to continually consider include dysautonomia, most notably POTS, nutritional deficiencies (e.g., ferritin, zinc, vitamin D, B12), and B6 toxicity.

23.4 A FOCUS ON CARDIAC DYSAUTONOMIA: POTS

23.4.1 Assessment

Orthostatic intolerance (OI) affects around 70% of children with Long COVID and includes postural orthostatic tachycardia syndrome (POTS), orthostatic tachycardia, and related conditions.[19,20] Symptoms can be non-specific and are not limited to light-headedness and improvement of symptoms when reclining, often leading to delayed diagnoses or being attributed to anxiety.[21] OI and POTS significantly impact the quality of life and are modifiable with medical management.

Table 23.1 Key Comorbidities and Differential Diagnoses

Symptom	Potential Comorbidities or Differential Diagnoses	Key Components of History, Examination, or Investigations
Fatigue **Post-Exertional Malaise**	Anaemia Nutrient deficiencies (iron, B12, folate) Sleep disorders (e.g., obstructive sleep apnoea, narcolepsy)	• Detailed sleep history, including screen for obstructive sleep apnoea (OSA) and allergic rhinitis • Supplements or medications that could be contributing to fatigue • Activity diary to identify energy patterns and triggers of malaise.[a]
Dizziness **Orthostatic intolerance**	Postural Orthostatic Tachycardia Syndrome (POTS) Sinus tachycardia syndrome Postural hypotension Vertigo Migraine Seizure disorders Other cardiac arrythmias	• Active stand test • Ambulatory blood pressure monitoring • Electrocardiogram • Halter monitor • Echocardiogram • Postural blood pressure • Electroencephalogram • Specialist review
Chest pain **Palpitations**	Pericarditis/Myocarditis Other cardiac causes (e.g., arrythmias, structural heart abnormalities) Costochondritis	• Cardiac magnetic resonance imaging • Troponin • Electrocardiogram • Echocardiogram • Clinical examination and pain elicitation
Shortness of breath **Cough** **Dyspnoea**	Asthma Persistent bacterial bronchitis Bronchiectasis POTS	• Timing of cough and triggers • Respiratory function test • +/− specialist for consideration of Cardiopulmonary Exercise Testing

Brain fog **Difficulties concentrating**	Attention deficit hyperactivity disorder Autism spectrum disorder Specific Learning difficulties Sleep disorders	• History usually adequate to distinguish causes
Headache[b]	Specific headache diagnoses Migraine Relative dehydration secondary to POTS	• Vision check • Consider need to refer to neurologist • Assess for POTS
Insomnia **Poor sleep quality**	Obesity Snoring Apnoea Poor sleep hygiene Primary sleep disorder Excess stimulants (e.g., caffeine)	• History of waking feeling unrefreshed or difficulty falling back to sleep • Paediatric sleep Questionnaire (PSQ) • Obstructive Sleep Apnoea (OSA-11) questionnaire
Gastrointestinal symptoms (nausea, abdominal pain, bloating, diarrhoea, constipation)	Coeliac disease Infective causes Inflammatory bowel disease Food intolerances Gastritis/Reflux disease/Gastrointestinal ulcer Gastroparesis/delayed gastric emptying Medications	• Coeliac screen +/– HLA genotype • Stool: Microbiological Stool Analysis, Faecal Multiplex PCR test, *Helicobacter pylori*, calprotectin • Symptom and food diary to identify dietary triggers with elimination trial • Gastric emptying study • Consider need for referral to gastroenterologist and/or dietitian
Rashes **Allergies** **Sinusitis** **Dermatographia**	Hay fever Chronic sinusitis Mast cell activation syndrome	• Allergen testing • Consider need for referral to immunologist
Recurrent infections	Primary immunodeficiency Primary ciliary dyskinesia	• Cell subsets • Immunoglobulin levels

[a] Triggers may be social, emotional, sensory, cognitive, or physical.

[b] Ensure headache has no red flags for malignancy.

BOX 23.5 COMMON INVESTIGATIONS FOR CYP WITH LONG COVID

This list is not exhaustive, and additional investigations may be needed

- Active stand test
- Electrocardiogram (ECG)
- Blood tests:

  - Baseline: Full Blood Examination (FBE); Urea, Electrolytes and Creatinine (UEC); Liver Function Tests (LFT); C-reactive protein (CRP); Erythrocyte Sedimentation Rate (ESR); nutritional assays (ferritin, folate, B12, B6, zinc, vitamin D); morning cortisol; glucose and HBA1C; thyroid studies; coeliac screen; fibrinogen
  - Consider where relevant: Epstein-Barr Virus (EBV); Cytomegalovirus (CMV) serology; D-dimer; immune phenotyping; Creatine Kinase (CK); metanephrines.

- Stool: Microbiological Stool Analysis, Faecal Multiplex PCR test, *Helicobacter pylori*, calprotectin
- Not often needed but may be helpful: chest x-ray; respiratory function testing; echocardiogram; 24-hour ECG; magnetic resonance imaging brain.

POTS is characterised by symptoms of OI for 3 months, together with a sustained excessive increase in heart rate on standing in the absence of postural hypotension (see Chapter 16).[22,23] Diagnostic criteria are not outlined for young children and heart rate criteria are debated for adolescents.[22] False negatives are common and repeat testing at different times is recommended. A tilt table test may aid diagnosis in complex cases, but the active stand test is simpler, validated and suitable for primary care.[21] Our experience is that a portion of CYP (and adults) will have signs and symptoms of POTS such as acrocyanosis and demonstrate functional improvement with management without reaching POTS criteria; therefore, the decision to manage POTS should take a holistic stance and not rely exclusively on heart rate criteria.

23.4.2 Management

The initial therapeutic approach frequently encompasses non-pharmacological strategies, which include substantially augmenting fluid and sodium in addition to dietary intake,[22] ensuring sufficient sleep quantity and quality, using compression garments as tolerated and raising the head of the bed (see Chapter 16).[22,23]

For many CYP with Long COVID and POTS, these modifications can provide significant benefits. However, pharmacological therapies are often necessary to further enhance functional capacity and can be pivotal in enabling participation in desired activities, such as attending school (see Table 23.2).[24,25]

23.4.3 Exercise, POTS, and Long COVID

Once pharmacological and non-pharmacological management of POTS has been optimised, consider if exercise aimed at enhancing muscle tone and cardiovascular efficiency, within the limits of the CYPs fatigue and PEM, is safe to initiate (see Chapter 11). This is best done under the guidance of an experienced clinician (e.g., exercise physiologist, physiotherapist). Any notion of "pushing through" should be avoided as could trigger a substantial and sustained increase in symptoms.[26,27] Instead, a cautious approach that is mindful of fluctuations in capacity and symptoms is critical.

23.5 A PRACTICAL APPROACH TO MANAGEMENT

All children should receive holistic care focused on improving quality of life and functional capacity, aiming for complete recovery. Priority symptoms identified by the child, family, or caregivers must be addressed early and systematically. While a multidisciplinary approach is ideal, practical challenges like financial or energy constraints may limit access to allied health services. In such cases, prioritising experts in PEM-informed care and utilising telehealth can reduce physical, social, and cognitive burdens, making care more sustainable for families.

A structured yet flexible management approach is essential, tailored to each child's unique presentation and priorities. This includes strategies for frequently reported symptoms and, where appropriate, evidence-based pharmaceutical options, as outlined in Table 23.2. This adaptable framework ensures care evolves alongside emerging evidence and individual needs, empowering children and their families to navigate recovery more effectively.

BOX 23.6   AN APPROACH TO INITIAL OR EARLY APPOINTMENTS

Assessment:

- Establish likelihood of Long COVID diagnosis.
- Understand current strengths, activity capacity, and engagement in school/study/work.

- Define current support network, including engagement in allied health, mental wellbeing supports and complementary medicine practitioners.
- Identify any other known conditions present and whether these are optimised or need specific additional attention (e.g., Asthma, ADHD, anxiety, depression).
- Review of systems and establish priority symptoms.
- Explore symptom fluctuations, impact of fatigue, presence or absence of PEM (or "crash"), cognitive difficulties (brain fog), temperature tolerance, cutaneous symptoms, and impact of posture on symptoms.
- Review investigations to date.
- Review medications and supplements.
- Consider hypermobility and need for Beighton scoring.

Management:

- Initiate symptom management where needed for fatigue, orthostatic intolerance, sleep, headaches, gastrointestinal disturbances, mast cell activation syndrome, or allergies.
- Determine if any further investigations are needed.

Education:

- Discuss PEM and management by pacing, POTS investigation (or diagnosis), self-management and triggers to avoid.
- Assist in determining appropriate time commitment to schooling/work/ extracurricular activities.
- Discuss COVID risk mitigation and action plan for reinfection.

23.6 PHARMACEUTICAL MANAGEMENT OPTIONS

Very few studies have been done in CYP to inform specific Long COVID pharmaceutical options. This is a critical area for more research, both for medications that may provide symptom relief, and those that may address the underlying driver or mechanism for long COVID. Table 23.2 outlines pharmaceuticals that can be considered for symptom management in Long COVID and POTS.

Table 23.2 Pharmacological and Non-Pharmacological Symptom Management Suitable for Paediatric Patients. Please Refer to Appropriate Paediatric Guidelines for Contra-indications, Interactions and Dosage.[22–25,28,29]

Symptom	Non-pharmacological	Pharmacological	Potential Additional Benefits
Established Therapies			
Pain	Warm/cold therapy	Paracetamol/ Non-Steroidal Anti-Inflammatory Drugs (NSAIDs) Gabapentin Tricyclic antidepressants	Sleep, mood
Sleep	Sleep hygiene	Melatonin Promethazine Cyproheptadine Clonidine Magnesium	Mood Headache Mast Cell Activation Syndrome (MCAS) and allergies
MCAS and Allergies	Trigger avoidance	Oral H1 antihistamine Famotidine (H2 antihistamine) Mast cell stabiliser (Montelukast, sodium cromoglycate or ketotifen) Antihistamine nasal spray and eye drops	Asthma Chronic sinusitis
Headache/ migraine	Craniocervical physiotherapy Avoid triggers and excessive sensory stimuli Pacing	Paracetamol/ NSAIDs Propranolol Cyproheptadine Triptan	POTS MCAS Sleep Nausea

Gastrointestinal symptoms	Low Fermentable Oligosaccharides, Disaccharides, Monosaccharides, and Polyols (FODMAP) diet Low histamine diet	Famotidine Probiotic (lactobacillus/ bifidobacterium)	MCAS Reflux, nausea Fatigue
Nausea	Small meals	Proton pump inhibitor Cyproheptadine Ondansetron Domperidone	Sleep
POTS and Orthostatic intolerance	Hyperhydration Salt loading (up to 3000 mg of sodium in electrolyte form) Compression Elevate bed head by 4–6 inches Small meals Avoid standing still and heat	Ivabradine Propranolol or other b-blockers Midodrine Fludrocortisone Pyridostigmine	Migraines Sleep
Emerging Therapies			
Fatigue and post-exertional malaise		Low dose naltrexone Guanfacine Modafinil	Fatigue Pain Brain fog
POTS		Intravenous immunoglobulin Intravenous saline infusion Stellate Ganglion Block	

Note: The evidence for these therapies is often extrapolated from research with adults.

23.7 CONCLUSION

Long COVID in CYP presents unique challenges, highlighting the need for a child-centred approach to diagnosis and management. The condition's wide-ranging symptoms and functional impacts demand tailored strategies that address medical and developmental needs. CYP deserve high-quality care, including appropriate prescribing to maximise their participation in daily life. Their voices must be central to the diagnostic process, ensuring their experiences are validated and their needs comprehensively addressed.

Preventing Long COVID is as critical as managing it. Reducing COVID-19 transmission through improved air quality measures, particularly in schools, and ensuring access to vaccination are essential strategies. These measures not only minimise the risk of acute infection but also help prevent long-term complications that disrupt education, social development, and family life.

Persistent stigma and gaps in healthcare knowledge continue to create barriers for CYP, reinforcing the urgency for education, advocacy, and inclusive care. By prioritising equitable, evidence-informed, and compassionate practices, we can empower CYP to recover, thrive, and regain a sense of normalcy. Addressing both prevention and management ensures a brighter future for affected children and their families, with opportunities for better health and full participation in life.

REFERENCES

1   Rao S, et al. Postacute sequelae of SARS-CoV-2 in children. Pediatrics. 2024;153:e2023062570. doi:10.1542/peds.2023-062570.

2   Toepfner N, et al. Long COVID in pediatrics—epidemiology, diagnosis, and management. Eur J Pediatr. 2024;183(4):1543–53. doi:10.1007/s00431-023-05360-y.

3   Ha EK, et al. Long COVID in children and adolescents: Prevalence, clinical manifestations, and management strategies. Clin Exp Pediatr. 2023;66:465–74. doi:10.3345/cep.2023.00472.

4   Jiang L, et al. A systematic review of persistent clinical features after SARS-CoV-2 in the pediatric population. Pediatrics. 2023;152:e2022060351. doi:10.1542/peds.2022-060351.

5   Buonsenso D, et al. Social stigma in children with Long COVID. Children. 2023;10(9):1518. doi:10.3390/children10091518.

6   World Health Organization (WHO). WHO clinical case definition update for post COVID-19 condition in children and adolescents [Internet]. Geneva: WHO; 2023 [cited 2025 Feb 7]. Available from: https://www.who.int/publications/i/item/WHO-2019-nCoV-Post-COVID-19-condition-CA-Clinical-case-definition-2023-1.

7   Peluso MJ, et al. Mechanisms of Long COVID and the path toward therapeutics. Cell. 2024;187:5500–29. doi:10.1016/j.cell.2024.07.054.

8 Davis HE, et al. Long COVID: Major findings, mechanisms and recommendations. Nat Rev Microbiol. 2023;21:133–46. doi:10.1038/s41579-022-00846-2.

9 Altmann DM, et al. The immunology of Long COVID. Nat Rev Immunol. 2023;23:618–34. doi:10.1038/s41577-023-00904-7.

10 Scoullar MJ, et al. Towards a cure for Long COVID: The strengthening case for persistently replicating SARS-CoV-2 as a driver of post-acute sequelae of COVID-19. Med J Aust. 2024;221:587–90. doi:10.5694/mja2.52517.

11 Proal AD, et al. SARS-CoV-2 reservoir in post-acute sequelae of COVID-19 (PASC). Nat Immunol. 2023;24:1616–27. doi:10.1038/s41590-023-01601-2.

12 Rothensteiner M, et al. Long COVID in children and adolescents: A critical review.Children. 11. Epub ahead of print 2024. doi:10.3390/children11080972.

13 Camporesi A, et al. Characteristics and predictors of Long Covid in children: A 3-year prospective cohort study. eClinicalMedicine. 76. Epub ahead of print 1 October 2024. doi:10.1016/j.eclinm.2024.102815.

14 Stephenson T, et al. A 24-month National Cohort Study examining long-term effects of COVID-19 in children and young people. Commun Med. 2024;4:255. doi:10.1038/s43856-024-00657-x.

15 Kikkenborg Berg S, et al. Long COVID symptoms in SARS-CoV-2-positive children aged 0–14 years and matched controls in Denmark (LongCOVIDKidsDK): A national, cross-sectional study. Lancet Child Adolesc Health. 2022;6:614–23. doi:10.1016/S2352-4642(22)00154-7.

16 Boufidou F, et al. SARS-CoV-2 reinfections and Long COVID in the post-omicron phase of the pandemic. Int J Mol Sci. 24. Epub ahead of print 2023. doi:10.3390/ijms241612962.

17 Razzaghi H, et al. Vaccine effectiveness against Long COVID in children. Pediatr. 153. Epub ahead of print 2024. doi:10.1542/peds.2023-064446.

18 Gross RS, et al. Characterizing Long COVID in children and adolescents. JAMA. Epub ahead of print 21 August 2024. doi:10.1001/jama.2024.12747.

19 Delogu AB, et al. Autonomic cardiac function in children and adolescents with Long COVID: A case-controlled study. Eur J Ped. 2024;183:5. doi:10.1007/s00431-024-05503-9.

20 Morrow AK, et al. Long-term COVID 19 sequelae in adolescents: The overlap with orthostatic intolerance and ME/CFS. Curr Pediatr Rep. 2022;10:31–44. doi:10.1007/s40124-022-00261-4.

21 Kavi L. Postural tachycardia syndrome and Long COVID: An update. Br J Gen Pract. 2022;72:8. doi:10.3399/bjgp22X718037.

22 Boris JR, et al. Pediatric postural orthostatic tachycardia syndrome: Where we stand. Pediatrics. 2022;150(1):e2021054945. doi:10.1542/peds.2021-054945.

23 Vernino S, et al. Postural Orthostatic Tachycardia Syndrome (POTS): State of the science and clinical care from a 2019 National Institutes of Health Expert Consensus Meeting - Part 1. Auton Neurosci 2021;235:102828. doi:10.1016/j.autneu.2021.102828.

24 Miller AJ, et al. Pharmacotherapy for postural tachycardia syndrome. Auton Neurosci 2018;215: 28–36. doi:10.1016/j.autneu.2018.04.008.

25 Spera FR, et al. Post-COVID postural orthostatic tachycardia syndrome and inappropriate sinus tachycardia in the pediatric population. Curr Clin Micro Rpt. 2024;11:115–25. doi:10.1007/s40588-024-00217-w.

26 Greenwood DC, et al. Physical, cognitive, and social triggers of symptom fluctuations in people living with Long COVID: An intensive longitudinal cohort study. Lancet Reg;46:101082. doi:10.1016/j.lanepe.2024.101082.

27 Appelman B, et al. Muscle abnormalities worsen after post-exertional malaise in Long COVID. Nat Commun 2024;15:17. doi:10.1038/s41467-023-44432-3.

28 Oskoui M, et al. Practice guideline update summary: Acute treatment of migraine in children and adolescents. Neurology 2019;93:487–99. doi:10.1212/WNL.0000000000008095.

29 Whitehouse WP, et al. Management of children and young people with headache. Arch Dis Child - Educ Amp Pract Ed 2017;102:58. doi:10.1136/archdischild-2016-311803.

Chapter 24

Long COVID in Culturally and Linguistically Diverse Communities

Danielle Hitch, Luna Amine, Kieva Richards, Angela Ma, and Farhana Dewan

---

BOX 24.1 LEARNING OBJECTIVES

By the end of this chapter, readers should be able to:

- Understand the challenges and barriers for people from CALD communities living with Long COVID.
- Apply cultural humility and privilege principles through reflective practice.
- Identify strategies for enhanced culturally sensitive rehabilitation.
- Develop strategies to improve communication and therapeutic relationships with people from CALD communities.

24.1 INTRODUCTION

Culture is a fundamental yet often underestimated social determinant of health that influences information processing, health perceptions, practices, and healthcare delivery.[1,2] It encompasses the knowledge, values, behaviours, and customs a society or group shares.[3] Health professionals must understand social and cultural factors affecting health and wellbeing to provide high-quality, effective, and tailored care.[4] Culturally responsive rehabilitation is, therefore, a professional and ethical priority.

People from Culturally and Linguistically Diverse (CALD) communities experience worse health outcomes from COVID-19 than those from the dominant culture, including higher infection rates, excess deaths, and lower vaccination levels.[5]

DOI: 10.4324/9781003528104-30

However, their Long COVID experiences remain largely unexplored.[6] This chapter introduces key concepts for culturally sensitive rehabilitation for Long COVID, explores facilitators and barriers, and proposes service- and system-level recommendations. It draws on narrative interviews with Australian CALD women with Long COVID, international evidence, and the authors' lived experience.

BOX 24.2   PRACTICE POINT

Reflecting on your cultural identity is key to engaging with cultural diversity. Use these prompts to write a brief statement about yourself:

- How would you describe your cultural background or ethnicity?
- Were you and your parents born in your current country of residence?
- What languages do you speak?
- What holidays, celebrations, or traditions do you celebrate?
- From your perspective, what makes someone a "good" person?
- What do you like or dislike about your cultural background or ethnicity?
- Have you experienced a positive and/or negative reaction based on your cultural background or ethnicity?

24.2 CULTURALLY RESPONSIVE LONG COVID REHABILITATION

Many terms describe rehabilitation that engages with and is responsive to the patient's cultural identity, including culturally relevant practice, cultural competence, and cultural safety.[7] Culturally relevant practice assesses systemic oppression's impact on communities and develops interventions to address it.[8] Cultural competence involves developing health professionals' knowledge and skills to support effective care for people from CALD backgrounds.[9] Cultural safety helps health professionals increase awareness of systemic inequities for CALD communities through recognising differences, decolonising practices, engaging with power dynamics, and fostering reflection.[10]

Cultural humility is crucial, regardless of your approach to culturally responsive rehabilitation. It is defined[11] as,

A process of self-reflection to understand personal and systemic biases and to develop and maintain respectful processes and relationships based on mutual

trust. Cultural humility involves humbly acknowledging oneself as a learner when it comes to understanding another's experience.

Healthcare systems have traditionally prioritised professional expertise and Western power hierarchies.[12] These approaches can hinder reflection on biases and the influence of health professionals' cultural backgrounds on care. A lack of cultural humility reinforces the dominance of Western science and evidence-based practices, sidelining traditional or alternative healthcare. Embracing cultural humility helps health professionals recognise limitations, address blind spots, and transform practice to be more culturally responsive.

Another key concept is understanding privilege, which "isn't about what you've gone through; it's about what you haven't had to go through."[13] In rehabilitation, privilege can impact the health profession – patient relationships in a range of ways, including ableism[14] and socioeconomic disparities between the two parties.[15] It also exists between health profession groups, with some holding more power within healthcare systems.[16] It also exists between health professionals and patients, with the former perceived to have knowledge and skills that hold more power in healthcare systems than lived experience. Privilege neglects experiences we haven't encountered and can lead to conscious or unconscious oppression of those perceived as "different."

Nixon's[17] metaphor for privilege and oppression (Figure 24.1) offers a framework for understanding its dimensions. The top of the coin represents privilege, while the bottom represents disadvantage, determined purely based on a person's identity. These positions are unearned but determined by who someone is. The illustration below captures this concept.

Unearned privileges often go unrecognised, while disadvantage is profoundly felt. Ignoring inequities from privilege invalidates the experiences of those facing systemic disadvantage, perpetuates inequality, and hinders change. Everyone interacts with multiple systems of inequality (e.g., elitism, racism, ableism, sexism) throughout their lives, highlighting how complex and intersectional these concepts are. Relative privilege and disadvantage in these systems do not cancel each other out. For example, a person with Long COVID may face a disadvantage as a CALD community member while being privileged by their social class.

Reflections on privilege may provoke discomfort and resistance by challenging beliefs about fairness, meritocracy, and identity. Recognising privilege confronts how inequality shapes advantages, which may evoke fear of blame or guilt for

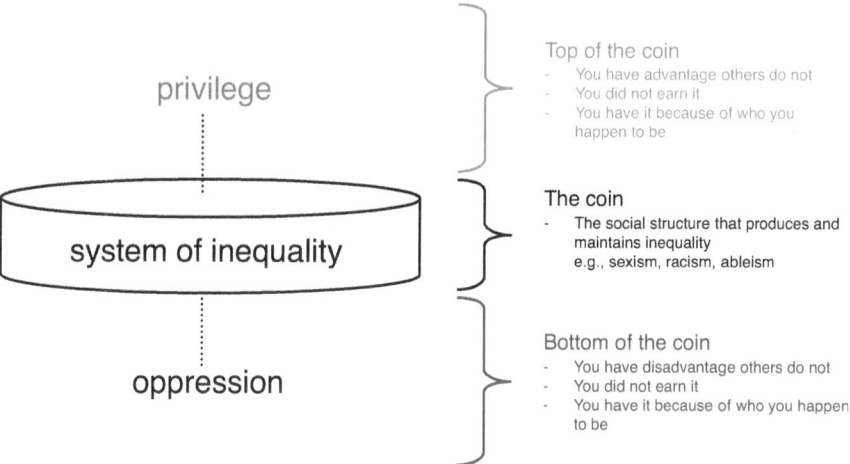

Figure 24.1 The coin model of privilege and critical allyship: implications for health.

Note: "The coin model of privilege and critical allyship: Implications for health" (https://bmcpublichealth.biomedcentral.com/articles/10.1186/s12889-019-7884-9/figures/1) by Stephanie Nixon (https://www.dlsph.utoronto.ca/faculty-profile/nixon-stephanie-a/) is licensed under CC BY 4.0 (https://creativecommons.org/licenses/by/4.0/), https://www.dlsph.utoronto.ca/faculty-profile/nixon-stephanie-a/https://creativecommons.org/licenses/by/4.0/).

unearned benefits. Resistance can also arise from reluctance to acknowledge how privilege perpetuates others' disadvantages, damage to self-perception or social standing, or exposure to unconscious biases. Despite these challenges, health professionals must reflect on their privilege and/or disadvantage to foster understanding and nonjudgemental dialogue around inequality.

BOX 24.3   PRACTICE POINT

Reflect on your identity across dimensions (e.g., gender, race, ability, socioeconomic status).

- Which dimensions are on the top or bottom of your coin?
- How do these dimensions influence your practice as a rehabilitation health professional?

People from CALD communities are often framed negatively as a "challenge" or "problem" in practice, placing blame on them instead of systemic contributors to health inequity. This perspective ignores the benefits of being from a CALD community. The following discussion takes a balanced view, exploring how culture can support and hinder people with Long COVID.

24.3 EXPERIENCES OF HEALTHCARE FOR PEOPLE FROM CALD COMMUNITIES WITH LONG COVID

The COVID-19 pandemic was unprecedented in scale, impacting every country and culture.[18] The global response transcended culture and language, particularly in its early stages.

> *Regardless of your belief or culture everyone came as one. They leave their culture, leave their religion and leave whatever they believe aside to make sure that they fight Covid. It was not a life experience where we think different and act different.*
>
> Research Participant

The pandemic's scope offers a universal context for Long COVID experiences: "I learned that COVID-19 had no respect to cultural background, ethnicity, age, skin, colour, no anything. No matter the language you speak, COVID-19 dealt with everybody in the same way." The lack of healthcare and other supports was considered universal: "The support's not there for anybody."

However, international research shows CALD communities face more healthcare access barriers than the dominant culture.[19] People with Long COVID report discrimination from healthcare providers, which is exacerbated by structural racism and health inequities[20] for CALD communities. Racial discrimination may also hinder transferring rehabilitation gains to daily life.

> *I just felt like my job security was being threatened because I felt like they believed I was going to be having some problems … [they had] perceptions around maybe not being up to the task or not able to do the job efficiently [because of my culture].*
>
> Research Participant

Racism is a significant barrier to equitable healthcare, with some CALD people with Long COVID anticipating it: "I'm black so I have a difference. You know? I feel like that most of the time. Some doctors could be racist … I feel like a lot." Their experiences often involve implicit, subtle, and conscious racism tied to stereotypes about CALD patients being less knowledgeable or capable.

There were moments when I felt racially stereotyped. Some healthcare providers made assumptions based on my background, which affected how seriously they took my concerns. This was frustrating and made me feel marginalised in my treatment. While I can't say for certain they were solely racially motivated, I do believe that my background contributed to the dismissals. It felt like my symptoms were not taken as seriously because of assumptions related to my race and cultural context. I felt assumptions were made that I might not understand medical terminology or that my symptoms were related to stress rather than being valid Long COVID concerns. There was also a perception that I might be less assertive or knowledgeable about my health, which influenced how seriously my symptoms were taken.

Research Participant

In our research, some people with Long COVID from the non-dominant culture acknowledged their privilege in being able to "pass" as white Australians, "Even though I'm not from Australia, I look and sound like I am." They believed this led to better treatment by health professionals and recognised it intersected with other aspects of their identity, "I was advantaged 'cause I'm white um so and because you know like cis."

However, they often noted the assumption that people with Long COVID are lazy: "So my cultural background is I'm English, born in New Zealand. I don't know how much is cultural, but I think generally, there has been like. 'Is this legitimate or are you just not wanting to work?'" This reflects cultural assumptions about work among Australians of European backgrounds, attributing unemployment and poverty to personal failings.[21] Therefore, cultural influences on rehabilitation may also affect people with Long COVID from the dominant local culture.

Migration status significantly influenced the experience of people with Long COVID from CALD communities. Recent arrivals may lack established health provider relationships and may face limited access to health services due to refugee or asylum seeker status.[22]

Coming in from another country, not quite so long ago, it made it much harder for me. I wasn't in the healthcare system or have Medicare when COVID hit, and I had to struggle to finance my medication.

Research Participant

For long-established migrants, marginalisation from the pandemic and Long COVID might reawaken negative migration experiences. One person shared how Long COVID emphasised her struggles to connect when she first arrived,

I realised how little support I have had. I didn't even know what a settlement service was like until I got to that job, and I was like, holy fuck, that exists! I had to do everything alone … so it was kind of coming to terms with how hard that was. That's confronting.

Research Participant

BOX 24.4   PRACTICE POINT

Children and grandchildren of migrants may belong to CALD communities through intergenerational transmission of languages, traditions, societal structures, and religions.

- How does your health service define CALD communities?
- Are country of birth and primary language the main criteria?
- How might this affect your work with subsequent generations of migrant families?

24.4 HEALTH LITERACY

Health literacy significantly affects the ability of CALD communities to access, understand, and use Long COVID information for decision-making and service navigation.[23] The complexity of Long COVID and uncertainty around its treatment present a challenge to developing credible patient information.[24] While CALD communities are often assumed to have low health literacy, the same currently applies to many health professionals in the case of Long COVID.[25]

Our interviewees identified beliefs about health and wellbeing as barriers to accessing rehabilitation. Some CALD communities may avoid services due to cultural values of independence or stigma around Long COVID. However, concerns often eased after accessing care.

Conversations about health in my culture can sometimes lean towards stigma, and the fear of speaking up to people to get help … I was scared that I was gonna be ostracised at that point. But then I found courage to speak up, and, you know, ask for help. When I accessed the health care, I was surprised by the support I got, which changed my perspective of feeling this stigma around speaking up sometimes.

Research Participant

"The way people greet each other can affect on this illness. For example, when you're shaking hands or kissing each other, it can increase the risk of virus transmission. But in different cultures, you can see, for example, they do not do shaking hands or kissing each other, so it [the risk] is lower"

"From our cultural background, we just take off our shoes when we go to our home and we don't use the shoes that we use to go to the shopping center, public toilet, everything. This is something we do here as well, and I think it was the thing that really helped me during the COVID"

"The first time when I actually got COVID, I was with my friend and using the same shisha together. We were about 10 people, and all of us actually got COVID at the same time from one place. So it was not a good thing, but again, this is something coming from my cultural background, to have shisha sometimes with friends"

Figure 24.2 Cultural influences on preventing COVID-19 transmission.

While general health literacy about Long COVID may be low, CALD communities possess significant culture-specific knowledge on minimising COVID-19 transmission. As shown below (Figure 24.2), our interviewees shared examples illustrating the persistence of culturally significant behaviours, which may both increase and decrease the risks of COVID-19 transmission.

Many people from CALD communities use lifestyle strategies and nutrition as first-line treatments for Long COVID. Herbal teas were popular across cultures, and evidence supports their use for respiratory conditions,[26,27] "I can remember, people believe that consuming herbal beverages can decrease the symptoms." People also described general recuperation strategies, "Proper nutrition, a bit of exercise, and then I was just giving myself some time to heal." A lifestyle strategies programme trial for Long COVID[28] showed improved quality of life, self-care, anxiety, and depression. Pre-pandemic evidence suggests plant-based diets may reduce systemic inflammation, which underlies many Long COVID symptoms.[29]

However, people from CALD communities with Long COVID also face widespread misinformation about their condition and COVID-19. Some of this is culturally focused, as one African woman described,

> *There was a general relief, general information then, but I feel this is false. Like, 'Oh, no, blacks can't have COVID with this, with that. And it's surprising many blacks had COVID and my country's belief was 'Don't worry, you're good. Just take water'. And so, it was just bad, because it happened and a lot of blacks were affected too.*

Research Participants

An African man was one of the first infected with COVID-19 in Wuhan but fully recovered.[30] This sparked rumours that black people were genetically immune to COVID-19, leading many to ignore public health orders and infection prevention practices.[31] This misinformation likely increased prevalence in black communities, contributing to high Long COVID rates.[31]

24.5 COMMUNICATION

Communication challenges due to language differences are often cited when working with CALD communities. The term "language barrier" has been critiqued for oversimplifying complex power dynamics between people using different languages.[32] It can also place responsibility on the person speaking the minority language rather than addressing systemic factors.[33] The following comment highlights the impact of language differences on the lived and rehabilitation experience of people with Long COVID.

> *English is my second language, and it did impact my care. Sometimes, I struggled to express my symptoms clearly, especially when I was feeling overwhelmed. This occasionally led to misunderstandings with healthcare providers, making it harder to communicate my needs effectively. My brain fog and cognitive symptoms affected me more significantly in English. When trying to express myself in my second language, it became even more challenging, especially during moments of confusion or fatigue. In my native language, I felt slightly more comfortable.*

Research Participant

Medical terminology and jargon can be barriers for CALD communities, leading to misunderstandings about assessment and treatment. Specialist terms may also cause unnecessary distress, as related by a health professional,

Before the Session

- Family or friends should not interpret, due to their relationship with the patient and to preserve the right to privacy.

- Ask the patient if they have preferences regarding interpreter age, gender, etc.

- Ensure technology is ready before telehealth sessions. Provide interpreters with a brief orientation if they are new to the platform.

- Briefly discuss session goals, terminology and expected content with the interpreter before meeting the patient.

- Schedule additional time for sessions involving interpreters to ensure thorough communication.

- Some languages have no written form and newer CALD communities may lack qualified interpreters. Report issues obtaining interpreters as a safety concern to your manager.

During the Session

- Use first-person language when speaking directly with the patient, e.g., 'How are you feeling today?' or 'Did you want to try that again?'

- Ask your patient, not the interpreter, about cultural practices or beliefs.

- When working with Deaf or non-verbal people using sign language, position the interpreter beside you and opposite the patient to make eye contact and observe body language.

- Use simple, clear language and pause often to support accurate interpretation. Avoid medical jargon and provide context for health terms

- Avoid complex terms, medical jargon or colloquialisms that may be hard to translate.

- Regularly confirm the patient understands the information provided.

- Provide translated plain language health information and culturally sensitive resources wherever possible as an alternative format to the interpreted discussion. Ensure readability levels are suitable for diverse populations

- Ensure interpreters are aware of, and adhere to, privacy and confidentiality standards.

After the Session

- Do not ask or document the interpreter's opinion of the client, even if offered.

- Give the interpreter feedback on their contribution to the session's success.

- Conversely, address interpreter performance concerns directly after the session with them and the contracted agency.

- Clearly document the use of an interpreter in the patient's record, including their name and language.

Figure 24.3 Recommendations for working with interpreters and people from CALD communities.

I phoned a lady to tell her that her PCR test was negative when I was redeployed to the Respiratory Clinic. Her record said she had lived in Australia for many years and didn't need an interpreter. Gave her the results and she got really distressed – crying and hyperventilating. I had to get her husband on the line to help. He said, "You told her it was negative, and negative means bad, so now she has the 'rona and she is old so she will die"! I quickly explained that she didn't have COVID-19. In future, I told people,' You DO NOT have COVID' before I told them the test result was negative.

Danielle

Interpreters play a key role in culturally responsive rehabilitation, supporting health professionals and people with Long COVID. The following recommendations for engaging with linguistic diversity[34] (Figure 24.3) promote respectful, effective communication for both parties.

24.6 RECOMMENDATIONS FOR CULTURALLY SENSITIVE LONG COVID REHABILITATION

The following recommendations draw on the authors' lived and professional experience and international evidence. They aim to ensure rehabilitation services deliver culturally sensitive care for people with Long COVID, promoting the best outcomes for all.

24.6.1 Actively Include Family and Community Members with the Patient's Permission

Family and cultural communities are crucial supports for many CALD people with Long COVID: "I had my family, they were really there for me, so I was just leaning on them because they provided support, both financially and emotionally for me. Oh yeah, that's what helped me recover." CALD communities offer culturally appropriate networks of support, including formal services and informal support, and are increasingly located online, enabling connections with peers in their country of origin.

My cultural background provided me with resilience and a strong support network, even if it was mainly online. It also helped me find community resources tailored to my experiences, which made me feel less isolated.

Research Participant

While healthcare systems often focus on individual health, involving family and engaging with the local cultural community improves prevention and treatment outcomes.[35] With consent, design inclusive strategies (e.g., family exercise activities) and enable peer engagement for those with Long COVID,

[She was] a church member. We connected, we talked about our experiences and what we could do to help ourselves and what we've actually been doing.

Research Participant

24.6.2 Demonstrate and Communicate Cultural Humility and Respect

Demonstrating cultural humility with CALD communities involves respecting cultural norms, such as addressing elders first or gender-specific communication preferences. Active listening and attention to non-verbal cues are crucial, as some cultures avoid direct disagreement despite reluctance to engage in a task. Using interpreters aids communication, but health professionals should develop direct communication over time. Listening to others share their cultural background, acknowledging knowledge limitations, and honouring diverse communication styles show cultural humility and strengthen therapeutic relationships.

24.6.3 Incorporate Traditional Healing Approaches Into Rehabilitation

Several traditional or cultural treatments show preliminary evidence for Long COVID symptom relief. Observational studies suggest acupuncture is safe and may provide symptomatic relief.[36] Some studies report positive outcomes from nutritional supplements and traditional Chinese medicine for gastrointestinal symptoms.[37] Limited evidence exists for other traditional, complementary, and integrative approaches, but more research is needed.[38] Asking CALD communities about their traditional healing methods provides insight into their health and enables health professionals to align rehabilitation with patients' healthcare beliefs.

24.6.4 Build Partnerships with Culturally Tailored Services

Culturally tailored health services address the specific needs of community groups, often focusing on chronic and complex conditions. Mainstream services may employ bilingual and bicultural health workers who are valued for their cultural skills and knowledge. These workers facilitate communication and understanding between services and communities where they share cultural experiences, focusing on building relationships rather than direct clinical care.[39] Formalising partnerships with culturally tailored services or health workers enhances rehabilitation services' cultural sensitivity.

24.6.5 Upskill the Rehabilitation Workforce for Working with People from CALD Communities

Provide training for health professionals in cultural humility, interpreter use, local/global contexts, health literacy, and intersectional awareness.[40] Offer practice-based materials and workshops on culture-specific Long COVID rehabilitation challenges and strategies. Build partnerships with CALD organisations to enable mutual learning and shared capacity building. Better knowledge of what services and supports are available to people from CALD communities also enables timely and responsive referrals for co-morbid conditions and other health issues (see Chapter 2).

24.6.6 Invest Resources to Support Better Rehabilitation for People with Long COVID from CALD Communities

Collecting quality data on the cultural and linguistic needs of people with Long COVID underpins better service planning. Ethnicity and language are often absent in clinical records, especially when patients are assumed to belong to the dominant culture. Understanding local communities supports investment in culturally sensitive materials, such as culture-specific examples, written information, and referrals to tailored services. While governments produce COVID-19 materials in multiple languages, few address Long COVID. A readily available library of resources in local languages streamlines culturally sensitive care and may already be available from governmental or culturally specific services.[41]

24.7 CONCLUSION

This chapter highlights the importance of culturally responsive rehabilitation for CALD communities with Long COVID. Recognising the impact of cultural identity on health behaviours and experiences, it addresses systemic barriers, including racism, migration challenges, and care inequities. Reflecting on privilege and adopting culturally informed approaches fosters trust, meaningful engagement, and respectful, relevant care. As healthcare systems tackle Long COVID's complexities, this chapter urges a commitment to addressing CALD communities' unique needs, ensuring all voices are heard and care is tailored to diverse realities.

24.8 ACKNOWLEDGEMENTS

The research study described in this chapter was supported by a 2023 Early or Mid-Career Research Award Grant from the Women's Health Research, Translation and Impact Network. The authors sincerely thank and acknowledge the contributions of the following clinician researchers to the research referred to in this chapter – Krishna Vakil, Atefeh Taghizadeh, Zarina Hau, Jiyoon Jung, Farhana Dewan, Jessie Wong, and Martha Tadros. The authors would also like to acknowledge the sharing of knowledge and discussions with Weenthunga Health Network that informed the development of Section 24.2.

REFERENCES

1 Chaturvedi S, et al. Are we reluctant to talk about cultural determinants? Indian J Med Res. 2011;133:361–63.

2 Levesque A, et al. The relationship between culture, health conceptions, and health practices. J Cross Cult Psychol. 2014;45:628–45. doi:10.1177/0022022113519855.

3 Heyes C. Culture. Curr Biol 2020, 30(20), R1246–50. doi:10.1016/j.cub.2020.08.086.

4 Constantinou CS, et al. Cultural competence in healthcare and healthcare education. Societies. 2022;12(6):178. doi:10.3390/soc12060178.

5 O'Donnell J, et al. Impacts of the COVID-19 pandemic on ethnically diverse communities. Popul Space Place. 2023;29:e2693. doi:10.1002/psp.2693.

6 Hossain MM, et al. Living with "Long COVID": A systematic review and meta-synthesis of qualitative evidence. PLoS One. 2023;18(2):e0281884. doi:10.1371/journal.pone.0281884.

7 Flaskerud JH. Cultural competence: What is it? Issues Ment Health Nurs. 2007;28(1):121–23. doi:10.1080/01612840600998154.

8 Van Voorhis RM. Culturally relevant practice: A framework for teaching the psychosocial dynamics of oppression. J Soc Work Educ. 1998;34(1):121–33. doi:10.1080/10437797.1998.10778910.

9 Galanti G-A. Culturally competent rehabilitation nursing. Rehabil Nurs. 2005;30(4):123–26. doi:10.1002/j.2048-7940.2005.tb00093.x.

10 Ramsden IM. Cultural safety and nursing education in Aotearoa and Te Waipounamu [Doctoral dissertation] [Internet]. Wellington: Victoria University of Wellington; 2002. Available from: https://www.croakey.org/wp-content/uploads/2017/08/RAMSDEN-I-Cultural-Safety_Full.pdfhttps://www.croakey.org/wp-content/uploads/2017/08/RAMSDEN-I-Cultural-Safety_Full.pdfhttps://www.croakey.org/wp-content/uploads/2017/08/RAMSDEN-I-Cultural-Safety_Full.pdf.

11 First Nations Health Authority of British Colombia (FNHA). (2023). Cultural safety and humility standard [Internet]. Vancouver: FNHA; [cited 2025 Feb 7]. Available at https://www.fnha.ca/wellness/wellness-and-the-first-nations-health-authority/cultural-safety-and-humility.

12 Currie G, et al. Inter-professional barriers and knowledge brokering in an organisational context: The case of healthcare. Organisation Studies. 2012;33(10):1333–61. doi:10.1177/0170840612457617.

13 Khan JF. A sermon on the project of whiteness … [Instagram post] [Internet]. *Instagram*; 2020 Jun 1 [cited 2025 Feb 7]. Available from: https://www.instagram.com/p/-CA3OB9fByeN/https://www.instagram.com/p/CA3OB9fByeN/https://www.instagram.com/p/CA3OB9fByeN/.

14 Hartley MT, et al. Ableism and able privilege: Integrating social justice concepts in rehabilitation education. Rehabil Res Policy Educ. 2024;38(2):123–35. doi:10.1177/0034355224123688710.1177/0034355224123688710.1177/00343552241236887.

15 Job C, et al. Health professionals' implicit bias of patients with low socioeconomic status (SES) and its effects on clinical decision-making: A scoping review. BMJ Open. 2024;14:e081723. doi:10.1136/bmjopen-2023-081723.

16 Ammann C, et al. Negotiating social differences and power geometries among healthcare professionals in a Swiss hospital. Gender Place Cult. 2020;28(12):1715–37. doi:10.1080/0966369X.2020.1847047.

17 Nixon SA. The coin model of privilege and critical allyship: Implications for health. BMC Public Health. 2019;19:1637. doi:10.1186/s12889-019-7884-9.

18 Feehan J, et al. Is COVID-19 the worst pandemic? Maturitas. 2021;149:56–58. doi:10.1016/j.maturitas.2021.02.001.

19 Henderson S, et al. Culturally and linguistically diverse peoples' knowledge of accessibility and utilisation of health services: Exploring the need for improvement in health service delivery. Aust J Prim Health. 2011;17(2):195–201. doi:10.1071/PY10065.

20 Berger Z, et al. Long COVID and health inequities: The role of primary care. Milbank Q. 2021;99(2):519–41. doi:10.1111/1468-0009.12505.

21 Rosenthal L, et al. Protestant work ethic's relation to intergroup and policy attitudes: A meta-analytic review. Eur J Soc Psychol. 2011;41(7):874–85. doi:10.1002/ejsp.832.

22 Novak A, et al. Identification, management and care of refugee patients at a metropolitan public health service: A healthcare worker perspective. Aust Health Rev. 2021;45:338–43. doi:10.1071/AH19200.

23 Rosenthal L, et al. Health literacy. J Community Hosp Intern Med Perspect. 2013;3(2):21217. doi:10.3402/jchimp.v3i2.21217.

24 Hodgson CL, et al. Long COVID – Unravelling a complex condition. Lancet. 2023;11(8):667–68. doi:10.1016/S2213-2600(23)00232.

25 Ojha S, et al. A quantitative evaluation of knowledge, perception, awareness, and preparedness of Long COVID among health professionals and students in India. J Radio Nurs. 2024;43(1):83–88. doi: 10.1016/j.jradnu.2023.10.005.

26 Timmer A, et al. Pelargonium sidoides extract for treating acute respiratory tract infections. Cochrane Database Syst Rev. 2013;(10):CD006323. doi:10.1002/14651858.CD006323.pub3.

27 Hu X-Y, et al. Andrographis paniculata (Chuān Xīn Lián) for symptomatic relief of acute respiratory tract infections in adults and children: A systematic review and meta-analysis. PLOS ONE. 2017;12(8):e0181780. doi: 10.1371/journal.pone.0181780.

28 Navas-Otero A, et al. A lifestyle adjustments program in Long COVID-19 improves symptomatic severity and quality of life: A randomised control trial. Patient Educ Couns. 2024;122:108180. doi:10.1016/j.pec.2024.108180.

29 Storz M. Lifestyle adjustments in Long-COVID management: Potential benefits of plant-based diets. Curr Nutr Rep. 2021;10(4):352–63. doi:10.1007/s13668-021-00369.

30 Laurencin CT, et al. The COVID-19 pandemic: A call to action to identify and address racial and ethnic disparities. J Racial Ethn Health Disparities. 2020;7(3):398–402. doi:10.1007/s40615-020-00756-0.

31 Glanton D. Column: Let's stop the spread — of the myth black people are immune to the coronavirus. *Chicago Tribune*; 2020 Mar 19 [cited 2025 Feb 7]. Available from: https://www.chicagotribune.com/columns/dahleen-glanton/ct-dahleen-glantoncoronavirus-black-immunity-myth-idris-elba-202003195auoqjzrmbcsphitbhpocth3qa-story.html.

32 Harzing A, et al. The language barrier and its implications for HQ-subsidiary relationships. Cross Cult Manag Int J. 2008;15(1):49–61. doi:10.1108/13527600810848827.

33 Amano T, et al. The manifold costs of being a non-native English speaker in science. PLoS Biol. 2023;21(7):e3002184. doi:10.1371/journal.pbio.3002184.

34 Victorian Government. Working with interpreters [Internet]. Melbourne: State Government of Victoria; [cited 2025 Feb 7]. Available from: https://www.vic.gov.au/guidelines-using-interpreting-services/working-interpreters.

35 Komaric N, et al. Two sides of the coin: Patient and provider perceptions of health care delivery to patients from culturally and linguistically diverse backgrounds. BMC Health Serv Res. 2012;12:322. doi:10.1186/1472-6963-12-322.

36 Williams JE. Acupuncture treatment of Long-COVID: A narrative review of selected case studies and review articles. Asian J Complement Altern Med. 2022;10(4):95–97. doi:0.53043/2347-3894.acam90042.

37 Gawey B, et al. The use of complementary and alternative medicine for the treatment of gastrointestinal symptoms in Long COVID: A systematic review. Ther Adv Chronic Dis. 2023;14:20406223231190548. doi:10.1177/20406223231190548.

38 Chen X, et al. Traditional, complementary and integrative medicine for fatigue post COVID-19 infection: A systematic review of randomised controlled trials. Integr Med Res. 2024;13(2):101039. doi:10.1016/j.imr.2024.101039.

39 Migrant Health Australia. Building on strength: Policy brief [Internet]. [Place unknown]: Migrant Health Australia; 2022 Jun [cited 2025 Feb 7]. Available from: https://culturaldiversityhealth.org.au/wp-content/uploads/2022/07/Building-on-Strength-Bilingual-and-Bicultural-Workforce-Policy-Brief.pdf.

40 Huish C, et al. Intercultural gaps in knowledge, skills and attitudes of public health professionals: A systematic review. J Public Health. 2023;45(Suppl 1):i35–i44. doi:10.1093/pubmed/fdac166.

41 Health Translations Victoria. Long COVID [Internet]. Melbourne: State Government of Victoria; [cited 2025 Feb 7]. Available from: https://www.healthtranslations.vic.gov.au/resources/long-covid-fact-sheet

Chapter 25

Long COVID in Rural and Remote Communities

Sandy Davies, Sumitha Gounden, Emily Armstrong, Martin Ferguson-Pell, and Danielle Hitch

---

BOX 25.1   LEARNING OBJECTIVES

By the end of this chapter, readers should be able to:

- Better understand the unique opportunities and challenges experienced by people with Long COVID and health professionals in rural and remote communities.
- Reflect on adapting models of care to local healthcare contexts by considering person-centred care, resource availability, and cultural appropriateness for rural populations.
- Appreciate innovative models of care and their potential applications to rural and remote communities.
- Identify practical and feasible strategies for service improvement and their application to the local context.

25.1 INTRODUCTION

Around 40% of the world's population lives in rural or remote communities,[1] yet they lack comparable healthcare access to their compatriots in urban areas. Chronic health workforce shortages in these areas are a serious global issue, with fewer health professionals available per capita as remoteness increases.[2] These inequities lead to poorer health outcomes and higher chronic disease rates for rural and remote populations.[3] We firmly believe that your location or postcode should not determine your health and wellbeing.

This chapter explores the unique experiences of people with Long COVID in rural and remote communities (hereafter rural), drawing on research and lived experience. Two case studies from Australia and Canada illustrate the potential for innovative

DOI: 10.4324/9781003528104-31

practices that improve accessibility for all marginalised and isolated people with Long COVID. Practical recommendations for service improvement are also provided, which recognise the limited resources available in many rural contexts.

25.2 THE CHALLENGES OF LIVING WITH LONG COVID IN RURAL COMMUNITIES

25.2.1 Limited Access to Specialist Services

Despite the benefits of rural living, geographical isolation poses many challenges to accessing healthcare. Local primary care providers (such as General Practitioners or GPs) are the main access point, but initial specialist consultation appointments can take months. There are also not enough visiting specialists to meet community needs, leading to extremely long waiting lists.[4] Government support schemes to access specialist care exist in some areas but cannot fill all the existing service gaps.

These problems impact rural people with Long COVID even more, given their need for management by multiple medical specialities. They often travel long distances and take time away from responsibilities to access care,[5] a burden that urban patients do not have to bear.

> *When the appointment date arrives, attending means an entire day off work, travelling an exhausting distance, only to be given a flurry of blood tests and told to come back again in 6–8 weeks.*
>
> Sandy

Many services shifted to telehealth early in the pandemic, which patients welcomed and found comparable to face-to-face appointments.[6] However, incentives for its use have largely been removed[7] and rural communities still face issues related to inconsistent internet access.[5]

> *Now telehealth is only available upon forceful insistence, presumably because in Australia, the Medicare Benefits Schedule rebate is not sufficient for a profitable practice. When your health is compromised, fighting for your right to care depletes every last reserve.*
>
> Sandy

25.2.2 Systemic Health Workforce Issues

Even when health services are available locally, rural and remote people with Long COVID are often poorly serviced due to systemic healthcare workforce issues.[8] Rural health professionals may also be marginalised from professional networks that support their Long COVID learning and practice.[9] While confident in community engagement and intersectoral partnerships, these practitioners report desiring better training in data-based decision-making and issues related to diversity, equity, and inclusion.[10] Consequently, they face additional barriers to upskilling in the rapidly evolving field of Long COVID.

> *Despite initially feeling patronised by my General Practitioner, as more and more information became available, he began to take the condition seriously. Despite months of multiple tests and his conclusion of post-viral fatigue, medical solutions were not forthcoming, only basic lifestyle advice like restricting exercise, rest, and being patient with yourself.*
>
> Sandy

There is a high turnover in rural health services for medicine, nursing, allied health, and mental health professionals, especially in small towns.[11] This significantly impacts continuity of care for people with Long COVID, as high GP turnover can lead to more emergency department visits, reduced access to timely appointments, and lower patient satisfaction.[12] Long COVID patients need "relationship-based care" with consistent access to professionals who know them well and can coordinate their complex care needs.[13] However, their options for finding the "right" professional in a rural area are far more limited.

25.2.3 **Marginalisation and Isolation**

People with Long COVID face significant marginalisation due to stigma and lack of recognition, as discussed in other chapters. This is particularly true for those in rural communities, who are isolated from others with the condition and have less voice in research, healthcare, and policy decisions.[7] Perceptions and knowledge about Long COVID in rural communities may also be a barrier to support.

> *I used to think menopause was a conversation stopper, then I acquired Long COVID. Mentioning post-viral fatigue is by far an even quicker way to clear the room, especially in a regional remote area. People refuse to believe it's a real thing. Once you mention Long COVID eye contact disappears and you can almost hear the 'whoosh' as people hurriedly scurry away…*
>
> *I was asked to present a paper at a conference, which should have been a career highlight and absolute joy. When I couldn't even muster the reserves for minimal follow through with participants after the event, I realised my Long COVID was indeed real, no matter how many naysayers and disbelievers existed in our remote regional area.*

I learned to only mention Long COVID in trusted circles and private social media support groups as the judgement, non-verbal cues and disbelief were palpable. When I would post about Long COVID on my business social media pages, people in my digital network would reach out via private message asking for advice for themselves, their spouse, their adult children or others in their circle impacted by Long COVID. Perceived stigma around the topic holds so much power that those who reached out never publicly supported my social media posts about Long COVID despite seeking my assistance privately.

Sandy

Many people with Long COVID seek peer support in online forums, often involving those in urban areas with better healthcare access. While helpful, the advice may not suit rural communities or their cultural contexts.

If it hadn't been for others in urban areas with better medical access sharing the information they received, my recovery would have taken even longer. However, my academic soul still struggles with the fact that I gained more beneficial information from social media than anywhere else.

Sandy

25.3 THE BENEFITS OF RURAL LIVING FOR HEALTH AND WELLBEING

Living in rural communities is often seen as a healthcare barrier. However, these contexts also offer benefits for people with Long COVID. A strengths-based approach can empower patients to exercise self-determination (see Chapter 20) by optimising existing resources, assets, and capabilities. Highlighting what people with Long COVID can do in rural settings, rather than what they can't do, better enables health professionals to foster dignity, inclusivity, and sustainable care.

Rural living nurtures close social connections and support networks, positively impacting health and wellbeing.[14] The social capital from these relationships enhances resources, strengthens community belonging, and amplifies the benefits of community belonging.[15] A slower pace of life reduces stress and sensory overstimulation, while lower air and noise pollution benefits respiratory and cardiovascular health. Significant evidence demonstrates that closer connections and regular engagement with natural environments promote health and wellbeing.[16] For First Nations and culturally connected peoples, these settings reinforce ties to land and traditions, supporting holistic health and wellbeing.

BOX 25.2   PRACTICE POINT

Identify the strengths, resources, assets, and opportunities in your closest rural or remote community. Consider how each can support people with Long COVID.

25.4 CASE STUDY: A HYBRID EARLY INTERVENTION MODEL OF CARE

The Western New South Wales Local Health District (WNSW-LHD) is the largest in the state and is home to the largest rural mental health service in Australia.[17] It covers an area of 246,672 square kilometres including rural and remote communities, which is around the size of Ghana or the United Kingdom. Its services include 3 major hospitals, 38 inpatient facilities, and 50 community health centres.[18] The area has over 276,000 residents, with 11% identifying as Aboriginal and/or Torres Strait Islander peoples (Figure 25.1).[1]

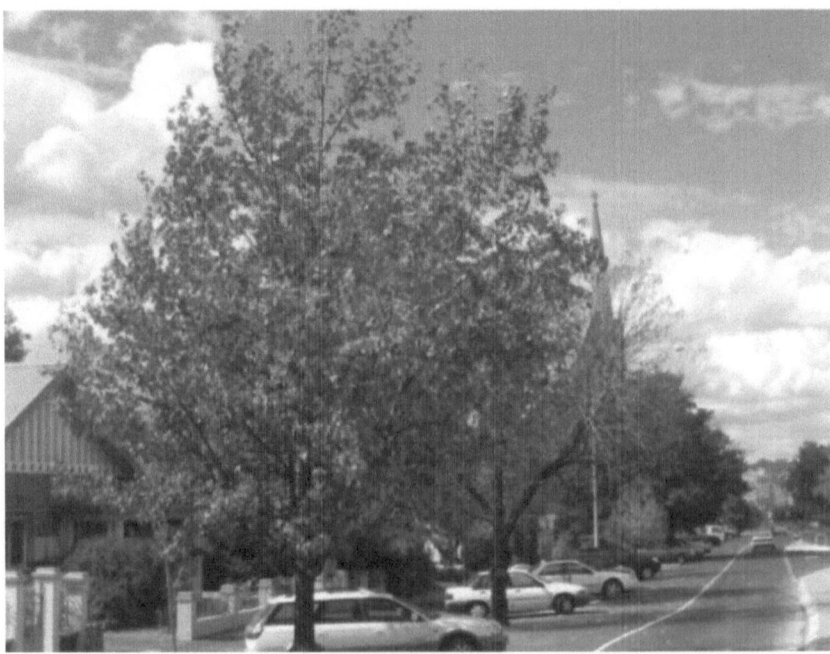

Figure 25.1 Autumn trees in Byng St, Orange NSW. Photograph by (WT-shared) Puzzlement at wts wikivoyage, CC BY-SA 4.0 <https://creativecommons.org/licenses/by-sa/4.0>, via Wikimedia Commons.

The Long COVID service targeted people with persistent symptoms >4 weeks post-COVID-19, reflecting an early rehabilitation approach. Community nurses identified ongoing issues during routine post-COVID welfare checks and referred patients to a rural rehabilitation physician who had special interest in Long COVID. Patients were triaged using the COVID-19 Yorkshire Rehabilitation Scale (C-19YRS)[19] and accepted if functionally disabled. Over time, patients were seen through a formal referral process from their GP and later the model expanded to include a community care team, integrated planned care service, and multidisciplinary cardiopulmonary rehabilitation team.

Patients were seen virtually and in person by the clinic and partner services, all receiving health coaching and care coordination. About 8% of patients in the integrated planned care service (n = 40) were referred to the Long COVID rehabilitation clinic, most of whom were female (n = 24, 65%). The clinic was well attended, with all but three referred patients receiving care. Over half the clinic patients (n = 20, 54%) reported complete symptom resolution and regained baseline functional status, typically after 1–3 care episodes (n = 22, 59%). As of April 2022, 20 Long COVID clinic patients remained enrolled in the integrated planned care service for ongoing health and psychosocial care. The following case study highlights the story of one person with Long COVID supported through this care model.

BOX 25.3   JIM'S STORY

"Jim"[2] is 28 years old and is a proud Wiradjuri man. He was a security guard and was exposed to COVID-19 in 2021 at his workplace by an infected courier driver from Sydney. Jim lives alone, but has strong family ties and regularly visits to his mother in a nearby town. After mild symptoms (fever, cough, and shortness of breath), Jim tested positive and was initially monitored via telehealth at home. Nine days later, his oxygen levels dropped significantly, leading to ICU admission with Type 1 Respiratory Failure secondary to COVID-19.

Jim was discharged from ICU after seven days with complex symptoms, including severe fatigue, persistent cough, shortness of breath, anosmia, excessive urination, and diarrhoea. He was referred to the Long COVID rehabilitation clinic about 5 weeks post-discharge and was again initially monitored via telehealth due to limited transport options. At the time, he experienced severe physical and cognitive fatigue, shortness of breath with mild exertion, reduced mobility, brain fog, poor sleep, anosmia, ageusia, continence issues, deconditioning, and social isolation, significantly limiting his daily life. Jim felt unwell and was unfit to work. As a casual contract worker, he continued receiving full salary with fortnightly medical certificates from the rehabilitation physician.

After two weeks, Jim attended the rehabilitation clinic for face-to-face assessment and goal setting. His rehabilitation goals were as follows: Short-Term Goals:

- Safely shower seated without experiencing breathlessness or extreme fatigue.
- Walk more than 100 metres without needing rest.

Long-Term Goals:

- Regain independence in self-care and home maintenance activities.
- Return to his job as a security guard.
- Walk 8 kilometres during his work shift without falling asleep or experiencing severe fatigue.
- Improved physical and cognitive health to reduce anxiety, build confidence, and improve self-efficacy.

Jim received multidisciplinary rehabilitation tailored to his personal rehabilitation goals (Figure 25.2).

Five months post-rehabilitation, Jim's 6-Minute Walk Test was 52% of the predicted value, highlighting his need for continued care. His recovery was gradual but promising, driven by his strong motivation to return to work and regain independence.

The case study showcases high-quality, evidence-based rehabilitation in a rural community, using a pragmatic, partnership-based model. This approach leverages existing services to address community needs, reducing patients' burden in organising and coordinating care. Early intervention may have prevented future service needs. Effective rural healthcare models emphasise community participation, interdisciplinary teamwork, and partnerships with health services[20] – an ideal combination for patients with Long COVID.

Fatigue Management & Energy Conservation
- Prescribed an over-toilet aid and shower chair to reduce falls risk.
- Educated on energy conservation techniques, like pacing and activity planning.
- Structured timetable to gradually increase daily activity levels and track progress.

Physical Rehabilitation
- Exercise program focusing on strength, balance and endurance (paced walking program, leg and arm strengthening exercises & aerobic fitness training)

Cognitive Rehabilitation
- Cognitive fatigue assessment, focusing on verbal versus written memory
- Practice computer use to increase sustained attention and reaction times
- Memory strategies and assistive tools to compensate for short term memory loss

Vocational Rehabilitation
- Referral to vocational rehabilitation providers to assist with a structured return-to-work plan

Psychosocial Interventions
- Support to reintegrate with family and community to reduce social isolation and improve emotional wellbeing
- Validation of lived experience and reassurance to reduce anxiety and stress.

Figure 25.2 Rehabilitation programme offered to "Jim."

BOX 25.4 PRACTICE POINT

How would your rehabilitation service deliver these interventions to someone like Jim? What partnerships or referral pathways would be needed? Reflect on the collaboration level between your service and others who might be involved in his care. Could the interface between services risk delays or disruptions to care continuity?

25.5 CASE STUDY TWO: BRIDGING THE DISTANCE – A TELEHEALTH MODEL FOR LONG COVID CARE IN RURAL ALBERTA

Alberta is one of the three Prairie Provinces occupying the centre of Canada. Characterised by vast, open plains in the south and east, the forests and rock of the Canadian Shield in the north, and the Rocky Mountains to the west, Albertans have ample environments in which to live. Three-quarters of the 4 million residents choose to live in the central corridor cities of Edmonton, Red Deer, and Calgary. However, approximately 1 million Albertans live in the rural parts of the province, which make up the majority of its 661,850 square kilometres. Given almost all the medical specialists in Alberta practice in either Edmonton or Calgary, rural Albertans often travel significant distances to receive specialist care (Figure 25.3).

In response to the influx of patients, Alberta Health Services established the Long COVID-19 Inter-Professional Outpatient Program (IPOP).[21] These three provincial public health clinics introduced an interdisciplinary approach combining primary care, medical specialty care, and allied health. While video appointments included rural patients, most rehabilitation sessions remained in-person due to complex presentations requiring specialised assessments unsuitable for telehealth (see Figure 25.4).

Persistent breathlessness at rest was the most common symptom reported by Albertans with Long COVID, alongside fatigue and brain fog. In late 2021, the University of Alberta's Rehabilitation Robotics Lab, the Breathe Easy program, and Alberta Health Services' Allied Health Office secured funding for a novel

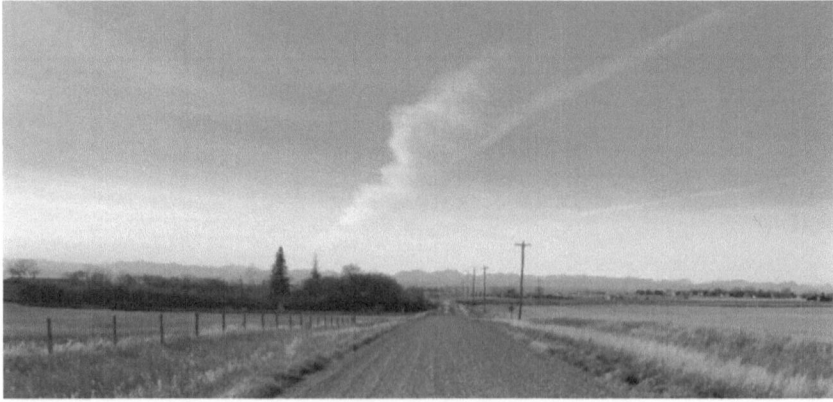

Figure 25.3 Rural Alberta. © 2020 Emily Armstrong.

CLINICAL PATHWAY FOR LONG COVID VIRTUAL ASSESSMENT

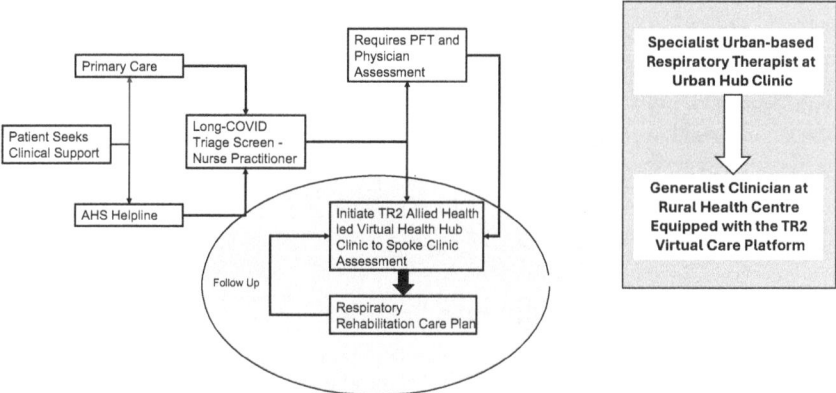

Figure 25.4 Clinical pathway for Long COVID virtual assessment.

telehealth model for rural Albertans with Long COVID (Figure 25.4). The model used a hub-and-spoke approach, where rural physiotherapists (spokes) conducted assessments guided by urban IPOP respiratory therapists (hub) and collaboratively implemented care plans (Figure 25.5).

25.5.1 Developing and Selecting the Right Technology

Technologies were developed to provide remote information to IPOP respiratory therapists comparable to in-person assessments. The Rehabilitation Robotics Lab led this effort during COVID-19 lockdowns, conducting much of the discovery and testing from home, which limited initial validation. Various remote breathlessness assessment options were identified; some, like pulse oximeters, adapted well to telehealth, while others, such as lung auscultation, were more challenging. Devices like the Mintii and digital Littmann stethoscopes faced practical issues, including clothing rustling. However, Health Canada approval delays further hindered progress.

Markerless Motion Capture (MMC), a telehealth technology, tracks movements like range of motion, balance, and sit-to-stand tests quantitatively. It breaks tests into stages for detailed analysis, capturing complexities in endurance, balance, and posture. Though many systems exist, few are validated or compared with 2D and 3D systems. MMC was crucial for Long COVID monitoring, detecting small changes often missed in chronic illness assessments. Quantitative systems provide strong evidence of progress, motivating health professionals and Long COVID patients to persist with rehabilitation for better outcomes. For example, the Putrino Lab at Mount Sinai demonstrated that monitoring heart rate variability may predict "flare-ups," fatigue, and brain fog.[22] This highlights the value of quantitative measures in monitoring and treating Long COVID symptoms, particularly in rehabilitation clinics.

The team made notable progress in remote breath tracking using stretch sensors embedded in breathing bands placed on the chest and diaphragm. These sensors measured breathing depth and frequency at rest and during exercise in people with Long COVID. By correlating oxygen saturation with breathing patterns, health professionals gained critical insights into respiratory status. Intense breathing with low oxygen levels indicated potential lung tissue damage, requiring further medical care.

25.5.2 Putting the Model Into Practice

The final technology package comprised a laptop with Zoom for videoconferencing and real-time data sharing, an MMC system, two breathing bands, a digital stethoscope, and a pulse oximeter. It enabled musculoskeletal capacity assessments, such as sit-to-stand, broken into component movement stages for detailed analysis; blood oxygen saturation at rest, during exercise, and after exercise; breathing frequency and depth at rest, during exercise, and after exercise; and lung sounds.

People with Long COVID were screened by the IPOP team using a clinical protocol (see Figure 25.5). Those with severe symptoms requiring spirometry received in-person assessments. Common assessments included the 6-Minute Walk Test, sit-to-stand, and upper torso palpation. Suitable patients attended local

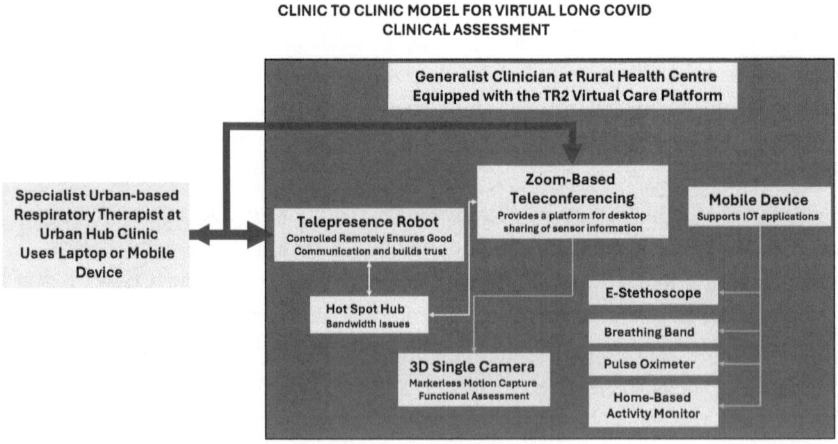

Figure 25.5 Clinic to clinic model for virtual Long COVID clinical assessment.

physiotherapy clinics equipped with the technology package, connecting via Zoom to IPOP respiratory therapists while supported by local physiotherapists.

This model utilises the greater availability of rural physiotherapists and affordable technologies to improve access to respiratory therapists and high-quality care for Long COVID patients. While technology identification and lab testing were completed, implementation funding was unavailable, and Alberta Health Services have since closed their IPOP clinics. Nonetheless, this case study highlights the potential of interdisciplinary models to deliver equitable care to rural and remote communities and monitor other patient groups, such as those with Chronic Obstructive Pulmonary Disease,[23] which is twice as common in Alberta's Indigenous communities. The thorough development of these technologies and clinical processes will allow for rapid implementation if funding arises.

BOX 25.5   PRACTICE POINT

What technology (if any) do you use in rehabilitation for people with Long COVID? What is your understanding of technology's role in rehabilitation? How would you rate your skills, knowledge, and comfort with using technology in practice?

25.6 PRACTICAL RECOMMENDATIONS FOR HEALTH PROFESSIONALS SUPPORTING PEOPLE WITH LONG COVID IN RURAL AND REMOTE AREAS

Both case studies highlight innovative rural practices, but these care models may not suit all communities. The following recommendations, based on research,[24–27] professional, and lived experience, suggest feasible options for rural or remote areas.

25.6.1 Develop a Community Strategy to Build Long COVID Capacity for Rural and Remote Health Professionals

- Supporting rural health professionals in understanding Long COVID and improving rehabilitation skills ensures patients receive quality care locally. The strategy should include:
  - Training and professional development in Long COVID management, with mentorship for junior professionals by experienced colleagues.

- Formalised partnerships between urban specialists, rural professionals, and community organisations to deliver care via agreed pathways.
- Integration with recruitment and retention strategies to promote workforce stability and sustainability.

25.6.2 Optimise Technology Integration Where Feasible

- Offer free training or a "buddy system" for health professionals, patients, and community members to use digital health solutions.
- Establish telehealth hubs with reliable internet, private spaces, and pre-set computers for health professionals and patients.
- Leverage telehealth for care delivery, professional development, community education, and peer support access.
- Use affordable technologies like pulse oximeters and digital stethoscopes for remote monitoring to minimise face-to-face visits.
- Schedule joint telehealth appointments with specialists to enhance shared care and team communication.

25.6.3 Identify and Strengthen Community Connections

- Map the social network available to people with Long COVID, including sources of emotional, practical, informational, financial, social, recreational, advocacy, cultural, or other forms of support. Contact services or organisations to gather details about their role and referral options. Collate this into a directory to provide a valuable resource for care options, collaboration, and partnerships.
- Peer support networks, led by people with Long COVID, can be hard to access in rural or remote areas. Health professionals can support their formation, provide venues or admin assistance, and facilitate connections with new members.
- Prioritise relationship-based care by ensuring consistent access to healthcare professionals familiar with the patient's history.

25.6.4 Enhance Information Sharing

- People with Long COVID may not know who or how to ask for help. Co-produce a guide to help them describe their situation, identify needs, and share this information within the local community.
- Establish mechanisms to ensure regular communication among all interdisciplinary care team members, particularly with the GP/Family Doctor. Promote

sharing information on effective strategies, tracking data, and assessment outcomes to avoid duplication or conflicting advice.

- Create shared resources (e.g., the service directory) as a central source of information.

25.6.5 Proactively Enable Access to Care Locally and Further Afield

- Ensure people with Long COVID access available financial supports, transportation assistance, or other available assistance for rural patients.
- Explore mobile or outreach service delivery to outlying communities.

25.6.6 Provide Culturally Inclusive and Stigma-Free Care

- Use participatory approaches to engage rural and Indigenous communities in health service design and delivery.
- Offer regular community education to promote help-seeking, raise awareness, and reduce stigma.
- Incorporate culturally appropriate care, including traditional healing practices where suitable.

Rural and remote communities, like Long COVID care, evolve over time. Regularly assessing these strategies ensures they remain effective and meet the local community's needs.

BOX 25.6 PRACTICE POINT

Choose one of the recommendations above and consider how it could be implemented in your local community.

25.7 CONCLUSION

The contents and case studies of this chapter describe options for providing better care and support for people with Long COVID living in rural communities. Sadly, their lived experiences to date have hindered recovery and negatively impacted their health and wellbeing,

During the hardest bits for me, it was a lonely isolating experience. I wish I could have had access to timely consultations, genuine care and beneficial advice from within our regional health services rather than being left to flail. My diagnosis and recovery were drawn out, lonely, stigmatising and isolating. I resolved to find my own solutions. I want better for others in the future.

Sandy

This chapter highlights the inequities faced by people with Long COVID in rural and remote communities, where geographical isolation and health system constraints worsen challenges. Case studies from New South Wales and Alberta demonstrate the value of integrated care through community partnerships and technology for high-quality care access. However, there are also many relatively low-cost strategies available for rapid implementation across diverse rural communities. We can, and must, do better for people with Long COVID in rural and remote communities.

NOTES

1   WNSW-LHD respectfully acknowledges the Traditional Owners of the Country through-out Western NSW, and their continuing connection to land, water, and community. It also acknowledges the resilience of these peoples, and that their spiritual connection to Country is the foundation of health, wellbeing, and healing. The authors also acknowledge the health professionals and programme managers of WNSW-LHD for their advocacy, dedica-tion, compassion, and culturally respectful collaborative care during an extremely challeng-ing time for our community.
2   This is a pseudonym.

REFERENCES

1 Siegel FR. Introduction. In: Cities and mega-cities. SpringerBriefs in geography. Cham: Springer; 2019. doi:10.1007/978-3-319-93166-1.
2 Stewart RA. Building a rural and remote health workforce: An overview of effective inter-ventions. Med J Aust. 2023;219. doi:10.5694/mja2.52033.
3 Disler RT, et al. Rural chronic disease research patterns in the United Kingdom, United States, Canada, Australia and New Zealand: A systematic integrative review. BMC Public Health. 2019;20. doi:10.1186/s12889-020-08912-1.
4 O'Sullivan BG, et al. Outreach specialists' use of video consultations in rural Victoria: A cross-sectional survey. Rural Remote Health. 2019;19(1):4544. doi:10.22605/RRH4544.
5 Erwin C, et al. Rural and remote communities: Unique ethical issues in the COVID-19 pan-demic. Am J Bioeth. 2020;20(7):117–20. doi:10.1080/15265161.2020.1764139.
6 Rasmussen B, et al. Patient preferences using telehealth during the COVID-19 pandemic in four Victorian tertiary hospital services. Intern Med J. 2022;52:763–69. doi:10.1111/imj.15726.

7 Shilane D, et al. Declining trends in telehealth utilization in the ongoing COVID-19 pandemic. J Telemed Telecare. 2023;1357633X231202284. doi:10.1177/1357633X231202284.

8 Thomas SL, et al. Ensuring equity of access to primary health care in rural and remote Australia: What core services should be locally available? Int J Equity Health. 2015;14:111. doi:10.1186/s12939-015-0228-1.

9 Kingstone T, et al. Finding the 'right' GP: A qualitative study of the experiences of people with Long-COVID. BJGP Open. 2020;4(5):1–12. doi:10.3399/bjgpopen20X101143.

10 Kett PM, et al. Competencies, training needs, and turnover among rural compared with urban local public health practitioners: 2021 Public Health Workforce Interests and Needs Survey. Am J Public Health. 2023;113(6):689–99. doi:10.2105/AJPH.2023.307273.

11 Cortie CH, et al. The Australian health workforce: Disproportionate shortfalls in small rural towns. Aust J Rural Health. 2024; 32: 538–46. doi:10.1111/ajr.13121.

12 Parisi R, et al. Predictors and population health outcomes of persistent high GP turnover in English general practices: A retrospective observational study. BMJ Qual Saf. 2023 Jul;32(7):394–403. doi:10.1136/bmjqs-2022-015353.

13 Atherton H, et al. Long COVID and the importance of the doctor-patient relationship. B J Gen Pract. 2021 Jan 28;71(703):54–55. doi:10.3399/bjgp21X714641.

14 Russell K, et al. Fostering community engagement, participation and empowerment for mental health of adults living in rural communities: A systematic review. Rural Remote Health. 2023;23(1):7438. doi:10.22605/RRH7438.

15 Arriola KJ, et al. Understanding the relationship between social capital, health, and well-being in a southern rural population. J Rural Health. 2024;40(1):162–72. doi:10.1111/jrh.12782.

16 Jimenez MP, et al. Associations between Nature Exposure and Health: A review of the evidence. Int J Environ Res Public Health. 2021;18(9):4790. doi:10.3390/ijerph18094790.

17 Western NSW Local Health District. Western NSW Local Health District (WNSWLHD) [Internet]. Sydney: NSW Government; [cited 2025 Feb 7]. Available from: https://www.nsw.gov.au/departments-and-agencies/wnswlhd.

18 Western NSW Local Health District. About us – Western NSW Local Health District (WNSWLHD) [Internet]. Sydney: NSW Government; [cited 2025 Feb 7]. Available from: https://www.nsw.gov.au/departments-and-agencies/wnswlhd/about-us.

19 O'Connor RJ, et al. The COVID-19 Yorkshire Rehabilitation Scale (C19-YRS): Application and psychometric analysis in a post-COVID-19 syndrome cohort. J Med Virol. 2022;94(3):1027–34. doi:10.1002/jmv.27415.

20 Strasser RP, et al N. Challenges of capacity and development for health system sustainability. Healthc Pap. 2018;17(3):18–27. doi:10.12927/hcpap.2018.25505.

21 Alberta Health Services. COVID-19 inpatient and outpatient pathways: Frequently asked questions [Internet]. Edmonton: Alberta Health Services; [cited 2025 Feb 7]. Available from: https://www.albertahealthservices.ca/assets/info/ppih/if-ppih-covid-19-ipop-faq.pdf.

22 Aitken A, et al. Smartphone-based monitoring of heart rate variability and resting heart rate predicts variability in symptom exacerbations in people with complex chronic illness, 28 November 2024, Preprint (Version 1), Research Square. Available at https://doi.org/10.21203/rs.3.rs-5423422/v1.

23 Camp P, et al. Prevalence of chronic obstructive pulmonary disease (COPD) in Indigenous/ First Nations communities in Canada: A random-sampled population study. Am J Respir Crit Care Med. 2019;199(2). doi:10.1164/ajrccm-conference.2019.199.1_MeetingAbstracts. A4872.

24 Houghton N, et al. Identifying access barriers faced by rural and dispersed communities to better address their needs: Implications and lessons learned for rural proofing for health in the Americas and beyond. Rural Remote Health. 2023;23:7822. doi:10.22605/RRH7822.

25 Dudley L, et al. COVID-19 preparedness and response in rural and remote areas: A scoping review. PLoS Glob Public Health. 2023;3(11):e0002602. doi:10.1371/journal.pgph.0002602.

26 Babawarun O, et al. Healthcare managerial challenges in rural and underserved areas: A review. World J Biol Pharm Health Sci. 2024;17(2):323–30. doi:10.30574/wjbphs.2024.17.2.0087.

27 Ohta R, et al. Rural health dialogue for the sustainability of help-seeking behaviors among older patients: Grounded theory approach. BMC Geriatr. 2023;23:674. doi:10.1186/s12877-023-04401-3.

Chapter 26

Gender and Long COVID

Shaping Experiences and Outcomes

Kristy Riley, Sara Holton, Rebecca Corva, Krishna Vakil, Elle Defèin, Catherine M. Bennett, and Danielle Hitch

---

BOX 26.1   LEARNING OBJECTIVES

By the end of this chapter, readers should be able to:

- Analyse how gender influences lived experiences, healthcare access, and treatment outcomes for people with Long COVID.
- Identify the unique challenges informal carers, predominantly women, face in balancing caregiving responsibilities and their own Long COVID recovery.
- Apply an intersectional perspective to understand how social determinants of health intersect with gender to shape Long COVID experiences.
- Develop strategies for implementing gender-sensitive and inclusive practices in rehabilitation services to ensure equitable and effective care.

26.1 INTRODUCTION[1]

Sex and gender significantly influence health and wellbeing[1] and are an integral aspect of living with Long COVID. They affect disease risks, survival, physiological responses, health behaviours, healthcare access, and treatment outcomes.[1,2] Women are twice as likely as other genders to develop Long COVID, but its impact on other gender identities is less well understood.[3]

DOI: 10.4324/9781003528104-32

This chapter provides health professionals with an overview of gender's role in Long COVID, drawing on over 100 narrative interviews with people living in Australia. It acknowledges Long COVID's impact on all genders and emphasises an intersectional perspective. This discussion focuses primarily on the experiences and outcomes of women, exploring the effects of this condition on their physiological responses and social roles. Finally, it proposes recommendations for gender-inclusive Long COVID services to ensure high quality and equitable care.

26.2 UNDERSTANDING LONG COVID IN UNDERREPRESENTED GENDERS

There are many gaps in our understanding of the experience of Long COVID for men, transgender, non-binary, gender-fluid, and other gender identities; however, limited evidence suggests these groups face additional challenges. One American study found transgender, non-binary, and genderqueer people (including agender, gender-fluid, and others) are more likely to develop Long COVID and experience more significant activity limitations.[3] However, the lack of routinely collected gender identity data in COVID-19 research limits understanding of potential health disparities.[4]

To date, no research has explicitly focused on men with Long COVID, who are almost always in the minority in multi-gender studies for this condition. However, interviews with men by the authors highlighted potentially distinctive aspects of their experience, with some reluctant to seek healthcare for fear of being perceived as "weak," "cause you don't want to feel like a sook.[2] You want to go, yeah, I'm going to get through this." Others described rushing recovery and disregarding advice to slow down and rest, "I probably pushed a little bit too hard in returning to work." In their haste to return to work, some men undertook activities that worsened their symptoms: "I was like getting into baths with bath salts at the end of the day just trying to cope with the muscle fatigue. But then, you've just got to keep on pushing."

Men are less likely than other genders to access healthcare services, possibly due to cultural and societal norms about masculinity and societal expectations to be "strong" and "independent."[5] Energy conservation and pacing are vital Long COVID management strategies, so these gender stereotypes may hinder men's recovery. Men are also more likely to experience severe acute illness and require intensive care,[6] both of which are risk factors for developing Long COVID. The lower prevalence of the condition in men may, therefore, partly result from underreporting due to their avoidance of treatment.

Further investigation to fill these knowledge gaps must adopt an intersectional perspective because people with Long COVID are more than their gender. Social and political health determinants and structural inequities shape health outcomes. An intersectional approach is vital for policies and treatments that address the multidimensional nature of Long COVID experiences.[7] Health professionals should be mindful of gender while recognising it is only one aspect of the person they treat.

BOX 26.2   PRACTICE POINT

Reflect on how your gender identity has shaped your experiences, perceptions, and interactions within the healthcare system as a provider and recipient of care.

26.3 WOMEN'S EXPERIENCES OF LONG COVID

While better understood than other genders' experiences, some evidence exists about the relationship between gender and rehabilitation participation for women.[8] A scoping review of international literature found generally lower rehabilitation participation rates for women with other conditions attributed to systemic barriers, biases, sociodemographic limitations, and personal challenges.[8] Across various diagnostic groups, women experienced less physical functional gain than men but comparable mental health and social outcomes.[8] Gender is, therefore, likely to influence Long COVID rehabilitation for women at multiple levels and in diverse ways.

26.3.1 Reproductive Health for Women with Long COVID

Women with Long COVID often report gender-specific symptoms. Common issues, particularly after the Omicron wave, include changes in menstruation, cycle length, increased pain, and heavier bleeding.[9–11] Women with severe Long COVID symptoms and/or elevated cortisol levels may face a higher risk of menstrual issues.[9–11] Stress and disruption from the COVID-19 pandemic have also contributed to menstrual irregularities in the general population but are significantly more common in women with a history of COVID-19.[12] Changes to long-established menstrual cycles and other reproductive health issues can cause significant distress and disruption to the daily lives of women.[13]

Women aged 50–60 years are eight times more likely to develop Long COVID than younger women,[14] with many approaching or experiencing menopause. They may encounter overlapping symptoms from these conditions, including joint pain, migraines, irritability, and brain fog. General Practitioners (GPs) play a pivotal role in differentiating these conditions and initiating appropriate treatment strategies. While Hormone Replacement Therapy is associated with a lower likelihood of mortality from COVID-19,[15] its role in Long COVID is yet to be determined.

Premenopausal women fare better during acute infection, though evidence for oestrogen's proposed protective effect remains inconclusive.[15] Perimenopausal women with Long COVID reportedly experience more frailty-related issues (e.g., fatigue, weakness, slower walking, lower physical activity) and more significant debility than perimenopausal women who recovered from COVID-19 or the public.[16] They may present to rehabilitation with lower physical function and activity levels than peers, with one woman noting, "Many of my Long COVID symptoms are of the menopause kind of thing … I'm just not as sharp."

"The Long COVID cognitive fatigue was nothing like the brain fog I'd experienced during perimenopause. Long COVID brain fog was like the menopausal version on steroids. It would not dissipate and actually felt heavily weighted"

"You're a hormonal woman with anxiety, go away"

It's a complete caricature. Why is it so easy to dismiss? Peri, menopausal, grumpy, over educated woman who doesn't feel she's entitled to somebody's attention? Like, no, I'm a human being who's suffering diminished life quality would like some answers, please"

"There was just no way through that barrier of I'm a 40-year-old woman with anxiety and possibly hypochondria"

"I feel like autoimmune conditions are like the new hysteria. Like 'Oh, women just get that and we don't know what to do about it.'"

Figure 26.1 Perimenopausal and menopausal women's lived experience of healthcare interactions.

Global research shows perimenopausal and menopausal women face stigma and discrimination due to gender-based stereotypes about their value to the community.[17–18] Societal perceptions of menopause are influenced by factors such as culture, education, and socioeconomic status.[19] The higher prevalence of Long COVID in women and historical responses to similar conditions can contribute to commonly reported experiences of disrespect and dismissal from health professionals (Figure 26.1).

26.3.2 Accessing and Engaging with Services and Support as a Woman with Long COVID

Gender-based attitudes towards women with Long COVID can hinder their efforts to engage in collaborative treatment decision-making. Many report proactively seeking information about the condition and treatments; however, health professionals often delayed action or onward referral for many months, "When I was still battling with it five months down the track, he finally referred me to [a Long COVID clinic]." When women's proactive efforts to engage in care meet resistance or minimisation, it discourages further support-seeking and participation in rehabilitation.

Women who self-advocate are often labelled as "difficult," "hypervigilant," or "pushy," and self-advocacy by women with Long COVID should not be a prerequisite for receiving care anyway, especially given its additional draw on limited physical and mental resources. Many were angry and frustrated at having to educate health professionals about the conditions, introducing an unfamiliar power dynamic to therapeutic relationships, "Actually I'm not going to sit here and educate you. I probably should for the poor person who comes after me, but it's not my job…." This was particularly true for women with experience in more established areas of healthcare, "I had a cancer scare and ended up in oncology world. Oh my god was it different – I got care which was collaborative. It highlighted a big difference in care and societies understanding."

BOX 26.3   PRACTICE POINT

How would you rate your current knowledge of Long COVID? Do you evaluate your patient's existing knowledge of their condition during assessment? How do you respond if your patient provides information or recommendations they have sourced themselves?

Women with Long COVID often regretted these lost opportunities for earlier intervention, as their persistence in seeking treatment was driven by a desire to prevent problems from becoming entrenched. They also reflected on the impact and costs of not receiving timely care on the broader community.

> *Where they're losing money that they could be saving it is when someone goes into the system and they have long COVID and they're spat back out and they go in and out, in and out, in and out. Every time we go to the GP (General Practitioner), we're taking $70 from Medicare ... I took probably $3,000 from Medicare and was not helped.*

Women disengage from Long COVID health services and support for various reasons, but a perceived lack of respect for their lived experience from health professionals was often the catalyst, "I recently walked out of a doctor's appointment, because I'm so sick of them not listening – I've been so patient and well behaved, it's so out of character for me." Health professionals who disregarded lived experience were seen as arrogant and uncaring, causing women to lose confidence in their skills. Such failures in therapeutic relationships had serious consequences for access to care, with one woman from a rural community opting to travel long distances to avoid her local health service,

> *It was so similar to when I had Guillain Barre... and [the doctors were] just like, 'Oh no, nup, nah, you don't have it'. I thought, how can you tell? ... so [service name] is not high on my list of places to go.*

BOX 26.4   PRACTICE POINT

Consider how you currently work with women with Long COVID and/or other conditions in your rehabilitation service.

- How might societal and cultural gender expectations impact their experience of your service?
- How do they influence your professional responsibilities and roles?
- What systemic changes would you propose to improve healthcare equity for women with Long COVID or similar conditions?
- How could you collaborate with others to address care gaps and health inequities for women?

26.4 INFORMAL CARERS AND LONG COVID

People with Long COVID may need support from informal (unpaid) carers or be carers themselves. Anyone can provide unpaid care to family, friends, or community members. However, 80% of informal carers are women, reflecting societal expectations and gender roles across many cultures.[20] Women aged 45–65 years are particularly affected, balancing work with caregiving responsibilities.[21] Many in this age group, coinciding with Long COVID's peak prevalence, are "compound carers" who care for multiple people, such as children and elderly parents.[22]

Long COVID detrimentally affects carer duties, impacting COVID-19 recovery in many ways. Motherhood, a highly valued yet demanding role for many women, may positively or adversely affect health and wellbeing.[23] Long COVID significantly impacts all parenting tasks, not just physically demanding ones, as described by one woman with young children, "I become breathless after reading a couple of pages of my kid's storybooks at night."

Experiences of acute COVID-19 infection can have lingering effects on mental health and wellbeing. One woman described being told to ween her baby early, which made her "feel terrible." She felt ongoing guilt and distress about being unable to contribute to childcare during quarantine, perceiving it as another example of failing as a mother. Mothering was a meaningful role in her life, but her COVID-19 experiences dented her self-efficacy and decreased her self-confidence going forward.

> Got a four year old, and a one year old, and that was pretty horrific. Hearing all of them crying …. not being able to see them, my husband breaking down and not being able to support him.

Another mother mentioned her need to be a "good mother" feeling her Long COVID symptoms hindered her from meeting this standard: "Makes it very hard to be a mother and supervise children and be a good parent, when you can't even be in the same room as them." In many cultures, mothers are expected to be attentive, loving, and devoted to their children, subordinating personal needs for their family's good.[24] They are acutely aware of Long COVID's impact on their children,

> My son constantly asks when I'll get better. He has unfortunately seen paramedics doing things to my heart and taking me away in an ambulance.

> *He's seen the most active member of the family become someone who lays in bed a lot.*

Mothers of children with disabilities felt extra pressure to maintain parenting duties, often lacking realistic alternatives, "If I'm too sick to look after my son and he's got care needs every day … you've just got to soldier on the best you can." This was exacerbated by experiences of trying to arrange alternative carers, which required significant but often fruitless effort,

> *I'm a single mum, I don't have family to help me…They managed to be able to get somebody in a week and a half later. But the person was completely and utterly useless … I had to keep getting up to actually show her 'this is where the back door is, this is where the power point is'. So, we battled on. I can't supervise my kids really properly. Can't engage with them really. There's been so much that I've needed help with.*

Parents with Long COVID, particularly those with young children, also face higher risks of reinfection (see Chapter 2) through exposure via family-related social contacts and environments.[25] For example, school environments may carry a higher risk of COVID-19 transmission, particularly when poorly ventilated and in physical activities like group singing and exercising.[26,27] They may also be exposed in their workplaces, and withdrawal from paid employment can have significant financial consequences for the entire family (see Chapter 20).

BOX 26.5   PRACTICE POINT

Do you discuss reinfection risks with people with Long COVID who are also parents? Could your rehabilitation service provide information about environmental interventions, such as High Efficiency Particulate Air filters and masking, to support Long COVID recovery?

The experiences and needs of the unpaid carers of children with Long COVID remain largely invisible, though some research is beginning to emerge. Long COVID in children has a profound impact on families, and these carers experience emotional strain, logistical challenges, and many systemic barriers.[28,29] The carers of young people with Long COVID may feel guilt and uncertainty about the help they are providing in the context of uncertainty around what best supports their child's health needs.

It has a flow on effect because the kids are anxious because they don't understand what's going on. It impacts their education, their health because mums are having to help them and stuff. That's a hell of a lot of pressure.

Many turned to online forums, private healthcare, or alternative therapies for support and solutions. They are best placed to observe and report the impact of symptoms like brain fog and fatigue on their child's life but often struggle with navigating healthcare systems and securing appropriate care. The mothers of children with Long COVID may also have the condition themselves, given the significant association between symptoms reported between both groups.[30]

While pacing and energy conservation are effective strategies for managing Long COVID, the carer duties of many women made them impossible to enact. Historically, self-prioritisation has been discouraged for women, and those perceived to put their own needs first are often judged harshly.[31] These stereotypes and expectations particularly harm recovery and management for women with Long COVID.

I don't think I knew the word for slow down. So, I probably didn't rest. I wonder if that means women are not allowed to rest, we are burned out prior to COVID hitting us from carrying so much load, and then when it hits us—bang? I wish I could warn people.

Long COVID also affects women's capacity to care for other family members, including elderly parents or relatives. This may involve assisting with daily activities, managing medication, coordinating care, providing emotional support, and navigating changing parent–child power dynamics.[32,33] Informal caregivers face burdens impacting their health and wellbeing, which, for people with Long COVID, is already compromised.[34]

I'm in the process of working out mums' estate ... I'm having difficulties focusing or not focusing, concentrating on doing the paperwork component or committing to doing that.

BOX 26.7 AMIRA'S[3] EXPERIENCE

There's so much individual focus on pacing and care and pressure on the individual from health professionals without much thought for how that would look and work for families. At times medical professionals have said "why does pacing seem so hard for you" and, as my beautiful sister-in-law said, "because I want to live my life."

Think about it, most of us get fed up with being home for a week when we have COVID or the flu, but this is now what happens to people with Long COVID. Our whole life is pacing, we lay around isolated most of our lives. It's not fun, it's boring, and it's probably the hardest thing you can do psychologically.

It also does not take into account that pacing means not living at times, like not attending family events. There's not enough family support to help with housework and I've had to abandon gardening. No assistance with attending appointments, school pickups, or activities for kids when a parent becomes unwell with Long COVID. Even for simple things, like if my son wants a friend over from school. The house needs to have the most basic level of tidiness, and that's hard with pacing for Long COVID.

You become invisible due to Long COVID. All the things and ways one would have community are gone, like school parents don't see you at the gates, neighbours don't see you out, you can't attend book club anymore, or the workplace drinks, or friends' parties. For most folks, it's out of sight, out of mind.

BOX 26.8 PRACTICE POINT

How do Amira's childcare responsibilities and family support impact her ability to use recommended pacing strategies? How could you foster discussions and actions around family-based support systems and realistic care plans to sustain (but adapt) her caregiving? How can rehabilitation plans address the ripple effects of Long COVID on the patient, their family, and community? What local or community resources can help Amira care for herself and others?

The impact of Long COVID on women extends to those for whom she provides care. The following commentary illustrates the number of people directly and indirectly affected when a woman has Long COVID.

26.5 RECOMMENDATIONS FOR GENDER INCLUSIVE LONG COVID CARE

Based on lived and professional experience and current evidence, we recommend the following actions for rehabilitation services to enable gender-inclusive Long COVID care. These aim to ensure all patients receive tailored, compassionate, and effective treatment, regardless of gender identity.

26.5.1 Upskill the Workforce on Gender Impacts in Long COVID

Train health professionals on recognising gender biases, vulnerabilities across genders, and gender intersections with other social determinants of health (e.g., ethnicity, socioeconomic, carer status).[3,35] Provide practice-based materials and workshops addressing gender-specific Long COVID rehabilitation challenges and strategies.

26.5.2 Embed Gender-Inclusive Practice Into Organisational Standards

Incorporate gender-sensitive practices, such as gender-neutral language, into policies, procedures, and guidelines.

26.5.3 Adopt an Open-Door Approach to Discussing Gender and Sexuality

Respect patient preferences and proceed only with explicit consent. If the person with Long COVID prefers not to discuss these topics, advise they are welcome to revisit them later. Ensure a safe, confidential, and welcoming environment for these conversations.

26.5.4 Ensure Rehabilitation Meets the Gender-Specific Needs of Each Person with Long COVID

Gender-specific interventions may address reproductive health for women or promote service engagement for men. Tailored approaches (e.g., women's cardiac rehabilitation groups) can enhance engagement, improve outcome and address cultural and societal gender expectations influencing recovery.

For example, health professionals could provide written "prescriptions" for rest or assistance with household tasks that specify rest periods or recommend outsourcing physically demanding activities. These documents can validate the need for support in the context of societal expectations and encourage co-parents and family members to share responsibilities. This strategy can also inform a structured framework for managing energy limitations and foster sustainable recovery strategies.

26.5.5 Include and Address Caregiving Duties in Rehabilitation Programmes

Provide targeted interventions for informal caregivers, focusing on women balancing caregiving, work, and Long COVID symptoms. Facilitate access to respite care, mental health support, and carer resources for people with Long COVID and their families.

26.5.6 Provide Accessible and Flexible Rehabilitation

Design services accommodating caregiving responsibilities with telehealth, flexible hours, and childcare support. Ensure geographic and financial accessibility through initiatives like outreach clinics in community facilities.

26.5.7 Community-Based Support and Peer Networks

Foster gender-inclusive peer support and community programmes to reduce isolation, mitigate marginalisation, and give practical support to Long COVID patients.

26.5.8 Data Collection and Research

Standardise gender identity data collection in Long COVID services and research to identify disparities and inform interventions. Include optional questions on sex, gender identity, and pronouns in intake forms. Include under-represented groups (e.g., men, transgender, non-binary, gender-fluid people) in research to understand their experiences.

BOX 26.9   PRACTICE POINT

Has your rehabilitation service implemented any recommended practices? Select one that is not currently in use and discuss with colleagues how to introduce it.

26.6 CONCLUSION

This chapter highlights the pivotal role of gender in Long COVID experiences and treatment. Women, the majority of those affected, face challenges intensified by societal expectations around caregiving and personal sacrifice. These are especially evident in caregiving roles, where demands often exceed energy limitations. Systemic barriers are the key drivers of health inequity and are compounded by our currently limited knowledge about the gender-specific needs of men, transgender, non-binary, and other gender identities. Adopting recommendations proposed for gender inclusive Long COVID care will support more effective care and better outcomes for all people with Long COVID.

NOTES

1   In this chapter, the terms 'man' and 'woman' refers to people assigned that gender at birth, with affirmed gender or identifying as that gender.
2   In Australian English, a 'sook' is a person perceived to be overly sensitive, who whines and complains about minor problems.
3   'Amira' is a pseudonym.

REFERENCES

1   Peters SAE, et al. Sex and gender reporting in global health: New editorial policies. BMJ Glob Health. 2018;3(4):e001038. doi:10.1136/bmjgh-2018-001038.
2   Cooper D, et al. Women, men, and health. In: Detels R, Karim QA, Baum F, editors. Oxford textbook of global public health. Oxford University Press; 2021. p. 415–30. doi:10.1093/med/9780198816805.003.0085.
3   Cohen J, et al. An intersectional analysis of Long COVID prevalence. Int J Equity Health. 2023;22(1):261. doi:10.1186/s12939-023-02072-5.
4   Babu TM, et al. Health equity necessitates the inclusion of gender identity data in COVID-19 clinical trials. Ann Epidemiol. 2023;85:3–5. doi:10.1016/j.annepidem.2023.06.024.
5   Vandello JA, et al. Precarious manhood and men's health disparities. In: Men's Health Equity. Routledge; 2019. p. 27–41. doi:10.4324/9781315167428-3.
6   Chaturvedi R, et al. COVID-19 complications in males and females: Recent developments. J Comp Eff Res. 2022;11(9):689–98. doi:10.2217/cer-2022-0027.
7   Ryan NE, et al. A call for a gender-responsive, intersectional approach to address COVID-19. Glob Public Health. 2020;15(9):1404–12. doi:10.1080/17441692.2020.1791214.
8   Ott J, et al. Scoping 'sex' and 'gender' in rehabilitation: (Mis)representations and effects. Int J Equity Health. 2022;21:179. doi:10.1186/s12939-022-01787-1.
9   Sakurada Y, et al. Clinical characteristics of female Long COVID patients with menstrual symptoms: A retrospective study from a Japanese outpatient clinic. J Psychosom Obstet Gynaecol. 2024;45(1):2305899. doi:10.1080/0167482X.2024.2305899.

10 Błażejewski G, et al. The impact of COVID-19 on the menstrual cycle in women. J Clin Med. 2023;12:4991. doi:10.3390/jcm12154991.

11 Lebar V, et al. The effect of COVID-19 on the menstrual cycle: A systematic review. J Clin Med. 2022;11:3800. doi:10.3390/jcm11133800.

12 Danesh L, et al. The effects of SARS-CoV-2 on menstruation. Reprod Biomed Online. 2021;43:769. doi:10.1016/j.rbmo.2021.08.014.

13 Pollack B, et al. Female reproductive health impacts of Long COVID and associated illnesses including ME/CFS, POTS, and connective tissue disorders: A literature review. Front Rehabil Sci. 2023;4:1122673. doi:10.3389/fresc.2023.1122673.

14 Akbari A, et al. Incidence and outcomes associated with menopausal status in COVID-19 patients: A systematic review and meta-analysis. Rev Bras Ginecol Obstet. 2023;45(12):e796–807. doi:10.1055/s-0043-1772595.

15 Sakulpaisal M, et al. The effects of exogenous estrogen in women with SAR-CoV-2 infection: A systematic review and meta-analysis. Hum Reprod. 2023;38(6):1111–23. doi:10.1093/humrep/dead074.

16 Navas-Otero A, et al. Characteristics of frailty in perimenopausal women with Long COVID-19. Healthcare. 2023;11(10):1468. doi:10.3390/healthcare11101468.

17 Li Q, et al. "They see me as mentally ill": The stigmatisation experiences of Chinese menopausal women in the family. BMC Womens Health. 2023;23. doi:10.1186/s12905-023-02193-5.

18 Rowson TS, et al. Hot topic: Examining discursive representations of menopause and work in the British media. Gender Work Organ. 2023. doi:10.1111/gwao.12889.

19 Dashti S, et al. Influencing factors on women's attitudes toward menopause: A systematic review. Menopause. 2021;28:1192–200. doi:10.1097/GME.0000000000001833.

20 Cascella Carbó GF, et al. Burden and gender inequalities around informal care. Investig Educ Enferm. 2020;38(1):e10. doi:10.17533/udea.iee.v38n1e10.

21 Oldridge L. Hidden care(e)rs: Supporting informal carers in the workplace. In: Nachmias S, Caven V, editors. Inequality and organisational practice. Cham: Palgrave Macmillan; 2019. p. 105–27. doi:10.1007/978-3-030-11647-7_5.

22 Wang F, et al. Health of aging families: Comparing compound and noncompound caregivers. Innov Aging. 2021;5:104. doi:10.1093/geroni/igab046.397.

23 Dehos F, et al. Time of change: Health effects of motherhood. IZA Discussion Paper No. 16942. doi:10.2139/ssrn.4805545.

24 Schmidt E, et al. What makes a good mother? Two decades of research reflecting social norms of motherhood. J Fam Theory Rev. 2022;15:57–77. doi:10.1111/jftr.12488.

25 Faux-Nightingale A, et al. Experiences and care needs of children with Long COVID: A qualitative study. BJGP Open. 2023;8. doi:10.3399/BJGPO.2023.0143.

26 Buonsenso D, et al. Clinical characteristics, activity levels and mental health problems in children with Long COVID: A survey of 510 children. Future Microbiol. 2022;17(8):577–88. doi:10.2217/fmb-2021-0285.

27 Bertran M, et al. Association between parents experiencing ongoing problems from COVID-19 and adolescents reporting Long COVID six months after a positive or negative SARS-CoV-2 PCR test: Prospective, national cohort study in England. SSRN Electron J. 2022. doi:10.2139/ssrn.4192732.

28 Downing L. Selfish Women. 1st ed. London: Routledge; 2019. doi:10.4324/9780429285349.

29 Ben-Isaac E, et al. When the physician becomes the caregiver: A review for physicians caring for their elder relatives. Pediatr Rev. 2021;42:405–13. doi:10.1542/pir.2020-002006.

30 Palacios J, et al. The experience of caring for an older relative in Chile: Going beyond the burden of care. Ageing Soc. 2020;42:1340–59. doi:10.1017/S0144686X20001567.

31 Kirvalidze M, et al. Variability in perceived burden and health trajectories among older caregivers: A population-based study in Sweden. J Epidemiol Community Health. 2022;77:125–32. doi:10.1136/jech-2022-219095.

32 Lindsay S, et al. Challenges with providing gender-sensitive care: Exploring experiences within pediatric rehabilitation hospital. Disabil Rehabil. 2020;44:891–89. doi:10.1080/09638288.2020.1781939.

33 Caughey AB, et al. USPSTF approach to addressing sex and gender when making recommendations for clinical preventive services. JAMA. 2021;326(19):1953–61. doi:10.1001/jama.2021.15731.

34 Ghisi GL, et al. Women-focused cardiovascular rehabilitation: An International Council of Cardiovascular Prevention and Rehabilitation Clinical Practice Guideline. Can J Cardiol. 2022;38(12):1786–98. doi:10.1016/j.cjca.2022.06.021.

35 Colantonio A. Sex and gender reporting in rehabilitation research: A commentary. Arch Phys Med Rehabil. 2023;104(8):1356–58. doi:10.1016/j.apmr.2023.03.034.

Chapter 27

The Social and Political Contexts of Long COVID

Deborah Lupton and Gemma Carey

BOX 27.1   LEARNING OBJECTIVES

By the end of this chapter, readers should be able to:

- Describe the social and political contexts of the lived experience of Long COVID.
- Explain how these contexts may have a detrimental impact on people with Long COVID.
- Highlight the important role played by the Long COVID patient community in advocating for better understanding and treatment from healthcare workers.

27.1 INTRODUCTION

From the beginning, Long COVID, like COVID itself, has been a social and political as well as a medical phenomenon. The management of both COVID and Long COVID is characterised by struggles for disadvantaged social groups to achieve recognition and better care. With rare exceptions, the management of the pandemic by governments and peak health bodies across the world has been chaotic, primarily driven by short-term political and economic imperatives and with little regard for supporting marginalised social groups.[1–3] Anti-science sentiment and denial of the continuing risks posed by COVID have begun to dominate government and public forums,[4] even while the World Health Organization still characterises COVID as a "pandemic" and waves of infection are still impacting countries around the world.[5] Continuing COVID infections and re-infections are placing greater numbers of people at risk of developing Long COVID.[6]

DOI: 10.4324/9781003528104-33

The COVID pandemic has brought many long-term struggles related to health inequalities and socioeconomic disadvantage into the spotlight. For this reason, the pandemic has been described as a "syndemic": a synthesis of an outbreak of infectious disease with other health conditions that are linked to socioeconomic disadvantage.[7] Long COVID could also be described as a syndemic. Members of certain social groups are at higher risk of developing Long COVID, due to a combination of inequalities and long-standing marginalisation. A UK-based study identified that people with multiple indicators of social disadvantage were more likely to experience prolonged symptoms of COVID-19.[8] One US study found that Long COVID was more common among adults under 65 years, women, American Indian or Alaska Native or other/multi race group, smokers, and people with a disability, depression, overweight, or obesity.[9] Other research from the United States found marked disparities in awareness of Long COVID among social groups of different race/ethnicities after controlling for education and income levels. While there was low overall awareness across the groups, awareness of the condition was lowest among Hispanic respondents with limited English proficiency, suggesting that they were missing out on educational materials about Long COVID.[10]

BOX 27.2 SYNDEMIC

The bio-social combination of illnesses, diseases, and socioeconomic vulnerabilities that synergistically interact to render a disease outbreak even more serious in certain social groups or populations.[7]

27.2 THE POWER OF PATIENT-GENERATED KNOWLEDGE

In many ways, the knowledge base and public awareness that has built up around Long COVID represents the power of patient communities to identify and name a novel health condition and to achieve medical recognition of it. These communities are often fighting ignorance and lack of interest among healthcare professionals. The initial discussions of what came to be known as "Long Haul COVID" or "Long COVID" began early in the pandemic, when some of the first people to have been infected by the novel coronavirus began to recognise that their symptoms were not improving weeks or months after the initial acute infection. Building on the social networking offered by online platforms and drawing on the "insider" expert knowledge of medical and allied health professionals who themselves were experiencing prolonged COVID symptoms, advocates and activists were quickly able to gain attention to their cause.[11–13]

Social media platforms such as Facebook and X/Twitter and other online forums and information sources were vital to this effort, enabling exchange of information quickly across the globe. As early as March 2020, patients began discussing their long-term symptoms after an acute COVID infection on social media. The term "long hauler" was first used on Facebook in April by a teacher in the United States, Amy Watson, who wore a trucker's cap in a selfie photo to refer to "long haul truckers" (those who work long shifts), as an analogy to the long-term illness she was experiencing. She realised that she was not recovering as she had expected and started a Facebook group as a support group for others in the same situation. Several other Facebook groups have since developed, some with thousands of members. There are numerous other groups on other social media platforms providing information and support to those with the condition.

Another key moment in the definition and public awareness of the condition was the first use of "Long COVID" as a hashtag on X/Twitter in May 2020 by patient activist and academic Elisa Perego. Perego argues that Long COVID may well have been the first illness created through patients finding each other on that platform (see Chapter 4).[13] By using online platforms such as social media, online surveys and making videos, and blog posts, patients were quickly able to collect and share evidence, and organise advocacy and activist efforts, even while they were struggling with the debilitating symptoms of Long COVID. For example, a video made by the "Long COVID SOS" advocacy group about their experiences, uploaded to YouTube in July 2020, received so much public attention that representatives from the group were invited to a meeting by the World Health Organization's COVID-19 response team.[13] Figure 27.1 shows a timeline of how these patient-led contributions led to heightened awareness and recognition of Long COVID as a major medical condition.

BOX 27.3 PRACTICE POINT

Reflect on your own attitudes as a health professional working with people with Long COVID. Do you accept their version of their illness and their lived experience expertise? Are you familiar with the latest patient-generated research on Long COVID? How might this inform your work with these patients?

Patient Contributions to Long COVID Knowledge

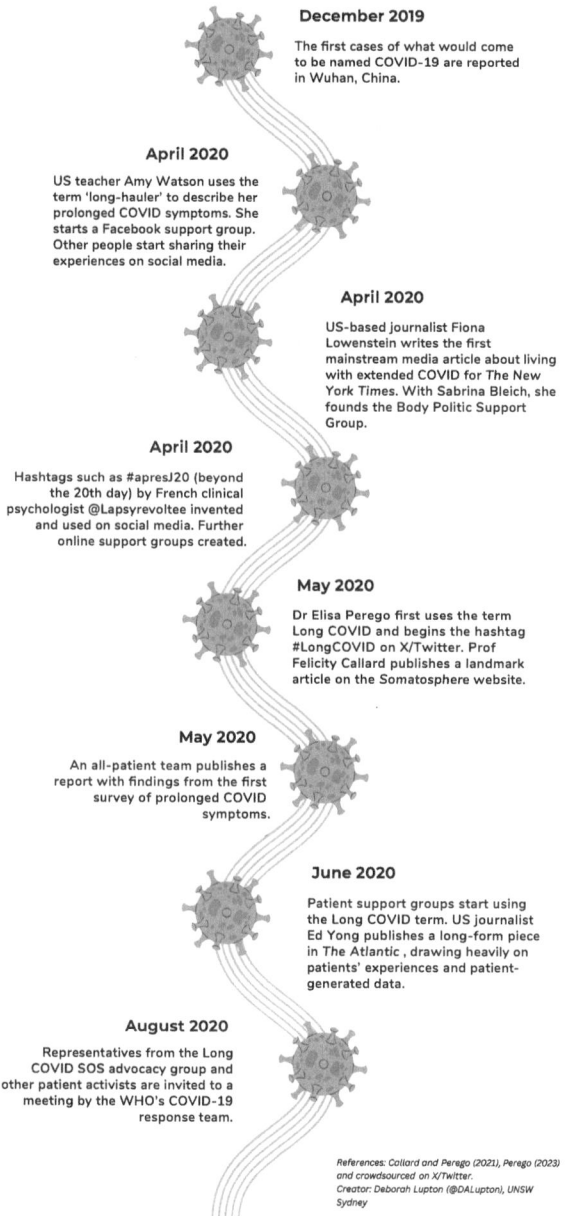

December 2019

The first cases of what would come to be named COVID-19 are reported in Wuhan, China.

April 2020

US teacher Amy Watson uses the term 'long-hauler' to describe her prolonged COVID symptoms. She starts a Facebook support group. Other people start sharing their experiences on social media.

April 2020

US-based journalist Fiona Lowenstein writes the first mainstream media article about living with extended COVID for The New York Times. With Sabrina Bleich, she founds the Body Politic Support Group.

April 2020

Hashtags such as #apresJ20 (beyond the 20th day) by French clinical psychologist @Lapsyrevoltee invented and used on social media. Further online support groups created.

May 2020

Dr Elisa Perego first uses the term Long COVID and begins the hashtag #LongCOVID on X/Twitter. Prof Felicity Callard publishes a landmark article on the Somatosphere website.

May 2020

An all-patient team publishes a report with findings from the first survey of prolonged COVID symptoms.

June 2020

Patient support groups start using the Long COVID term. US journalist Ed Yong publishes a long-form piece in The Atlantic , drawing heavily on patients' experiences and patient-generated data.

August 2020

Representatives from the Long COVID SOS advocacy group and other patient activists are invited to a meeting by the WHO's COVID-19 response team.

References: Callard and Perego (2021), Perego (2023) and crowdsourced on X/Twitter.
Creator: Deborah Lupton (@DALupton), UNSW Sydney

Figure 27.1 Patient contributions to Long COVID knowledge. © 2024 Deborah Lupton.

27.3 THE LIVED EXPERIENCE OF LONG COVID

Numerous studies have demonstrated the impacts on quality of life and social relationships experienced by people with Long COVID. They can often feel too unwell to take an active part in everyday tasks or study, contribute to family and friendship relationships, and engage in the leisure, exercise, and social activities that they once enjoyed.[14] Consequently, loneliness and feelings of social isolation are common.[15] People with Long COVID face major challenges to their identities, sense of self and social roles caused by the chronic nature of Long COVID and its uncertain prognosis.[16,17] Their work can be severely disrupted, leading to loss of employment, diminished income, and financial distress.[15,18] People with Long COVID have faced intense discrimination from both the medical profession and their friends and family.[19,20] Due to a lack of validation from others, they frequently experience self-doubt about the nature and severity of their illness,[21] as well as feelings of shame and social stigma.[22,23]

BOX 27.4   SOCIAL STIGMA

The discrimination and prejudice directed towards people or social groups by others in society. People who are the targets of social stigma often feel devalued and marginalised by others, even feeling they are outcasts.[24]

27.4 THE CRISIS OF EXPERTISE

There has been a "crisis of expertise" around issues of diagnosing and treating Long COVID.[25] Numerous studies have demonstrated that medical support is often still inadequate for people with Long COVID. Several years into the pandemic, many people with Long COVID continue to report experiencing difficulties in finding appropriate healthcare or healthcare practitioners who take their health problems seriously. These problems are largely due to medical ignorance and power imbalances in the healthcare system.[11,25,26] People seeking help have often been treated with "medical gaslighting" and told that "it's all in their heads," leading to feeling betrayed by the medical profession.[23,25] Even those people with Long COVID who are medical practitioners or other healthcare professionals have had to fight against disbelief from others in the healthcare system when seeking validation of their illness.[27]

Diagnosis of Long COVID has proved a particularly fraught area – both in the early stages of the pandemic and into the current era. Early confusion among medical professionals is unsurprising, given the novelty of COVID-19 itself. However, the pandemic has continued to spread globally, with infections and reinfections leading to growing numbers of people experiencing long-term symptoms after their acute illnesses. Even at this later stage of the pandemic, expert bodies have differed in how they are defining the condition of Long COVID and have used often clashing assumptions when doing so. It has been difficult to establish a clear biomarker for Long COVID, and the list of associated symptoms is long. As a consequence, medical practitioners frequently dispute people with Long COVID's claims to serious illness or disability.[28] Long COVID has been often characterised as a "mental illness" or "psychogenic" condition in the medical literature.[28] Some psychiatrists have even made comparisons with "hysteria" and "neurasthenia" (see, for example, a controversial opinion piece by Little and colleagues).[29]

27.5 MINORITISED COMMUNITIES AND LONG COVID

Entrenched socioeconomic disadvantaged and marginalisation intensifies the social impacts of Long COVID. Intersectional analyses indicate that women, some people of colour, sexual and gender minorities, and those without university degrees are more likely to have Long COVID and experience activity limitations due to the condition.[30] A UK study[31] included people with Long COVID from ethnically minoritised and other minoritised communities. These participants, who were already experiencing health inequalities, were further facing misrecognition, invalidation, and uncertainty. This was particularly the case for the process and categorisation of Long COVID diagnosis. Research investigating Black Americans' experiences of Long COVID found that social disadvantage interfered with symptom management and many participants experienced lack of acknowledgement from others concerning their illness.[32]

A problem with this kind of characterisation is that people outside the category of "women," or those from ethnic/racial minorities who are also under-recognised in Long COVID diagnoses, are excluded from adequate healthcare and social support.[25,28,31] The higher numbers of women reporting Long COVID symptoms compared with men have led medical experts to suggest that these responses are consistent with entrenched medical sexism and misogyny, similar to how "hysteria" and "neurasthenia" were defined as "women's problems" in earlier eras.[28]

27.6 PATIENT ACTIVISM INITIATIVES

In the absence of health promotion or prevention expertise, patient activist groups have engaged in public campaigns to raise awareness of the risks of poor COVID management and the importance of recognising how continuing infections can affect the body. One example is the International Long COVID Awareness initiative,[33] involving patients, healthcare providers, and allies. Members of this community activist group have created videos and graphics for posters, social media, and stickers as open access resources downloadable from their website, as well as links to related merchandise, such as pins, wristbands, t-shirts, and caps, designed and sold by members of the Long COVID community (see Figure 27.2 for an example).

This group has created Long COVID Awareness month (March every year) and International Long COVID Awareness Day (15 March every year) to organise advocacy and activism efforts, including protests and online activities. Their work seeks to draw attention to the need to prevent Long COVID with strong COVID protections, such as mass masking, testing, and the provision of clean air infrastructure. It also addresses the lack of medical care, treatments, and welfare support for people with Long COVID, as well as the discrimination, marginalisation, and stigma they experience. The Long COVID tricolour awareness ribbon (shown in the graphic in Figure 27.2), designed by first wave Long COVID patient Tracey Thompson, features grey to represent loss and grief, teal for hope and support, and black for loneliness and isolation. These activities have gone at least some way to highlighting the social impacts of Long COVID among the general population in a context in which public health messaging about the condition is extremely limited.

BOX 27.5   PRACTICE POINT

How can you contribute to and amplify patient initiatives to raise awareness of Long COVID among the communities or co-workers with whom you interact as part of your professional practice?

27.7 THE IMPORTANCE OF THE "LONG COVID" TERMINOLOGY

Despite all these patient-led initiatives, there is concerning evidence that hard-won recognition of the social and health impacts of Long COVID achieved since the outbreak of the pandemic is beginning to erode. Over time, the social trajectory of Long COVID has changed dramatically. Adopting the term Long COVID has provided a sense of identity for people living with the condition. The visibility of this term in the news media and the medical literature due to patient activism has transformed how it is perceived among clinicians and policymakers.[34] However, there is still evidence of a backlash from some medical and public health authorities who claim

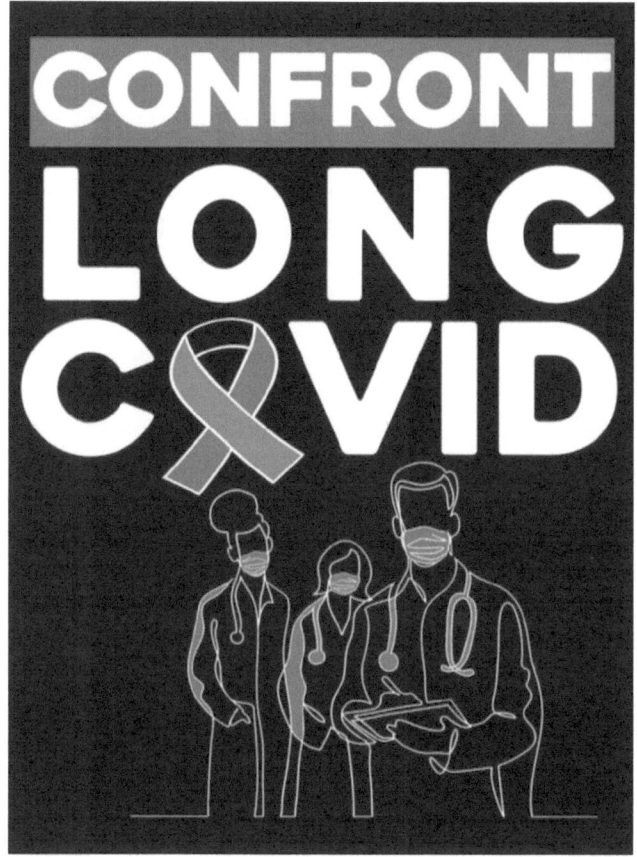

Figure 27.2 Activist graphic showing the tricolour Long COVID awareness ribbon. "Confront-Med" by Long COVID Awareness is licensed under CC0 1.0 Universal (https://creativecommons.org/publicdomain/zero/1.0/).

that Long COVID is no different from any other post-viral condition.[35] Furthermore, several medical professionals and government agencies have made the decision to replace the term Long COVID with medicalised terms such as "post-acute sequelae of COVID"[36]: thereby denying the patient-made and preferred terminology for their own condition.

These processes have been described as "medical silencing," in which members of the medical profession and other healthcare workers use their authority to prevent people from marginalised groups to be able to have a voice and find the help and support they need. Medical silencing is often combined with other forms of discrimination such as racism and misogyny.[37] People with contested or invisible health conditions have frequently been subjected to this form of abuse of medical authority.[37-39] Across the years of the pandemic, medical silencing has limited the scope of patient agency. Medical silencing has undermined Long COVID communities' attempts to demonstrate the expert knowledge they have accumulated from years of generating information about their own condition, sharing it with other patients, the medical profession, and the broader community, and advocating for better recognition, research, and therapies. The power and authority held by the medical profession has proved to be a constant and persistent barrier to achieving these objectives.

In a sociopolitical climate in which the risks of the continuing COVID-19 pandemic are routinely ignored by governments, healthcare systems, and public health agencies, it is likely that the number of people living with Long COVID will continue to grow. As demonstrated in this chapter, existing socioeconomic disadvantage is magnified by the experience of living with Long COVID. Until health professionals can listen more carefully and openly to people with Long COVID, acknowledge their expertise and authority on their own illness and work with them to achieve better healthcare and support, people with Long COVID are likely to face continuing discrimination, stigma, and marginalisation. Part of this process is recognising and acknowledging the social and political contexts in which people with under-diagnosed and under-recognised illnesses are routinely treated in healthcare settings and working to challenge these continuing inequalities.

27.8 LIVED EXPERIENCE COMMENTARY: GEMMA CAREY

I suffered with a form of Long COVID for approximately three years. Even as a Professor of Public Health, I struggled to find answers, appropriate medical care and support for my disabling condition. I was given many incorrect diagnoses, which often placed my physical symptoms (including chronic pain and seizures) in a psychological framing. So called 'functional' diagnoses plague Long Covid patients; the poor medical understanding of the condition to date has led much of the medical profession to re-tread 'hysteria' narratives of disease.

The experiences of having Long COVID and the stories of other patients I heard while embedded in the Long COVID community will mark me for life. Critically, I have learnt that the severity of the disease is matched by social, political and medical ostracism. Few other diseases leave individuals so severely disabled and sick that they are bedbound, unable to tolerate so much as a shard of light or the physical presence of another person, while subject to systemic attacks for being 'fakers', or having very serious physical symptoms dismissed as psychosomatic.

The broader political project of silencing the chronic aspects of the pandemic is translating into different forms of abuse for people with Long COVID, ranging from medical gaslighting to intimate and family violence. It is not uncommon, for example, for the families of bedbound Long Covid patients to believe broader social and medical narratives of psychosomatic illness and withhold basic food and hygiene from severely bedbound patients in an effort to get their family member to walk. Some people with Long COVID have been subjected to intimate partner violence.[40] Here we see that political inaction combined with societal desires to 'move on' from COVID risks the lives of people with Long COVID. If I as a privileged middle class, tertiary educated woman experience both interpersonal and systemic gaslighting, the experiences of those who are marginalised or individuals with cross cutting, or intersectional, marginalities are no doubt devastatingly exclusionary. This is particularly concerning when we know the burden of Long COVID falls disproportionately on these individuals and communities.

As pointed out earlier in this chapter, while those with Long COVID are discriminated against and met with a paucity of understanding of their condition, they nonetheless have demonstrated considerable agency and action around their own disease. The Long COVID community is informed, knowledgeable about their condition and increasingly organised; an extraordinary achievement for a collective in which having less than one functional hour a day is not uncommon.[41] This knowledge creation and social rights movement is driven predominately by necessity. In the absence of good medical support, online groups and networks have become the main place in which individuals share information about experiences, treatments and potential avenues for cure. Many people receive more information about their condition and how to manage it from such sources than they do from formalised healthcare.[42] We would do well to listen and listen deeply to these online forums, as well as individuals who have Long COVID.

These online groups, and the considerable knowledge and disease expertise contained within them, now form an important resource not just for individuals, but for those working in healthcare. There is a long history in a range of research fields that has demonstrated that patient experiences are critical to understanding and treating diseases: never more so when a disease is poorly understood or new, such as Long COVID. This began in the HIV pandemic and can be seen today in the disability justice movement, both of which have fought fiercely for the principles of 'nothing about us without us'.[43,44]

Critically, these two rights movements have demonstrated that we need to see patients with complex or emerging diseases as 'peers' in the scientific and medical processes. The need for this is twofold. First, the severity of suffering amongst those of us with Long Covid means that time is of the essence; many are too sick, or their quality of life is too poor, to wait for treatments to emerge from traditional 'top-down' practices of medicine, randomised control trials nor the time it takes to move from clinical research to practice, which is on average seventeen years.[45] Second, both the HIV and disability rights movements have shown that an absence of lived experience knowledge leads to treatments, support programs and other interventions are that more likely to be associated with harms.[46]

At present, there is little engagement with this community by healthcare workers or clinical researchers. The movement of information remains largely one way – from 'experts' to 'patients'. The missed opportunities here are substantial. I did not recover from Long COVID because of the advice or care of my many and highly qualified specialists. I recovered because of the information and advice shared within online Long COVID communities. Due to my own educational and financial privilege I was able to act on this information and advice. From the learnings of an online community, I recovered from severely bedbound to remission.

A recovery like that is both rare and expensive. A more systematic engagement and uptake of the knowledge emerging in these groups would see us achieve not just better treatment programs, but ones that are accessible to a wider range of individuals. As someone who has made this journey, I know the stakes are high. Within the online Long COVID community I saw deaths every week, often resulting from suicide or lack of access to basic supports such as healthcare and housing. These deaths are rarely if ever recorded as COVID or even Long COVID deaths, attributed instead to something 'downstream' of their infection. The truth of these fatalities is inscribed only in the online messages they leave behind, as the silent and silenced part of the COVID epidemic continues to grow.

Gemma

BOX 27.6 PRACTICE POINT

As a clinician, how can you practice understanding and empathy towards people with Long COVID who seek your professional help?

27.9 EPILOGUE

Professor Gemma Carey died in November 2024. Her invaluable contribution to this chapter was written only a few months before her death, in the brief period of time where her health had improved. She is greatly missed by her colleagues and members of the Long COVID community.

REFERENCES

1 Independent Panel for Pandemic Preparedness and Response. COVID-19: Make it the last pandemic [Internet]. Geneva: Independent Panel for Pandemic Preparedness and Response; 2021 May [cited 2025 Feb 7]. Available from: https://theindependentpanel.org/wp-content/uploads/2021/05/COVID-19-Make-it-the-Last-Pandemic_final.pdf.

2 Lupton D. COVID societies: Theorising the coronavirus crisis. Abingdon: Routledge; 2022.

3 Feldman JM, et al. US public health after COVID-19: Learning from the failures of the hollow state and racial capitalism. BMJ. 2024;384:e076969. doi:10.1136/bmj-2023-076969

4 Morris RD. How denialist amplification spread COVID misinformation and undermined the credibility of public health science. J Public Health Policy. 2024;45(1):114–25. doi:10.1057/s41271-023-00451-4.

5 World Health Organization (WHO). WHO Coronavirus (COVID-19) Dashboard [Internet]. Geneva: WHO; 2021 [cited 2024 Dec 12]. Available from: https://data.who.int/dashboards/covid19/deaths?n=c.

6 Al-Aly Z, et al. Long COVID science, research and policy. Nat Med. 2024;30:2148–64. doi:10.1038/s41591-024-03173-6.

7 McGowan VJ, et al. COVID-19 mortality and deprivation: Pandemic, syndemic, and endemic health inequalities. Lancet Public Health. 2022;7(11): e966–75. doi:10.1016/S2468-2667(22)00223-7.

8 Cheetham NJ, et al. Social determinants of recovery from ongoing symptoms following COVID-19 in two UK longitudinal studies: A prospective cohort study. medRxiv 2023.12.21.23300125. doi:10.1101/2023.12.21.23300125.

9 Nguyen KH, et al. Prevalence and factors associated with Long COVID symptoms among US adults. Vaccines. 2024;12(1):99. doi:10.3390/vaccines12010099.

10 Fisher KA, et al. Long COVID awareness and receipt of medical care: A survey among populations at risk for disparities. Front Public Health. 2024;12. doi:10.3389/fpubh.2024.1360341.

11 Rushforth A, et al. Long COVID – the illness narratives. Soc Sci Med. 2021;286:114326. doi:10.1016/j.socscimed.2021.114326

12 Perego E, et al. Why we need to keep using the patient-made term "Long COVID" [Internet]. BMJ Opinion; 2020 Oct 1 [cited 2025 Feb 7]. Available from: https://blogs.bmj.com/bmj/2020/10/01/why-we-need-to-keep-using-the-patient-made-term-long-covid/

13 Callard F, et al. How and why patients made Long COVID. Soc Sci Med [Internet]. 2021;268:113426. doi:10.1016/j.socscimed.2020.113426.

14 Robertson MM, et al. The epidemiology of long coronavirus disease in US adults. Clin Infect Dis. 2023;76(9):1636–45. doi:10.1093/cid/ciac961.

15 Sawano M, et al. Long COVID characteristics and experience: A descriptive study from the Yale LISTEN Research Cohort. Am J Med 2024;S0002–9343(24)00238-9. doi:10.1016/j.amjmed.2024.04.015.

16 Fang C, et al. "I am just a shadow of who I used to be"—exploring existential loss of identity among people living with chronic conditions of Long COVID. Sociol Health Illn. 2024;46(1): 59–77. doi:10.1111/1467-9566.13690.

17 Spence NJ, et al. Getting back to normal? Identity and role disruptions among adults with Long COVID. Sociol Health Illn. 2023;45(4):914–34. doi:10.1111/1467-9566.13628.

18 Hossain MM, et al. Living with "Long COVID": A systematic review and meta-synthesis of qualitative evidence. PLoS One. 2023;18(2):e0281884. doi:10.1371/journal.pone.0281884.

19 Samper-Pardo M, et al. The emotional well-being of Long COVID patients in relation to their symptoms, social support, and stigmatization in social and health services: A qualitative study. BMC Psychiatry. 2023;23(1):68. doi:10.1186/s12888-022-04497-8.

20 Baz SA, et al. "I don't know what to do or where to go": Experiences of accessing healthcare support from the perspectives of people living with Long COVID and healthcare professionals: A qualitative study in Bradford, UK. Health Expect. 2023;26(1):542–54. doi:10.1111/hex.13687.

21 Clutterbuck D, et al. Barriers to healthcare access: Findings from a co-produced Long COVID case-finding study. medRxiv 2024.01.03.24300767. doi:10.1101/2024.01.03.24300767.

22 Callan C, et al. "I can't cope with multiple inputs": A qualitative study of the lived experience of 'brain fog' after COVID-19. BMJ Open. 2022;12(2):e056366. doi:10.1136/bmjopen-2021-056366.

23 Au L, et al. Long COVID and medical gaslighting: Dismissal, delayed diagnosis, and deferred treatment. SSM Qual Res Health. 2022;2:100167. doi:10.1016/j.ssmqr.2022.100167.

24 Goffman E. Stigma: Notes on the management of spoiled identity. New York: Simon and Schuster; 2009.

25 Eyal G, et al. What's in a name? Contrasting the politics of post-COVID symptoms across three countries. Cienc Public Soc. 2024;1(1):3–22. doi:10.31235/osf.io/juxag.

26 Greenhalgh T, et al. What is quality in Long COVID care? Lessons from a national quality improvement collaborative and multi-site ethnography. BMC Med 2024;22:159. doi:10.1186/s12916-024-03371-6.

27 Gorna R, et al. Long COVID guidelines need to reflect lived experience. Lancet. 2021;397(10273):455–57. doi:10.1016/S0140-6736(20)32705-7.

28 Barker KK, et al. The long tail of COVID and the tale of Long COVID: Diagnostic construction and the management of ignorance. Sociol Health Illn. 2024;46(S1):189–207. doi:10.1111/1467-9566.13599.

29 Little J, et al. Long COVID–Can we deny a diagnosis without denying a person's reality? Australas Psychiatry. 2024;32(1):44–46. doi:10.1177/10398562231222809.

30 Cohen J, et al. An intersectional analysis of Long COVID prevalence. Int J Equity Health. 2023;22(1). doi:10.1186/s12939-023-02072-5.

31 Mullard J, et al. "You're just a guinea pig": Exploring the barriers and impacts of living with Long COVID-19: A view from the undiagnosed. Sociol Health Illn. 2024;46(8):1602–25. doi:10.1111/1467-9566.13795.

32 Bergmans RS, et al. "I'm still here, I'm alive and breathing": The experience of Black Americans with Long COVID. J Clin Nurs. 2024;33(1):162–177. doi:10.1111/jocn.16733.

33 Long COVID Awareness. Long COVID Awareness: Information, advocacy, and support [Internet]. [Place unknown]: Long COVID Awareness; [cited 2025 Feb 7]. Available from: https://www.longcovidawareness.life/.

34 Kaplan K, Mendenhall E. Framing Long COVID through patient activism in the United States: Patient, provider, academic, and policymaker views. Soc Sci Med. 2024;350:116901. doi:10.1016/j.socscimed.2024.116901.

35 Lupton D. Why scrapping the term 'Long COVID' would be harmful for people with this condition [Internet]. *The Conversation*; 2023 Oct 5 [cited 2025 Feb 7]. Available from: https://theconversation.com/why-scrapping-the-term-long-covid-would-be-harmful-for-people-with-the-condition-225880.

36 Parotto M, et al. Post-acute sequelae of COVID-19: Understanding and addressing the burden of multisystem manifestations. Lancet Respir Med. 2023;11(8):739–54. doi:10.1016/S2213-2600(23)00239-4.

37 Dhairyawan R. The medical practice of silencing. Lancet. 2021;398(10298):382–83. doi:10.1016/S0140-6736(21)01659-7.

38 de Boer ML. Epistemic in/justice in patient participation. A discourse analysis of the Dutch ME/CFS Health Council advisory process. Sociol Health Illn. 2021;43(6):1335–54. doi:10.1111/1467-9566.13301.

39 Carel H, et al. Epistemic injustice in medicine and healthcare. In: The Routledge handbook of epistemic injustice. Abingdon: Routledge; 2017. p. 336–46.

40 Fitz-Gibbon K, et al. Disconnected and insecure: The intersection between experiences of Long COVID and intimate partner violence. Melbourne: Monash University; 2024.

41 Carlile O, et al. Impact of Long COVID on health-related quality of life: An OpenSAFELY population cohort study using patient-reported outcome measures (OpenPROMPT). Lancet Reg Health Eur. 2024;40:100908. doi:10.1016/j.lanepe.2024.100908.

42 Russell D, et al. Support amid uncertainty: Long COVID illness experiences and the role of online communities. SSM Qual Res Health. 2022 Oct 4;2:100177. doi:10.1016/j.ssmqr.2022.100177.

43 Bass E. To end a plague: America's fight to defeat AIDS in Africa. MA: MIT Press; 2022.

44 Charlton JI. Nothing about us without us: Disability oppression and empowerment. Cambridge: University of California Press; 1998.

45 Morris ZS, et al. The answer is 17 years, what is the question: Understanding time lags in translational research. J R Soc Med. 2011;104(12):510–20. doi:10.1258/jrsm.2011.110180.

46 Shakespeare T. Recognising lived experience is essential to empowering disabled patients. BMJ 2022;378:o2359. doi:10.1136/bmj.o2359.

SECTION SEVEN
CONCLUSION

Chapter 28

The Future of Long COVID

Unanswered Questions and Emerging Trends

Elle O'Brien, Joanne Wrench, and Danielle Hitch

BOX 28.1 LEARNING OUTCOMES

By the end of this chapter, readers should be able to:

- Describe key priorities for Long COVID research within a prioritisation framework.
- Understand key barriers and limitations to Long COVID research and translation into practice.
- Outline best practice principles for research to support sustainable improvement in Long COVID care and outcomes.

28.1 INTRODUCTION

Almost all research papers, discussion forums and guidelines on Long COVID highlight this condition's significant unknowns and complexity. When developing this book, we intended to flip this discussion: what *do* we know, and how can we apply this information to improving the lives of people with Long COVID? Drawing on rehabilitation principles and evidence from other chronic conditions, combined with the latest Long COVID evidence, has shown us how much can be done – and how much more there is to do. This chapter examines what's next, where we are headed and what we should prioritise for Long COVID research and care.

DOI: 10.4324/9781003528104-35

BOX 28.2   PRACTICE POINT

What have you learnt or reflected upon while reading this book? How will this new knowledge influence your practice as a rehabilitation health professional?

28.2 CURRENT UNDERSTANDINGS OF LONG COVID REHABILITATION

28.2.1 Long COVID is a Multifaceted and Systemic Physiological Condition

Chapters in the first section of this textbook described the history, characteristics, and boundaries of Long COVID as a health condition. Patient-led advocacy played a pivotal role in naming and raising awareness of Long COVID, with online communities driving research, policy changes, and public recognition. The most reported symptoms include fatigue, cognitive dysfunction, and Post-Exertional Malaise (PEM); however, this condition can impact every body system and structure. Symptoms can persist for months or even years and profoundly impact physical and mental health, wellbeing, and participation in daily life.

Long COVID shares similarities with other Post-Acute Infection Syndromes (PAIS) but is distinguished by its unique viral origin, lack of specific biomarkers, and fluctuating nature, which complicate diagnosis and management. Comparisons with conditions like Myalgic Encephalitis/Chronic Fatigue Syndrome not only reveal shared experiences of stigma, delayed diagnoses, and systemic inequities but also highlight the importance of patient-centred care and early intervention. Contributing factors for the symptoms and functional problems experienced by people with Long COVID include immune dysregulation, viral persistence, genetic predisposition, and socioeconomic determinants, with its prevalence influenced by factors like infection severity, vaccination status, and variant type.

28.2.2 Long COVID Identification and Planning Requires Collaborative Approaches that Leverage Big Data and Implement Tailored Outcome Measures

In the second section of this book, chapters explored how the identification of Long COVID requires a multifaceted approach, integrating patient-centred care, collaborative efforts, and innovative data strategies. Long COVID's systemic nature necessitates a clinical approach to diagnosis, which also depends on engagement by diverse stakeholders (including General Practitioners (GPs), specialists, other health professionals, and people with Long COVID). Big data analytics can harness the power of large datasets to refine diagnostic criteria, uncover risk factors, and identify disparities in care. Effective planning is based on implementing outcome measures that balance objective data with patient-reported outcomes, capturing lived experiences to ensure tailored and meaningful care. Shared decision-making is central to Long COVID rehabilitation, fostering trust and motivation by setting goals that align with personal values. Strategies like SMART goals and mind mapping enable adaptability in the face of fluctuating symptoms, which promotes resilience and supports progress.

28.2.3 Interdisciplinary Long COVID Teams are Best Placed to Deliver Holistic, High Quality and Person-Centred Care

Section 3 described the interdisciplinary Long COVID teams that apply a collaborative, person-centred approach to managing Long COVID's complex, multisystem nature. GPs play a key coordinating role, ensuring continuity of care and facilitating timely referrals to specialists for expert support around specific medical symptoms. Allied health professionals play a vital role in symptom management, rehabilitation, and restoring functional capacity. Together, the rehabilitation team integrates medical and allied health expertise with lived experience expertise to promote recovery and improve quality of life. While integrated care models are available, they are often hampered by systemic barriers, including fragmented healthcare systems, inequitable access, and lack of clinician expertise, highlighting the need for systemic reform. Effective interdisciplinary care for Long COVID prioritises inclusivity, patient education, and flexible service delivery, such as telehealth, to deliver tailored, comprehensive care.

28.2.4 Effective Long COVID Rehabilitation Employs Diverse Strategies to Enhance Participation in Daily Life

In Section 4, chapters provide intervention and management strategies addressing Long COVID's complex and variable symptoms. Key rehabilitation approaches include pacing, energy conservation, cognitive and psychological interventions, symptom and heart rate monitoring, nutritional interventions, personalised and safe activity and exercise, and respiratory muscle training. These strategies also incorporate activity modification, assistive technology, and environmental adaptations. Intervention and management planning must consider the interplay between health conditions, personal factors, and environmental influences to ensure care aligns with patients' lived experiences and functional goals.

Long COVID intervention and management strategies also encompass support for co-occurring conditions, particularly dysautonomia (most commonly Postural Orthostatic Tachycardia Syndrome or POTS). Management of POTS typically includes a combination of hydration, compression garments, pharmacological interventions, and closely monitored physical activity. However, evidence-based treatments for Long COVID are still emerging, and current practice is underpinned by respect and validation of lived experience and shared decision-making practices.

28.2.5 Long COVID Models of Care Integrate Multiple Services and Health Professions in Diverse Settings

Section 5 highlighted that models of care for Long COVID are evolving to meet the complex needs of people with this condition, offering interdisciplinary, person-centred approaches across hospital, allied health, community, and primary care settings. Hospital models address acute and long-term management but face challenges due to funding disparities and barriers at the interface with community-based care. Allied health models leverage interdisciplinary expertise to provide integrated and evidence-informed care and hold the potential for rapid scale up and dissemination. Community and primary care models focus on accessibility by integrating telehealth and GP-led clinics to address geographical and financial barriers. Workforce shortages, evolving evidence, and a lack of standardised guidelines can make delivering these services difficult.

Self-determination and self-management are critical aspects of Long COVID rehabilitation because they empower patients to take an active role in their care and implement intervention and management strategies in their daily lives. All the models of care presented in this book are affected by the broader economic impacts of the COVID-19 pandemic and Long COVID, including decreased health-related quality of life at the community and population level, lower workforce participation and productivity, and increased healthcare utilisation. Integrated financial support systems and policies to reduce cost and administrative burdens are needed to ensure both the viability and sustainability of Long COVID care.

28.2.6 Specific Populations Experience Distinctive Challenges when Living with Long COVID

The final section covers a range of key influencing Long COVID care and outcomes for specific populations. Intensive Care Unit survivors with Long COVID often experience persistent physical, cognitive, and psychological impairments, requiring early intervention and personalised rehabilitation strategies. Children and young people face unique developmental and health risks, highlighting the need for child-centred, multidisciplinary care that addresses stigma and developmental needs. Culturally and linguistically diverse (CALD) communities face systemic barriers to care, with effective management requiring cultural humility, inclusive practices, and partnerships with CALD organisations. In rural and remote communities, geographical isolation and healthcare shortages exacerbate access issues, but innovative telerehabilitation and community-driven models show promise in bridging these gaps. Gender disparities in Long COVID prevalence and care reveal the impact of societal norms, with women disproportionately affected and often dismissed, necessitating gender-sensitive approaches to research and treatment. Overall, the sociology of Long COVID underscores the condition's deep entanglement with systemic inequalities, stigma, and health professional gaslighting. In this context, patient-led activism has raised awareness and advocated for improved care.

28.3 UNANSWERED QUESTIONS

Living with Long COVID is an exercise in navigating uncertainty. Each day when I wake up, I do not know whether the hours ahead will be filled with energy and a relative sense of normality, or with an unrelenting cavalcade of symptoms that leave me incapacitated.

Elle

Many areas of the Long COVID map remain blank or briefly sketched. As Al-Aly and Topol[1] discuss, numerous factors associated with this condition contribute to this level of uncertainty. Long COVID's complexity stems from diverse presentations and likely multiple biological mechanisms. Limited consensus on definitions, diagnostic criteria, and trial endpoints, along with inadequate surveillance of long-term consequences and insufficient research funding for PAIS, contribute to this uncertainty. Stigma, discrimination, and a societal push to "move on" also marginalise those affected. The pandemic's unprecedented scale means everyone is at risk. However, the diverse contributing factors for Long COVID mean it often feels like "everything, everywhere, all at once."

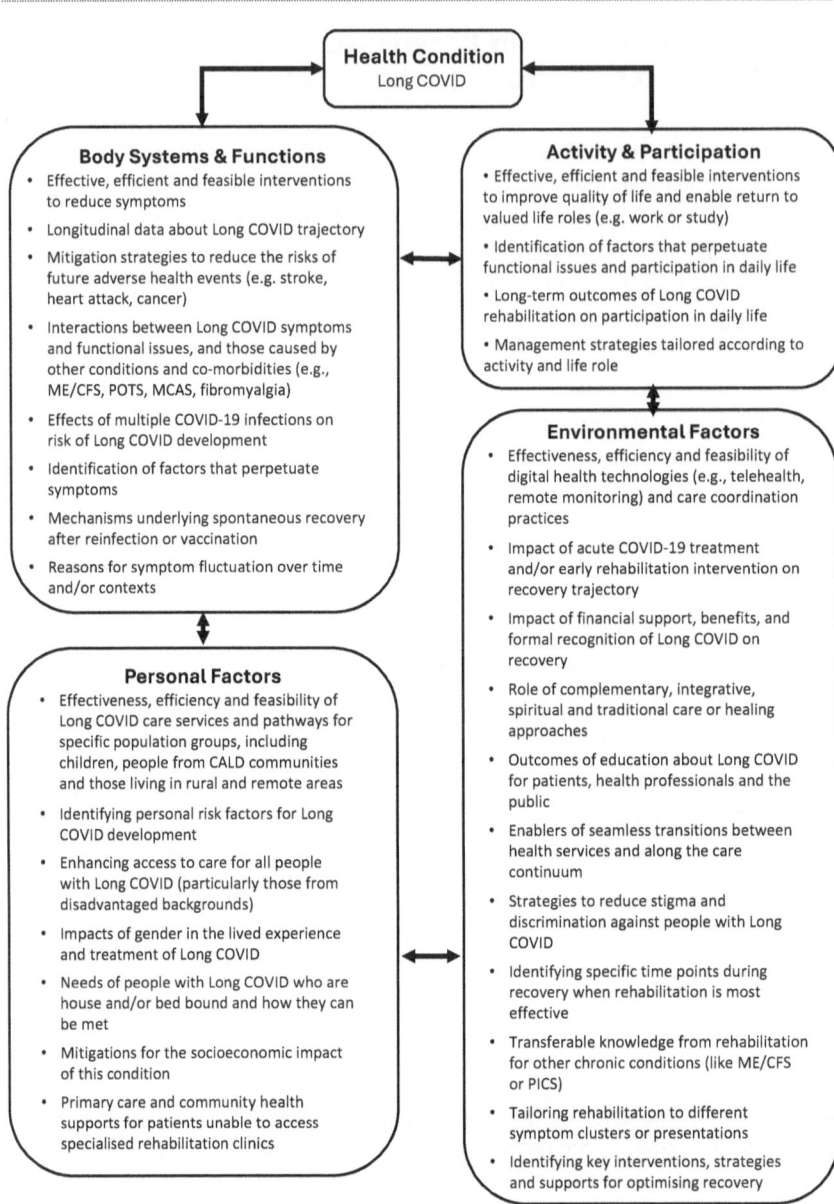

Figure 28.1 Unanswered questions about Long COVID rehabilitation.

In the face of such uncertainty, people with Long COVID may try interventions they doubt, simply to do *something*.

> *At my worst, I was housebound, but my doctor had nothing to offer. I was devastated. I resorted to taking unproven supplements and medications based on nothing but anecdote, trying expensive and dangerous "snake oil" remedies because doing nothing was unthinkable.*
>
> Elle

While the many unanswered questions are essential, how they are identified and prioritised is critical. The James Lind Priority Setting Partnerships approach (The Alliance)[2] exemplifies how to identify and prioritise unanswered but meaningful questions in healthcare. Patients, carers, and clinicians collaborate to identify key questions about their condition or field, using a rigorous methodology to prioritise research topics. The Alliance spent four months in 2020 and 2021 conducting surveys and workshops to identify research priorities with hospitals and non-hospitalised Long COVID patients, carers, and health professionals.[3] Other groups have also used multistep processes, including surveys, literature reviews, workshops, and contributions from working groups[4–7] to identify priorities and research questions with multiple stakeholders.

Many research priorities and questions relate to pathophysiology, diagnostics (particularly biomarkers), and pharmaceutical treatments. They reflect a primarily biomedical perspective, which may or may not align with lived experience.

BOX 28.3 PRACTICE POINT

Previous chapters have encouraged reflection on your thoughts and attitudes about Long COVID. Consider what else you want to know about Long COVID. What unanswered questions do you have about Long COVID as a rehabilitation health professional?

These priorities are interdependent, with the answers to some research questions contributing to the solution of others. For example, investigating strategies to reduce stigma and discrimination against people with Long COVID will also address enhanced access to care for all patients. This underscores the need for basic, applied, and health services researchers to work together and learn from each other's research programmes.

At this stage, there are many more questions than answers, and our gaps in knowledge have a profound impact on the lives of patients like me. Although researchers are rightly focussing on the diagnosis, treatment, epidemiology, and pathophysiology of Long COVID, they are a long way from answering the questions at the forefront of my mind: How long will this last? Will I ever be able to think clearly again, or work full-time, or dance with my friends? If I recover, will I spend the rest of my life afraid of reinfection, jumping at the sound of a rasping cough? What's happening to me? Why me?

Ellen

In rehabilitation, the research focuses on improving function and quality of life rather than solely "curing" the condition. How do you choose which questions to answer when there are so many? That depends primarily on the goals of the person with Long COVID, who is also informed by the health profession and service setting. Based on our lived and health professional experience with Long COVID, here are the priorities we would like to address in the coming 5–10 years (Figure 28.1).

BOX 28.4   CASE STUDY: THE VICTORIAN POST-ACUTE COVID STUDY (VPACS) GROUP

VPACS was formed in 2021 as Victoria, Australia, experienced increasing COVID-19 infections. Spearheaded by the Chief Surgeon of Victoria, Prof. David Watters, the group brings together researchers, clinicians, and policymakers to enhance collaboration, drive innovation, and support a targeted and unified collective for advocacy.[8] Members have been recruited from a wide range of backgrounds, including lived experience experts, major universities, leading research institutes, and primary and tertiary clinicians from most health networks in the state. Policymakers from the Victorian Health Department also attend to support the translation of the group's work into policy and reform.

The group meets monthly online, hosting interdisciplinary discussions spanning research, policy, and data linkage opportunities. Each meeting includes presentations from early career and established researchers and a discussion centred on the group's strategic initiatives and collaborations.

In 2023, VPACS coordinated a Long COVID scientific conference sponsored by the Department of Health, which offered opportunities for cutting-edge Australian research to be presented in partnership with lived experience perspectives. Papers from this conference were subsequently published in a special supplement of the *Medical Journal of Australia*,[9] and research collaborations between members have had success with major national research grants. A partnership was also established with the Victorian Agency for Health Information to support access to government databases for several data linkage projects. The textbook editors also met via VPACS, and other group members are chapter co-authors.

Given the unknowns of Long COVID, the group exemplifies the benefit of bringing lived experience experts, researchers, policymakers, and clinicians together to quickly identify gaps and new opportunities and translate research rapidly into practice. Grassroots communities of practice like VPACS are particularly adept at empowering and supporting local stakeholders to share their knowledge and experience in the service of contextually relevant solutions and sustainable improvements in practice.

28.4 FINDING ANSWERS AND SOLVING PROBLEMS

28.4.1 Long COVID Research

The first research study of Long COVID appeared in May 2020 and was a cross-sectional study conducted by Patient-Led Research for COVID-19.[10] Despite many unanswered questions, research about this condition has been slowly advancing and consolidating. In just five years, progress has been made in answering key questions about the causes of Long COVID, as discussed in Chapter 2. However, there remains no definitive answer, and the causes of Long COVID are likely multifactorial and dependent on individual context. Untangling "cause" from "effect" will likely take many years and require sustained, international collaboration between researchers.

Research on COVID-19 was initially produced at an unprecedented pace, revealing both the potential for rapid scientific output and the pitfalls of lowered standards of evidence for publication. Some studies published early in the pandemic carried a high risk of bias, reflecting the urgency to understand a novel condition and the constraints imposed by pandemic restrictions, which limited researchers' ability to complete studies.[11] Female researchers were particularly affected by disruptions such as homeschooling and increased family responsibilities.[12] The evolving nature of COVID-19 and Long COVID means much of the early evidence is now less applicable. Despite this, these studies remain essential sources of evidence to drive future research.

BOX 28.5   PRACTICE POINT

The LitCOV database (https://www.ncbi.nlm.nih.gov/research/coronavirus/) is a valuable resource for keeping up with developments. Considering the discussion above, how relevant can the findings be to your practice?

The complexities of Long COVID have exposed significant challenges to long established research methodologies, particularly regarding the development and use of appropriate control groups. Control groups are essential in Long COVID research to identify its unique characteristics compared to other conditions, validate the relationship between symptoms, identify risk factors, and evaluate treatments with methodological rigour. Without control groups, research findings may be biased or incomplete, hindering the development of effective interventions.

Inefficiencies in clinical trial design are common in COVID-19 research, with most adopting interventional or placebo controls while excluding key confounders like social connections.[13] Using historical data as control benchmarks also raises concerns because of the pandemic's broad impact on health, wellbeing, and social determinants. Population norms established for standardised outcome measures may need to be revisited and interpreted cautiously if used as a comparison group.[14]

The scientific foundation of treatment is a shared priority for health professionals and people with Long COVID alike:

> *One of the hardest parts about having Long COVID is discovering that there are no validated interventions or cures and that most off-label treatments are guesswork at best.*

> Elle

Including participants with undetected or misclassified COVID-19 threatens the reliability of control groups over time, as does contamination caused by differing COVID-19 variants, which have distinct presentations and recovery trajectories, necessitating variant-specific control groups. Symptom clusters and phenotypes further highlight the need for methodologies that capture constellations of symptoms rather than focusing on individual ones. In this area, current Long COVID research often falls short. Addressing these challenges through nuanced methods can deepen understanding of Long COVID and offer valuable insights and innovations for other chronic and complex conditions.

The meaningful inclusion of people with Long COVID in rehabilitation care and research has been a recurring theme throughout this book. In the absence of professional guidance, people with this condition come up with their own solutions, which also offer potential targets for research. The activism and engagement of the Long COVID community as a social movement, as described in Chapter 4, provides a solid foundation for patient-led and driven research that will help everyone reach our shared vision for greater equity, less disability and distress, and better health and wellbeing outcomes.

> *I have spent much of my limited energy over the last three years trawling through research articles, online seminars, and every other available resource trying to figure out how to recover. As someone who is studying science at university, it has been exciting and encouraging to see how quickly the research is progressing. But, as a patient, it has been heart-breaking to see how little we still know.*
>
> Elle

Given the multitude of potential research topics and priority areas, general principles of best practice in Long COVID research provide a much-needed general framework for future studies. The following recommendations (Figure 28.2) are drawn from current evidence[15–19] and the authors' professional and lived experience.

28.5 THE FUTURE OF LONG COVID REHABILITATION

As demonstrated in this textbook, the future of Long COVID rehabilitation is promising. A firm foundation for evidence-based practice has emerged in just five short years. Significant challenges remain for clinical research and knowledge translation into practice. Identifying and implementing effective, efficient, and feasible interventions requires health systems to adapt in response to emerging research and lived experience evidence. The COVID-19 pandemic highlighted the capacity of health services to implement innovation rapidly, so there is no doubt that the sorts of change advocated for in this book are possible. Based on international experience, positive change in Long COVID rehabilitation will depend on adaptive and responsive organisational structures, well-functioning

1. Authentic, Meaningful & Equitable Engagement	2. Refine & Standardise Definitions	3. Appropriate & Robust Methodologies
• **Involve patients as partners:** Ensure relevance and validity by collaborating with patients at all stages of the research process, from question formulation to dissemination. • **Engage the broader community:** Use participatory citizen-science methodologies, enabling community members with and without Long COVID to shape and contribute to research. • **Inclusive participation:** Ensure representation from diverse demographics, including marginalised groups and children. • **Encourage broad collaboration:** Incorporate perspectives from caregivers, health professionals, and researchers to develop comprehensive research priorities. • **Promote patient-centred frameworks:** Create research agendas solely reflecting patient needs, independent of other stakeholder priorities.	• **Adopt a unified definition or description of Long COVID:** Prioritise consensus around the definition of Long COVID to standardise research outcomes, clinical practices, and communication among healthcare professionals. • **Engage with variability:** Recognise and synthesise existing definitions across studies to include a wide range of symptoms and contexts.	• **Embed theoretical frameworks:** Ground research in established frameworks to ensure a structured approach, comprehensive perspective and enhanced translation. • **Select the best method for the research question:** The question must drive study design, rather than perceptions of methodological rigour or value. • **Mixed methods approaches:** Combine qualitative and quantitative data to capture the complex and multifaceted nature of Long COVID experiences. • **Validate outcome measures with Long COVID populations:** Develop and validate instruments to enable comparisons across populations and consolidation of findings.

4. Adapt to Pandemic Driven Societal Changes	5. Long Term Planning	6. Improved Data Synthesis & Sharing
• **Flexible recruitment strategies:** Adapt recruitment methods to engage diverse groups. • **Ethical adaptations:** Modify consent processes for online environments to ensure participant understanding. • **Context-specific documentation:** Acknowledge the unique local and temporal conditions shaping research findings and report these factors for broader applicability. • **Use online research methods:** Use virtual recruitment and data collection methods to provide a COVID safe environment for research participation.	• **Sustain research efforts:** Advocate for ongoing, stable funding that supports multi-institutional or international collaborations between research institutes. • **Focus on long-term outcomes:** Consider study time frames and whether they reflect the ongoing lived experience of Long COVID. • **Manage resource constraints:** Balance research activities with other demands on healthcare systems, ensuring sustained support for investigators. • **Ensure translatability:** Prioritise low cost, accessible interventions to support scalability.	• **Integrate Findings:** Prioritise synthesis of evidence from diverse sources to consolidate knowledge and inform global strategies. • **Promote Open Access:** Ensure research outcomes are accessible to inform broader public health strategies and enhance understanding of Long COVID. • **Improve data analysis:** Conduct analysis on sub-groups (such as sex) to gain a more nuanced picture.

Figure 28.2 Recommendations for best practice in Long COVID research.

communication systems, investment and commitment from the workforce, a shared understanding of purpose and goals, accessible and cost-effective treatments, and professional networks that facilitate collaboration and creativity.[20]

The future of Long COVID rehabilitation will also depend on engagement in policy and frameworks at the systems level. Mechanisms to link lived experience experts, researchers, clinicians, and decision-makers (like VPACS) are invaluable to getting evidence into practice. Connections between people with Long COVID and policymakers are critical because conflict between stakeholder groups is a barrier to coherent and coordinated service responses.[21]

> *At about the same time as I was floored by my diagnosis and disablement, Australia's Chief Health Officer declared, 'We're not seeing a major picture of long COVID.'... according to the Chief Health Officer's research and calculations and policy recommendations, I do not exist.*
> Submission 072, Australian Government' Sick and Tired' Inquiry[22]

Frameworks and models of care for Long COVID research need to span acute, sub-acute, and community care settings because action (or inaction) at all these stages of the patient journey impacts the development of, and potential recovery from, this condition.[23] They may also need to encompass other sectors (such as education, government, industry, and technology) to adequately address the complex social and political determinants of health that impact the lives of people with Long COVID. An opportunity, therefore, exists to create inclusive and truly integrated frameworks and models of care that diminish siloing and take a genuinely holistic approach to health and wellbeing.

Technological advances may also provide powerful tools for understanding and managing Long COVID. Several chapters in this book have illustrated the role of telehealth in increasing access to rehabilitation, and the accessibility of these platforms is constantly improving.[24] Wearable technology (such as smart watches, smart rings, and smart patches) is increasingly used for physiological monitoring and offers an accurate and low burden option for many people with Long COVID.[25] Artificial intelligence applications are also being developed to support self-management by enabling the prediction and prevention of PEM episodes and supporting clinical decision-making.[26,27] While some ethical issues and affordability barriers are yet to be resolved, health professionals should upskill in these technologies to provide their patients with the best possible care.

Finally, and perhaps most importantly, the future of Long COVID rehabilitation will require greater awareness of the condition itself. While rehabilitation aims to prevent the negative impacts of existing conditions, health professionals also have an obligation to focus on primary prevention to avoid the development of Long COVID in the first place.[28] Currently, Long COVID prevention public health campaigns are rare as governments and health officials promote a "return to normal."

28.6 CONCLUSION

We acknowledge the prospect of future breakthroughs makes little difference to the current lives of people with Long COVID. More rehabilitation options are now available than ever before as the field moves from "What is Long COVID?" to "What can we do about Long COVID?" The contents of this textbook provide new insights and multiple strategies for health professionals to take positive action on Long COVID and tackle this most wicked of problems.

Long COVID is a mercurial condition that provokes a wide range of sometimes conflicting perspectives. All these views and experiences are valid, and many have been acknowledged and included in this textbook. Despite different views at times, every Long COVID patient, family member, researcher, and health professional ultimately strives towards the same goal – the best possible outcomes for every person living with Long COVID.

> *Even if a cure cannot be found, developing treatments that enhance patients' quality of life and eliminate the need for risky self-experimentation is crucial. It is encouraging that diseases once considered debilitating can now be managed with relatively minor interventions, and this progress makes me hopeful that one day a simple pill might be all I need to manage my Long COVID. I am optimistic that one day we will be able to answer many questions but, for now, there is still a long way to go.*
>
> Elle

REFERENCES

1 Al-Aly Z, et al. Solving the puzzle of Long COVID. Science. 2024;383:830–32. doi:10.1126/science.adl0867.

2 James Lind Alliance (JLA). About Priority Setting Partnerships (PSPs) [Internet]. London: National Institute for Health Research (NIHR); [cited 2025 Feb 7]. Available from:. https://www.jla.nihr.ac.uk/about-priority-setting-partnerships

3 Houchen-Wolloff L, et al. Joint patient and clinician priority setting to identify 10 key research questions regarding the long-term sequelae of COVID-19. Thorax. 2022;77(7):717–20. doi:10.1136/thoraxjnl-2021-218582.

4 Grant A, et al. Four years in: What are the research priorities for Long COVID? A research priority-setting partnership between people with lived experience, carers, clinicians and researchers. Health Expect. 2024;27:e70072. doi:10.1111/hex.70072.

5 Kennedy AB, et al. Wonderings to research questions: Engaging patients in Long COVID research prioritisation within a learning health system. Learn Health Sys. 2024;8(Suppl. 1): e10410. doi:10.1002/lrh2.10410.

6 Ziegler S, et al. Long COVID citizen scientists: Developing a needs-based research agenda by persons affected by Long COVID. The Patient. 2022;15(5):565–76. doi:10.1007/s40271-022-00579-7.

7 O'Brien KK, et al. A framework of research priorities in COVID rehabilitation from the Rehabilitation Science Research Network for COVID: An international consultation involving qualitative and quantitative research. Disabil Rehabil. 2024 Jul 24. doi:10.1080/09638288.2024.2382904.

8 Tippett E, et al. Post-acute COVID-19 condition (PACC): A perspective on collaborative Australian research imperatives and primary health models of care. Aust J Prim Health. 2023;29(4):293–95. doi:10.1071/PY22009.

9 Watters, DA, et al. Long COVID in Victoria. Med J Aust. 2024;221(9 Suppl):S3–S4. doi:10.5694/mja2.52467.

10 Quinn TJ, et al. Following the science? Comparison of methodological and reporting quality of COVID-19 and other research from the first wave of the pandemic. BMC Med. 2021;19(1):46. doi:10.1186/s12916-021-01920-x.

11 Houchen-Wolloff L, et al. Joint patient and clinician priority setting to identify 10 key research questions regarding the long-term sequelae of COVID-19. Thorax. 2022;77:717–20. doi:10.1136/thoraxjnl-2022-218994. doi:10.1136/thoraxjnl-2021-218582.

12 Kwon E, et al. The effect of the COVID-19 pandemic on gendered research productivity and its correlates. J Informetrics. 2023;17(1):101380. doi:10.1016/j.joi.2023.101380.

13 Zhao MZ, et al. Evaluating the methodology of studies conducted during the global COVID-19 pandemic: A systematic review of randomised controlled trials. J Integr Med. 2021;19(4):317–26. doi:10.1016/j.joim.2021.03.003.

14 Jia R, et al. Mental health in the UK during the COVID-19 pandemic: Cross-sectional analyses from a community cohort study. BMJ Open. 2020;10(9):e040620. doi:10.1136/bmjopen-2020-040620.

15 Kennedy AB, et al. Wonderings to research questions: Engaging patients in Long COVID research prioritisation within a learning health system. Learn Health Syst. 2024;8(Suppl. 1): e10410. doi:10.1002/lrh2.10410.

16 Davis HE, et al. Long COVID: Major findings, mechanisms and recommendations. Nat Rev Microbiol. 2023;21(3):133–46. doi:10.1038/s41579-022-00846-2.

17 Ziegler S, et al. Long COVID citizen scientists: Developing a needs-based research agenda by persons affected by Long COVID. Patient. 2022;15:565–76. doi:10.1007/s40271-022-00579-7.

18 De las Salas R, et al. A scoping study of the emerging definition of 'Long COVID-19': Implications for future research and clinical practice. Inplasy Protocol 202290122. 2022. doi:10.37766/inplasy2022.9.0122.

19 Hitch D, et al. Occupational being during the COVID-19 pandemic. In: Kara H, Khoo S, editors. Researching in the age of COVID-19 Vol 2: Volume II: Care and resilience. Bristol University Press; 2020. p. 111–20. doi:10.2307/j.ctv18dvt4f.15.

20 Gautier L, et al. Hospital governance during the COVID-19 pandemic: A multiple-country case study. Health Syst Reform. 2023;9(1):e2173551. doi:10.1080/23288604.2023.2173551.

21 Hitch D et al. Equity amidst uncertainty: A comparative critique of multiple stakeholder perspectives about health equity for people with Long COVID. In: Lupton D, editor. The social impacts of Long COVID. Cham: Springer/Palgrave Macmillan; [forthcoming 2025].

22 Parliament of Australia. Inquiry into Long COVID and repeated COVID infections [Internet]. Canberra: Parliament of Australia; [cited 2025 Feb 7]. Available from: https://www.aph.gov.au/Parliamentary_Business//Committees/House/Health_Aged_Care_and_Sport/LongandrepeatedCOVID.

23 O'Brien KK, et al. Conceptual framework of episodic disability in the context of Long COVID: Findings from a community-engaged international qualitative study. medRxiv 2024. doi:10.1101/2024.05.28.24308048.

24 Yasini M, et al. Digital connecting for health, an open platform based on data integration and standards to adopt digital and telehealth solutions in the healthcare ecosystem. Stud Health Technol Inform. 2023;309:116–20.

25 Babu M, et al. Wearable devices: Implications for precision medicine and the future of health care. Annu Rev Med. 2024;75:401–15. doi:10.1146/annurev-med-052422-020437.

26 Ahmad I, et al. A survey on the role of artificial intelligence in managing Long COVID. Front Artif Intell. 2024;6:1292466. doi:10.3389/frai.2023.1292466.

27 Amjad A et al. A review on innovation in healthcare sector (Telehealth) through artificial intelligence. Sustainability 2023;15(8):6655. doi:10.3390/su15086655.

28 AbdulRaheem Y. Unveiling the significance and challenges of integrating prevention levels in healthcare practice. J Prim Care Community Health. 2023;14:1–6. doi:10.1177/21501319231186500.

Index